Medical Mini Review Series in Gastroenterology and Hepatology

Efficient Refresher for the Busy Clinical Gastroenterologist

Edited by

A.B.R. Thomson and N. Chande

www.giandhepatology.com

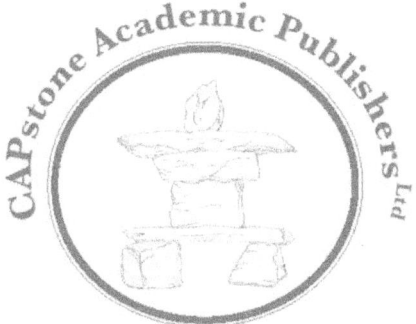

CAPstone (Canadian Academic Publishers Ltd) is a not-for-profit company dedicated to the use of the power of education for the betterment of all persons everywhere.

"The Democratization of Knowledge"

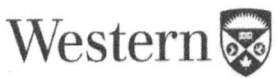

MINI UPDATE

MINI UPDATE

Schulich
MEDICINE & DENTISTRY

Western

Western

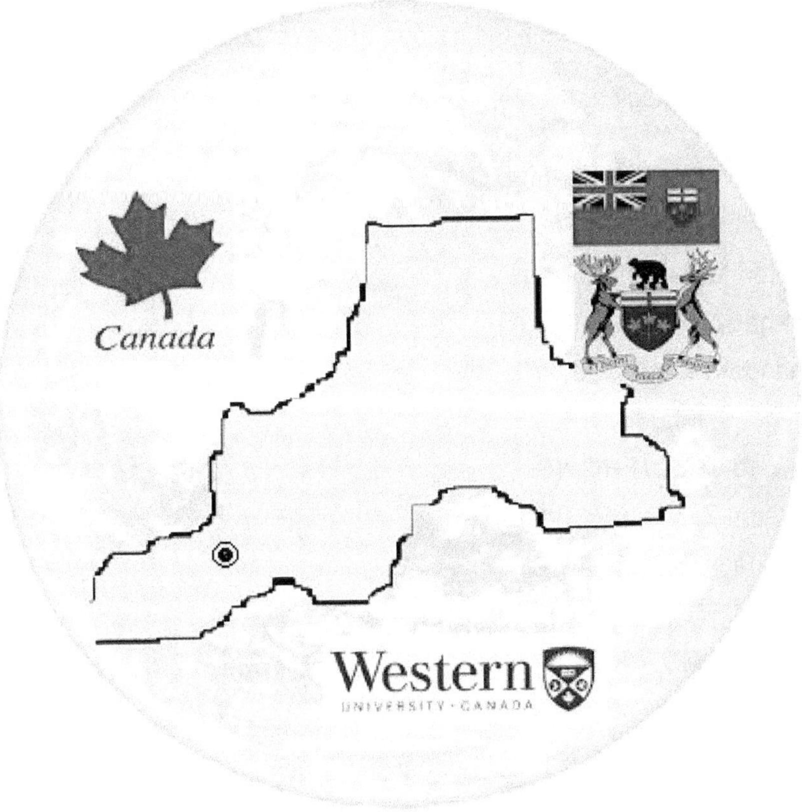

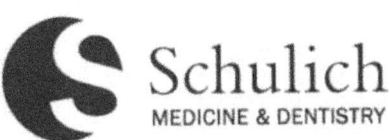

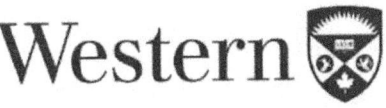

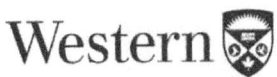

MINI UPDATE

The editors wish to thank the trainee and staff contributors who maintain the excellence of the Division of Gastroenterology at Western University.

Aljawad M, MD, FRCP(C)

Aljudaibi B, MD FRCP(C)

Beaton M, MD, FRCP(C)

Chande N, MD FRCPC (C)

Chandok N, MD, FRCP(C)

Gregor J, MD, FRCP(C)

Howard J, MD, FRCP(C

Kassam Z, MD, FRCP(C)

Khanna N, MD, FRCP(C)

Mosli M, MD, FRCP(C)

Ponich T, MD, FRCP(C)

Sey M, MD, FRCP(C)

Thomson ABR, MD, PhD, FRCP(C)

Wells M, MD, FRCP(C)

Wilson A, MD, FRCP(C)

Woodcock N, RD

Yan B, MD, FRCP(C)

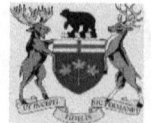

MINI UPDATE

Editor Biographies

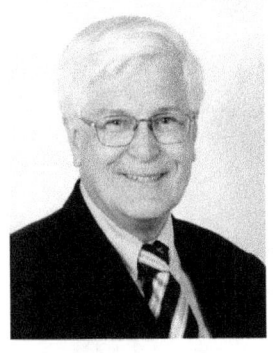

Dr. Alan Thomson has been President of the Canadian Association of Gastroenterology, a member of the Bockus Society, two-term Governor for Western Canada for the American College of Gastroenterology, winner of the prestigious University Cup in 2001, a recipient of the Gold Medal in Medicine of the Royal College of Physicians and Surgeons (Canada), Chief Royal College examiner in Gastroenterology, Director of the Division of Gastroenterology, three-time Teacher of the Year at the University of Alberta, Award for Excellence in Mentoring Graduate Students and Postdoctoral Fellows, and awarded Distinguished University Professor. Dr. Thomson is a Distinguished Emeritus University Professor, University of Alberta, and is currently an Adjunct Professor at Western University.

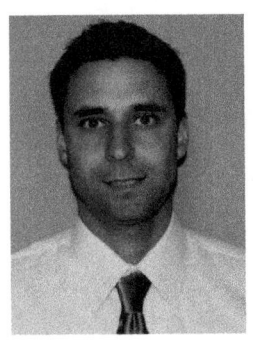

Dr. Nilesh Chande is an Associate Professor of Medicine in the Division of Gastroenterology at Western University, London, Ontario, Canada. He is the Director of the Gastroenterology Training Program and has interests in inflammatory bowel disease, general gastroenterology, and medical education.

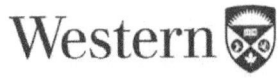

MINI UPDATE

As physicians, learning is life-long.

This book is dedicated to our trainees and

To the patients whom they will care for,

And care about.

Alan Thomson

For Shannon and our children who keep my mind on the

important things in life.

Nilesh Chande

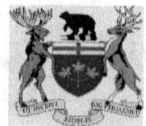

MINI UPDATE

Table of Contents

BACKGROUND	**1**
An Introduction to CT Scanning of the Abdomen *Zahra Kassam*	3
ESOPHAGUS	**33**
Eosinophilic Esophagitis *Nitin Khanna*	35
Esophageal Cancer *Mahmoud Mosli*	55
STOMACH	**71**
Gastritis & Gastropathies *Melanie Beaton*	73
Acid Secretion and Cytoprotection *Bandar Aljudaibi*	103
Management of Non-Variceal Upper GI Bleeding *Jamie Gregor*	125
Bariatric Surgery for the Gastroenterologist *Michael Sey*	171
Management and Risk of Interruption of Anti-Thrombotics for Endoscopic Procedure *Mohammed Aljawad*	199
Helicobacter Pylori Infection and Its Associated Diseases *Malcolm Wells*	221
Paraneoplastic Syndromes in Gastric Adenocarcinoma *Aze Wilson*	267
SMALL BOWEL	**277**
Bile Secretion and the Enterohepatic Circulation *Michael Sey*	279
IBD and Pregnancy *Mahmoud Mosli*	295
European evidence-based consensus on the prevention, diagnosis and management of opportunistic infections in IBD *Aze Wilson*	301
COLON	**311**
Clostridium Difficile Infection *Mohammed Aljawad*	313
Hereditary Colon Cancer: FAP and HNPCC *Brian Yan*	333
LIVER, HEPATOBILIARY TREE AND GALLBLADDER	**385**
Liver Diseases in Pregnancy *Michael Sey*	387
Acute Liver Failure *Aze Wilson*	419

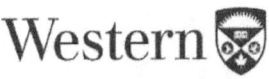

MINI UPDATE

Liver Transplantation *Natasha Chandok*	449
De Novo Malignancy in the Liver Transplantation Recipient *Natasha Chandok*	489
Minimal Hepatic Encephalopathy *Malcolm Wells*	509
Benign and Malignant Liver Mass Lesions *Mahmoud H Mosli*	527

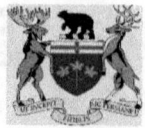

BACKGROUND

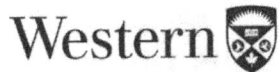

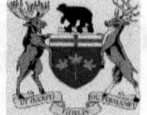

MINI UPDATE

An Introduction to CT Scanning of the Abdomen

Zahra Kassam

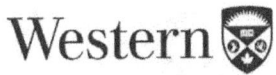

CT SCANNING OF THE ABDOMEN

Overview

- Brief introduction to Computed Tomography and basics of interpretation
- Pre-test anatomy
- Discussion of common protocols
- Unknown cases and answers
- Post-test anatomy

INTRODUCTION TO COMPUTED TOMOGRAPHY

CT Scanners

- Historically single detectors, only able to acquire one row of data at a time
  - Very slow – could take up to 30 minutes per scan
- Advent of multi-detector scanners has enabled rapid image acquisition
  - Parallel rows (64) of x-ray detectors
  - Each row records data independently as gantry rotates
  - Can image a larger patient volume in each rotation
  - Allows fast reconstruction in different thicknesses and planes
  - Allows multiphasic imaging (arterial, portal venous, delayed) and angiography

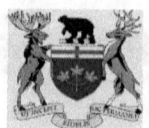

CT SCANNING OF THE ABDOMEN

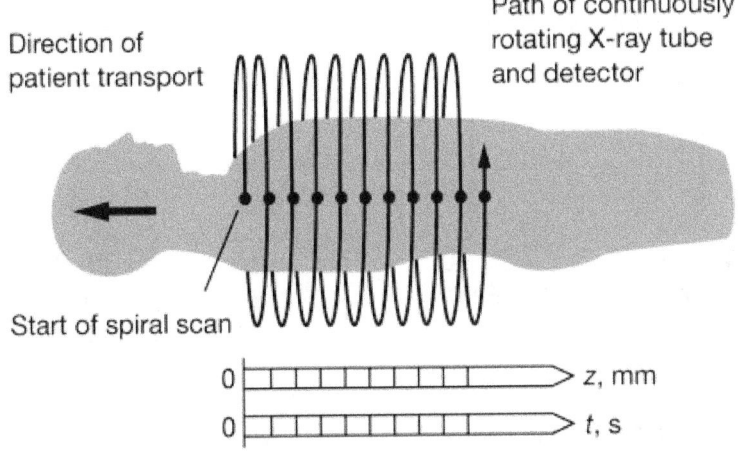

Source: Eur Heart J 2005;7 suppl G: G4-G12.

Measuring densities
- Radiography and Computed Tomography measure four basic densities:
  - Air
  - Fat
  - Water / soft tissue
  - Bone
- The denser a structure, the more likely it is to attenuate x-rays
- CT uses "Hounsfield Units" (HU) to describe relative densities
  - This is an arbitrary form of measurement based on relative X-ray attenuation value (CT number)
- Water is arbitrarily assigned a value of 0 HU
  - Positive integers are denser than water (e.g. muscle, bone)

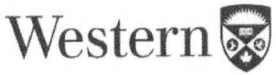

CT SCANNING OF THE ABDOMEN

- Negative integers are less dense than water (e.g. fat, air)

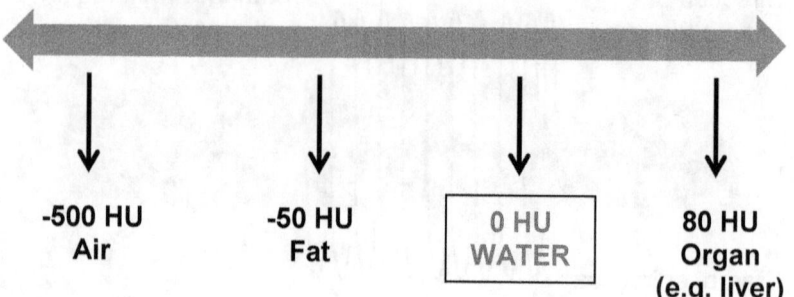

-500 HU
Air

-50 HU
Fat

0 HU
WATER

80 HU
Organ
(e.g. liver)

"Windows"

- Window width (WW)
  - Range of CT numbers displayed on the grey scale
    "Narrow" – only a few shades (densities) displayed
    "Wide" – many shades (densities) displayed
  - Each value below the defined range is black, above the defined range is white
  - Windows are defined arbitrarily, depending on what structures are being evaluated
  - Separate windows for looking at bone, lung, liver, soft tissue
  - The window settings are applied to the acquired data set
    (No need to re-scan the patient)
- Window level (WL)
  - Value around which the width is centered
- Common WW/WL:
  - Soft tissue: 450/50
  - Liver: 150/50
  - Lung: 1500/500
  - Bone: 2000/600

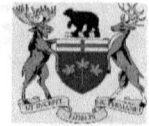

CT SCANNING OF THE ABDOMEN

Contrast

- Intrinsic contrast
  - Naturally occurring differences in density between normal structures in the body
    Air, Fat, Water / Soft tissue, Bone
  - Allows radiologist to distinguish between various tissues

- Extrinsic contrast
  - Intravascular
  - Enteric
  - Intracavitary (e.g. cystogram, sinogram)
  - Positive/negative agents
    e.g. water vs. barium

WHAT DO I LOOK FOR?
Lung bases –

- Nodules
- Air space disease
- Scarring
- Pleural/pericardial effusion
- Atelectasis
- Airways

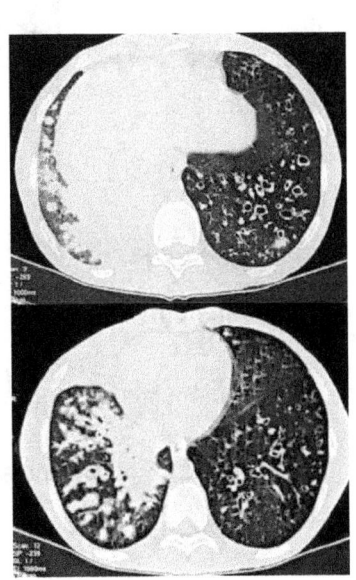

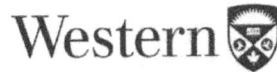

CT SCANNING OF THE ABDOMEN

Liver
- Size
- Attenuation
- Enhancement
- Lesions
- Capsule, surface
- Portal veins
- Hepatic veins
- Hepatic arteries

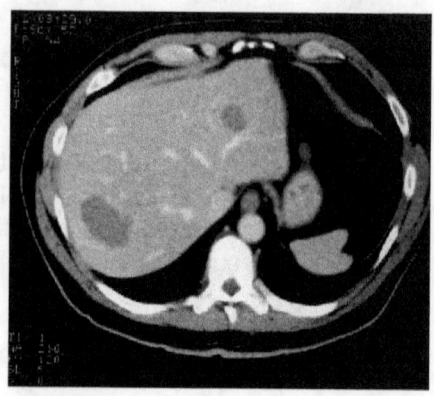

Biliary tree, gallbladder
- Bile duct dilatation
- Intraductal lesions
- Epithelial thickening
- Distention/thickening of GB
- Pericholecystic fluid
- Calculi
- Strictures

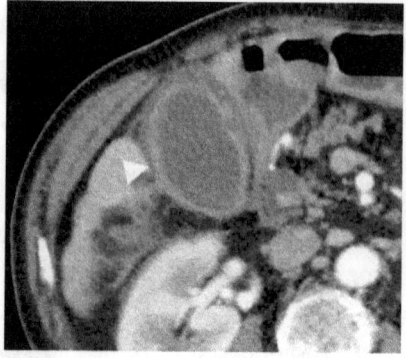

Inflamed gallbladder, with hyperemia and irregularity of the gallbladder wall. This was consistent with acute cholecystitis at surgery.

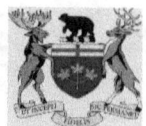

CT SCANNING OF THE ABDOMEN

Spleen
- Size
- Enhancement
- Splenules
- Splenic vein
- Splenic artery
- Perisplenic fluid

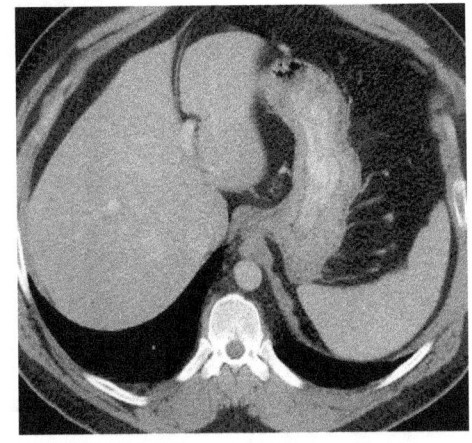

Pancreas (arrowhead)
- Size, position
  - Beware anomalies such as annular pancreas, ectopic pancreas
- Enhancement
- Pancreatic duct
- Nodes
- Fluid
- Inflammation

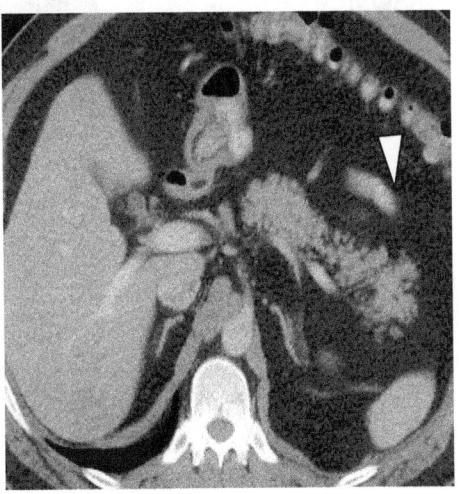

CT SCANNING OF THE ABDOMEN

Kidneys
- Size
- Position
- Enhancement
- Obstruction
- Lesions
- Perinephric spaces

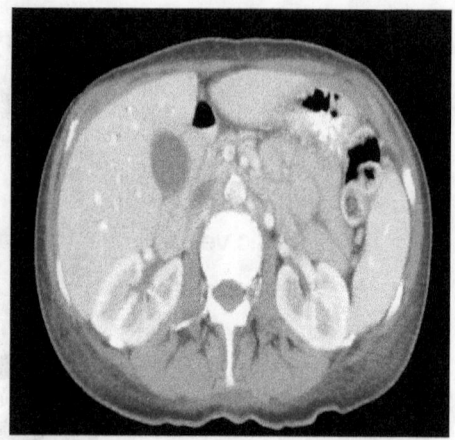

Stomach, small & large bowel
- Position
- Distention
- Wall thickening
- Fold thickness
- Mesentery
- Enhancement

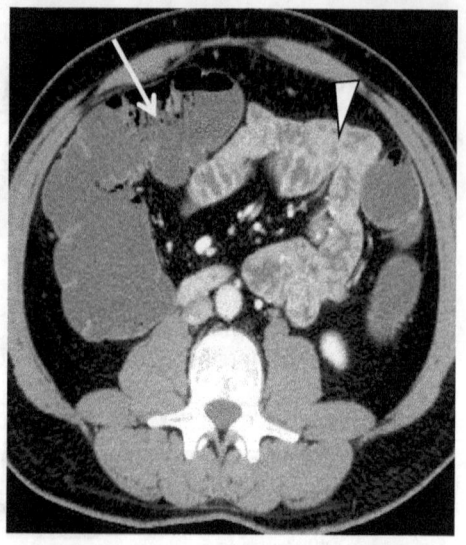

Normal large and small bowel (large bowel – arrow; small bowel – arrowhead).

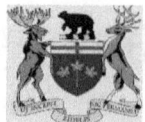

CT SCANNING OF THE ABDOMEN

COMMON PROTOCOLS AND WHEN THEY ARE USED

- Non-contrast CT:
  - Acute intraperitoneal or retroperitoneal hemorrhage
  - Calcification
  - Patient not suitable candidate for contrast
- Single phase IV contrast
  - Most routine indications
- Multiphasic IV contrast
  - Liver lesions
    +/- non-contrast, arterial, portal venous, delay
  - Renal masses
    Non-contrast, corticomedullary, nephrographic, excretory

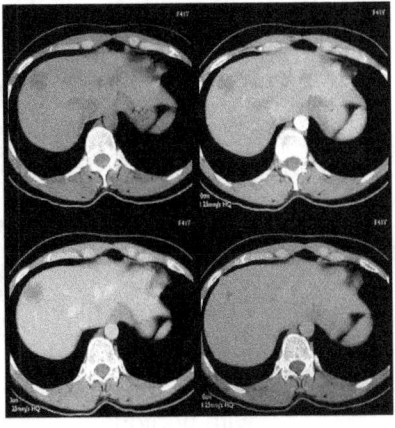

Multiphasic CT for evaluation of a liver mass. This multiphasic study confirmed a hepatic hemangioma.

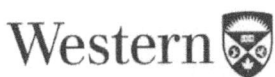

CT SCANNING OF THE ABDOMEN

Common protocols – Oral contrast

- o Positive oral contrast (hypaque)
    - Appears dense on CT
    - Abscess (helps differentiate fluid-containing bowel from extraluminal fluid)
    - Certain cancers with peritoneal metastases, e.g. ovarian
    - Other indications (variable)

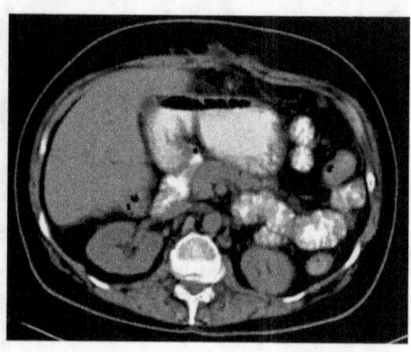

Positive (bright) oral contrast

- o Negative oral contrast (water/milk)
    - Bowel wall – mucosal abnormality
      Crohn disease
    - Pancreatic masses
      Distends duodenum and makes ampulla more visible
    - Bowel obstruction
      Intrinsic negative oral contrast – bowel secretes fluid in setting of obstruction (no need to administer

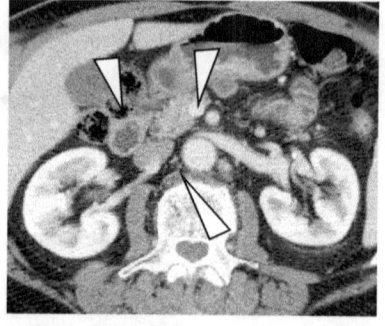

Negative oral contrast (water) was used in this case to distend the stomach. There is an ulcerated gastric carcinoma along the lesser curvature (arrowheads).

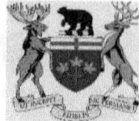

CT SCANNING OF THE ABDOMEN

additional contrast, may add to patient discomfort)

ESOPHAGUS

Boerhaave Syndrome

- o Spontaneous distal esophageal perforation following vomiting or straining (increase in IABP)
- o Typically left lateral wall of distal esophagus, just above GEJ
  - Vertically oriented full-thickness linear tear
  - Left side more vulnerable due to lack of supporting mediastinal structures
- o Untreated, 70% mortality rate Mediastinitis

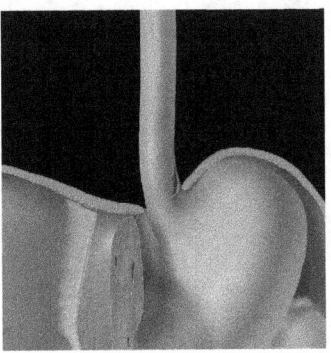

Source: Amirsys / Stat Dx

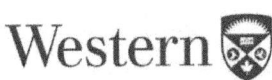

CT SCANNING OF THE ABDOMEN

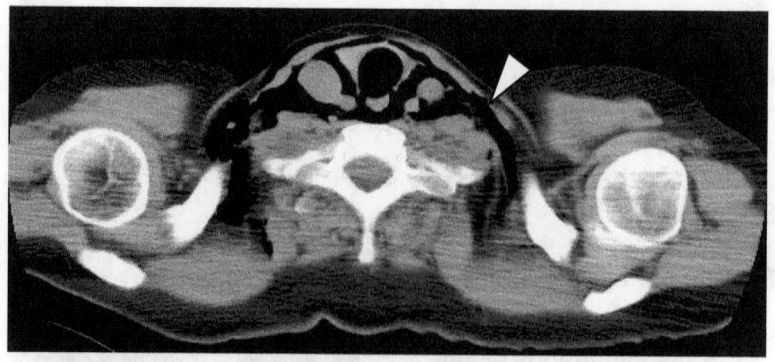

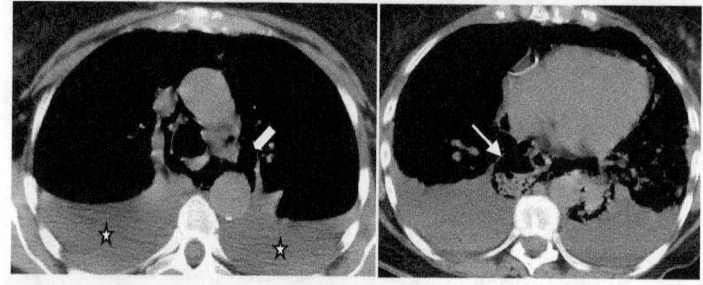

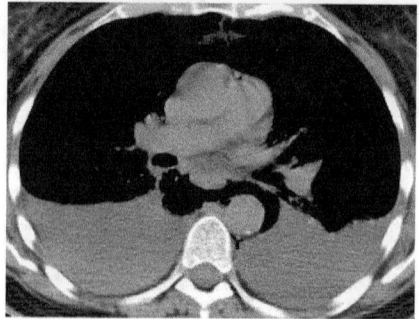

Boerhaave syndrome in this patient resulted in severe subcutaneous gas (arrowhead), pneumomedastinum (thick arrow), and bilateral pleural effusions (stars). The esophagus is markedly enlarged (thin arrow) – this patient is at high risk for mediastinitis.

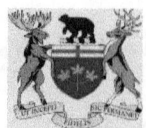

CT SCANNING OF THE ABDOMEN

GALLBLADDER

Acute Cholecystitis

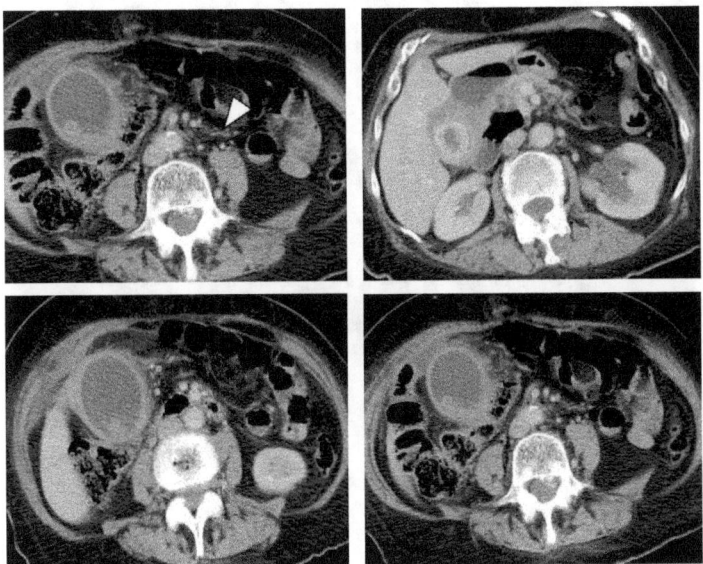

Distended gallbladder containing multiple calculi (arrowhead points to largest calculus). Gallbladder walls are thickened and show marked enhancement. There is also pericholecystic free fluid.

Gallbladder Carcinoma

- Epithelial malignancy arising from GB mucosa
- Commonly a large mass *infiltrating* from GB fossa into liver (GB has no capsule)
- May also be polypoid, intraluminal
- Calcified stones or porcelain GB
- Early invasion of liver/porta, early nodal dissemination
- DDx = differential diagnosis

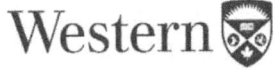

CT SCANNING OF THE ABDOMEN

- Metastatic disease (melanoma notorious but commonly goes to GB wall)
- Chronic cholecystitis

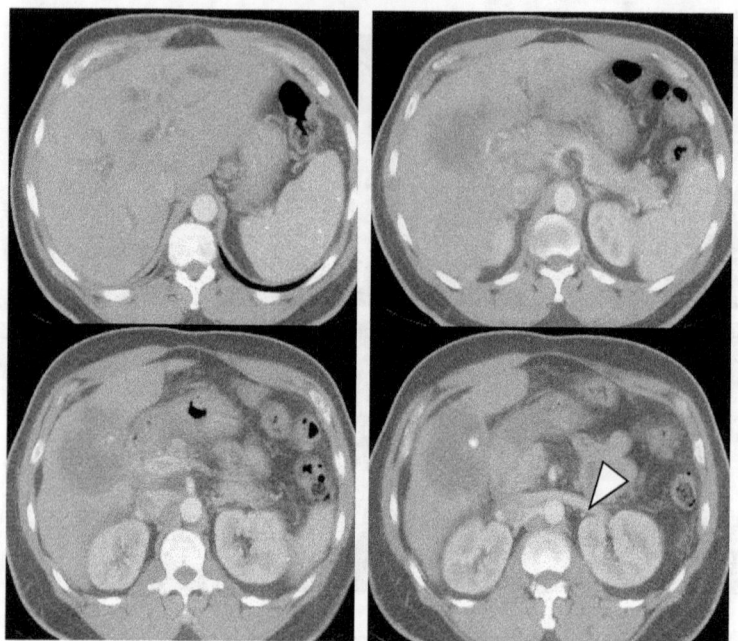

Gallbladder carcinoma. Large, poorly marginated hepatic mass causing intrahepatic biliary distention. Gallbladder is not visible in this patient, as it has been destroyed by the tumor. There was no history of cholecystectomy. A residual gallbladder calculus (arrowhead) provides a clue to the diagnosis.

PANCREAS

Acute pancreatitis

- o Inflammatory changes around pancreas
  - Soft tissue stranding
  - Fluid (simple or hemorrhagic, free or contained)
  - Ill-defined tissue planes

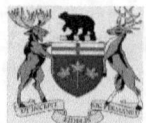

CT SCANNING OF THE ABDOMEN

- o Pancreatic enhancement
  - Necrosis Hemorrhage
- o Secondary changes
  - Gastric outlet obstruction
  - Venous thrombosis (splenic/SMV/confluence)
  - Pseudocysts
- o Potential causes
  - Gallstones
  - CBD calculus
  - Annular pancreas

Abbreviations: CBD, common bile duct; SMV, superior mesenteric vein

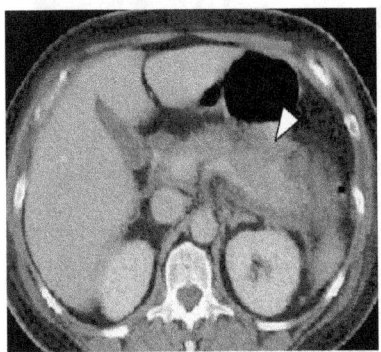 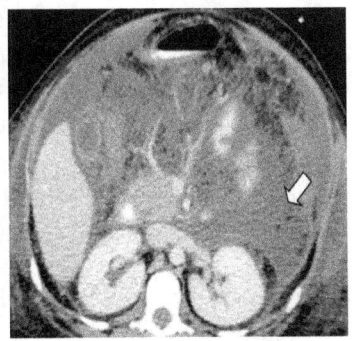

Inflamed, edematous pancreas with fluid in the anterior pararenal space (arrowhead). Marked ascites in the lower abdomen (arrows)

BILE DUCTS

Cholangiocarcinoma
- o Malignancy of biliary epithelium
- o Classification:
  - Intrahepatic
    Central or hilar
    - Klatskin

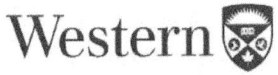

CT SCANNING OF THE ABDOMEN

Peripheral
- Exophytic
- Polypoid
- Infiltrative
- Extrahepatic

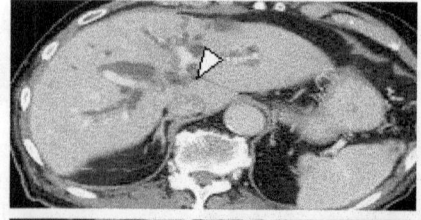
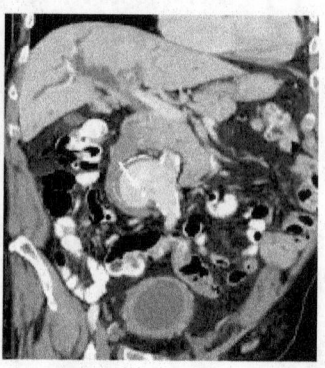
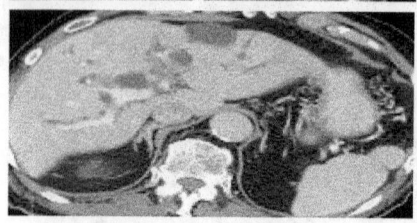

Axial images demonstrate intrahepatic biliary ductal dilatation. There is narrowing of the left portal vein at the liver hilus (arrowhead). Coronal image depicts an incidental abdominal aortic aneurysm (arrow).

Imaging Features of Cholangiocarcinoma
- Can be very subtle
- Infiltrative growth pattern, insinuates along and around structures
- Fibrous composition
  - May show *delayed enhancement* 10-15 min post injection
- Narrows tubular structures
  - Portal vein – look for thrombus
  - Hepatic artery – "sawtooth" pattern
  - Biliary strictures
- CT
  - Mild PV enhancement, may be more conspicuous on delayed

SMALL BOWEL

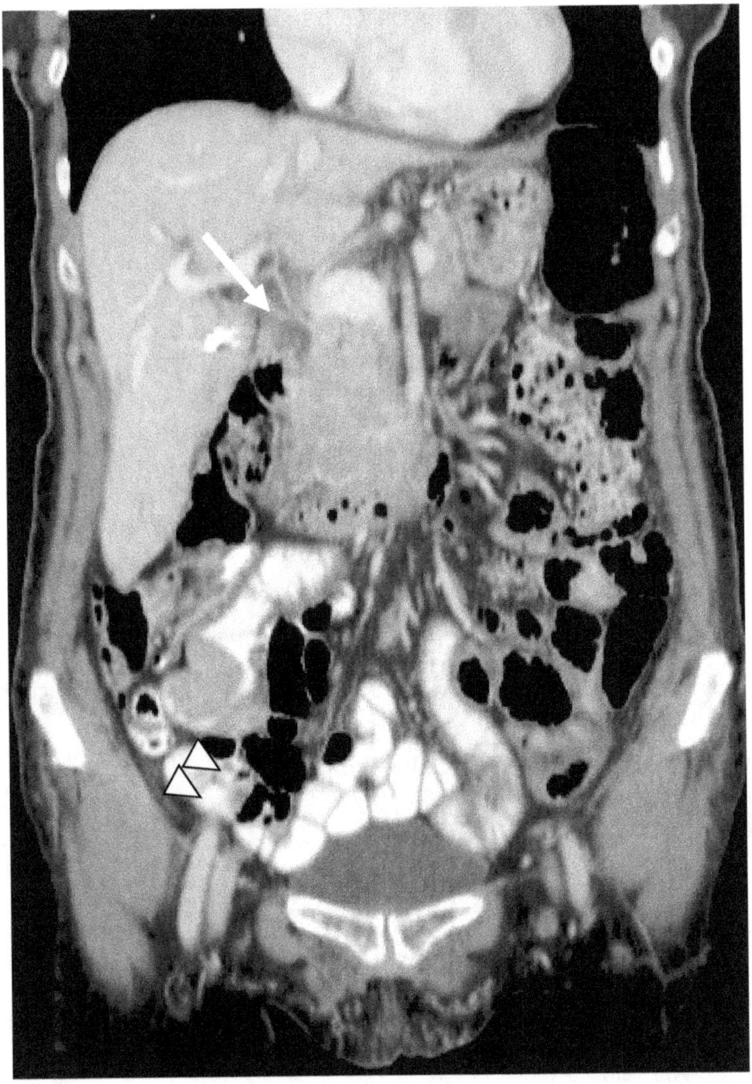

Small bowel lymphoma. Focal thickening of the distal small bowel (arrowheads) with nodal mass in the mesentery (arrow).

Small bowel (SB) Lymphoma

- Bull's eye or target lesion on barium study
- Classification:
  - Infiltrative
  - Polypoid
  - Nodular
  - Endoexoenteric
  - Mesenteric

  - Infiltrative most common
  - Mesenteric: "sandwich sign" – tumor grows around vessels without obstructing them; vessels are "sandwiched" between the tumor

- May be seen in celiac disease/sprue
- Now considered most common malignant SB tumor
  - 50% primary, 50% secondary
  - Mostly NHL, B-cell lymphoma
- Common sites
  - Stomach>SB>colon>esophagus
  - Ileum>jejunum>duodenum

Abbreviation: NHL, Non-Hodkins lymphoma

Mesenteric Panniculitis

- Mesenteric inflammatory disorder, unknown etiology
  - Chronic abdominal pain
- Fibrofatty mesenteric mass that surrounds mesenteric vessels but preserves a *fat halo* around vessels
  - Misty mesentery, small mesenteric LN
- Most commonly root of SB mesentery

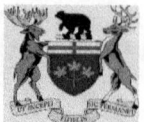

CT SCANNING OF THE ABDOMEN

- o Chronic inflammation, fat necrosis/fibrosis
- o Types:
  - Mesenteric panniculitis (inflammatory, fat necrosis)
  - Mesenteric lipodystrophy (less inflammatory)
  - Retractile mesenteritis (fibrosis/retraction)
- o May coexist with malignancy
  - Lymphoma, breast, lung, colon, melanoma
- o Differential diagnosis DDx:
  - Lymphoma
  - Carcinoid
  - Fibromatosis
  - Metastases

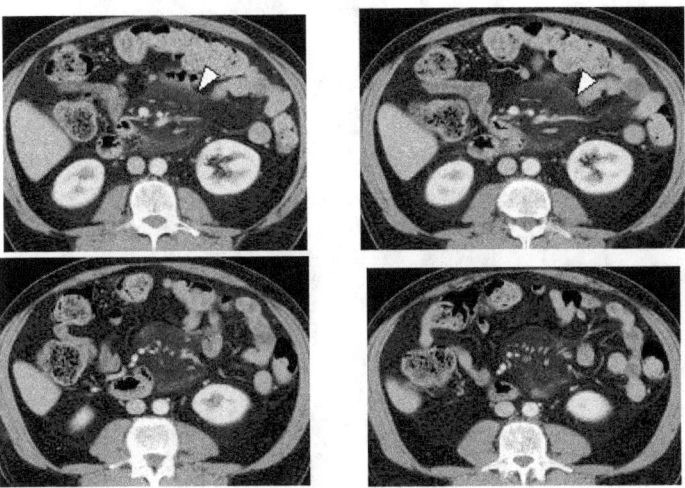

Mesenteric panniculitis. Soft tissue permeation/stranding (arrowhead) of the root of the small bowel mesentery in this patient with chronic abdominal pain.

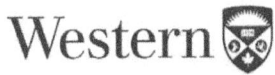

CT SCANNING OF THE ABDOMEN

Ileocolic Intussusception

- In adults, often due to a lead point, e.g. small bowel mass
- Intussusceptum (lead point) telescopes into intussuscipiens (colon), "dragging" along some of the small bowel mesentery with it
- On CT, fat density is visible within the intussuscipiens (usually colon)
- Patient may present with bowel obstruction

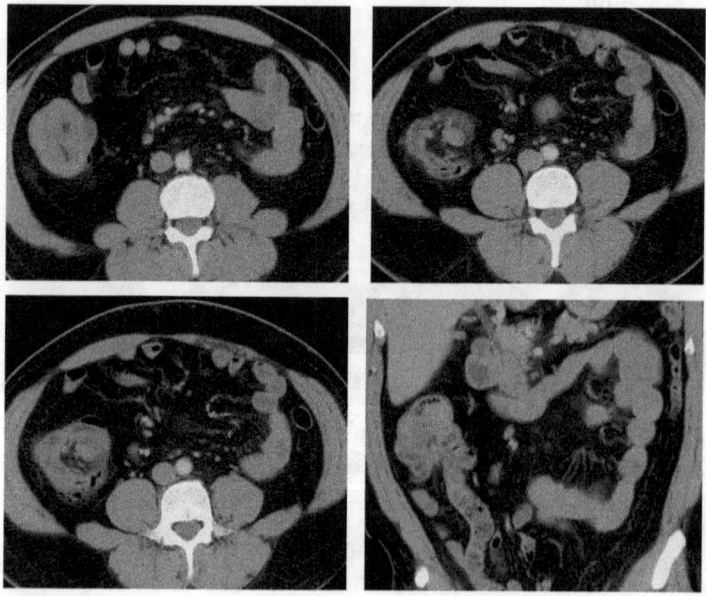

Ileocolic intussusception. Terminal ileum (arrowhead) has dragged small bowel mesentery with it into the proximal colon (therefore fat density is visible within the colonic lumen - arrow).

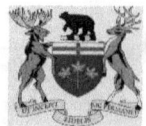

CT SCANNING OF THE ABDOMEN

Perforated carcinoma, transverse colon

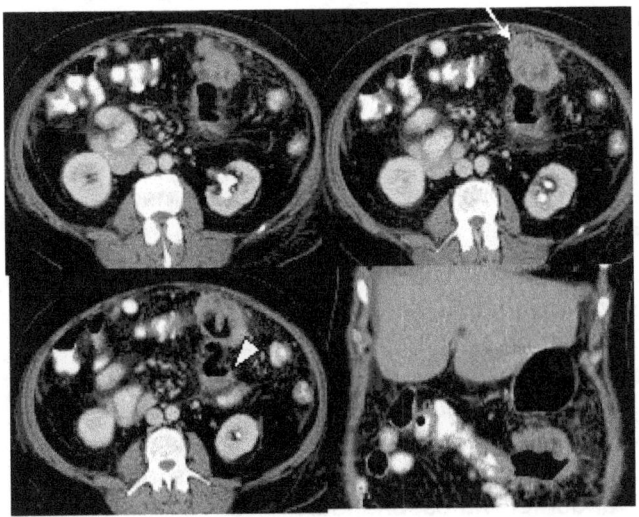

Large mass containing air, contiguous with the transverse colon, consistent with adenocarcinoma (arrow). The lower right image depicts the air within the tumor (arrowhead).

Sigmoid Volvulus

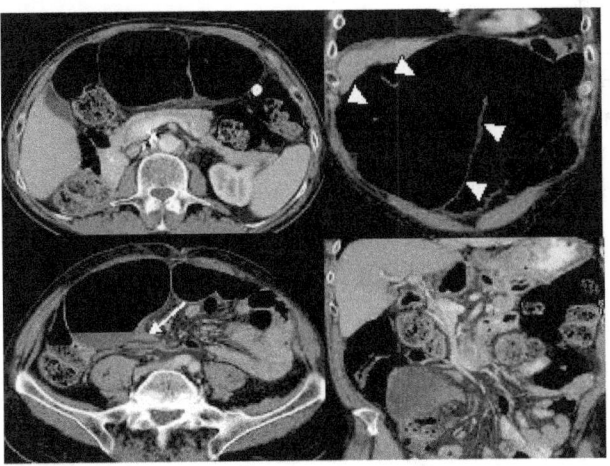

CT SCANNING OF THE ABDOMEN

CT images demonstrate a dilated loop of sigmoid colon, with a 'bird's beak" appearance on CT (arrow), and a "U-shaped" obstructed loop (arrowheads). These findings are diagnostic for volvulus.

Pneumatosis Intestinalis
- o   Air within the bowel wall, usually due to a mucosal defect
- o   Causes:
  - "Benign"
    Steroid therapy (weakens bowel mucosa)
    Intrinsic soft tissue disease (e.g. scleroderma, mixed connective tissue disorder)
    Asthma/COPD (positive pressure ventilation extends outside bronchus and tracks into abdomen via esophageal hiatus)
    Pneumomediastinum (tracks as above)
    Recent gastric intubation (air tracking through a small, iatrogenic mucosal defect)
    Ulcer disease
    Recent endoscopy
  - "Malignant"
    Ischemic gut
    Intestinal obstruction with strangulation
    Infection with gas forming organisms
    Trauma
    Ingestion of corrosive agents
    Toxic megacolon

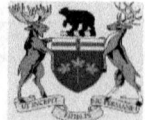

CT SCANNING OF THE ABDOMEN

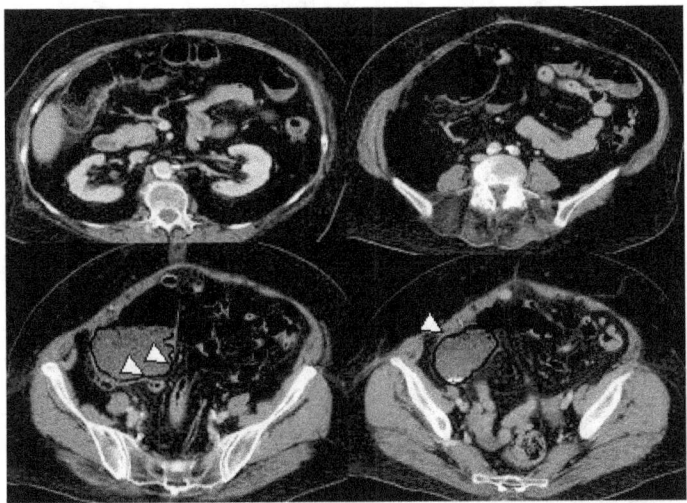

Air within the bowel wall (arrowheads), consistent with pneumatosis intestinalis.

APPENDIX

Acute Appendicitis

- Distended appendix, diameter >6 mm
- Mural enhancement
- +/- appendicolith (appears dense)
- Thickened cecal walls (arrowhead sign)
- Periappendiceal free fluid, abscess
- Position of the appendix is *variable* ileocecal valve or TI first, and work backward
- Important to localize appendix for surgical approach

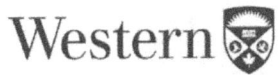

CT SCANNING OF THE ABDOMEN

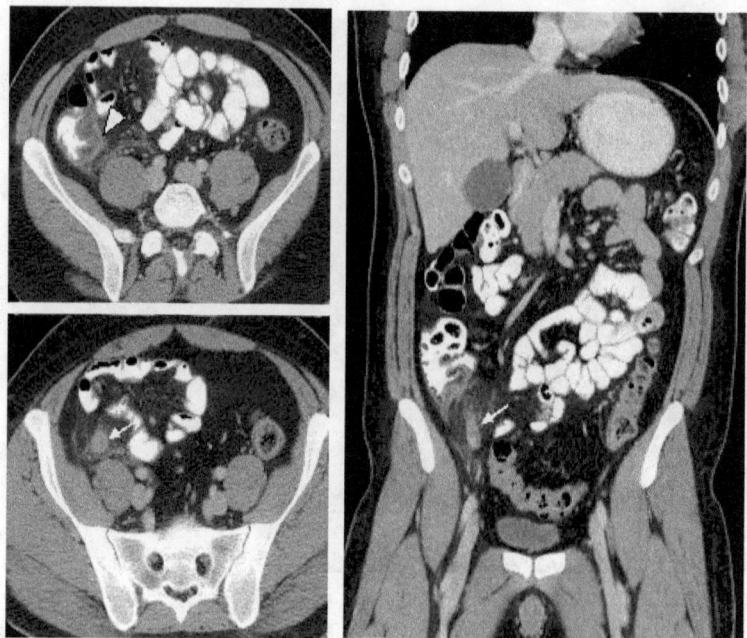

Acute appendicitis. Thickened medial cecal wall (arrowhead sign); dilated appendix (arrow)

Anatomy – Self Test

- Give the anatomical site or organ indicated by the numbered arrows in each case.

CT SCANNING OF THE ABDOMEN

Image 1

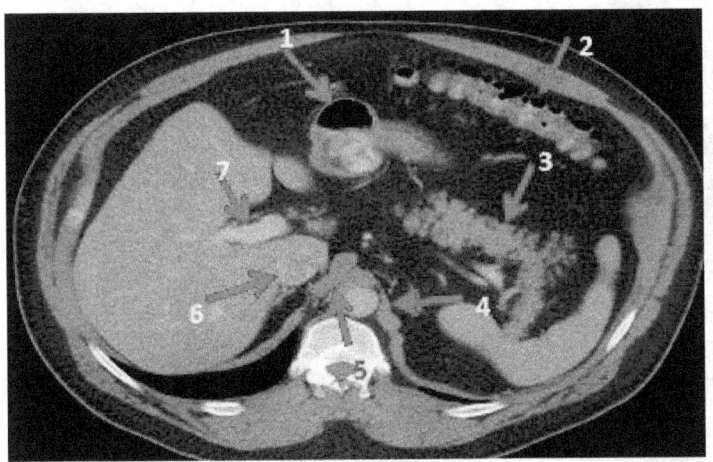

Image 2

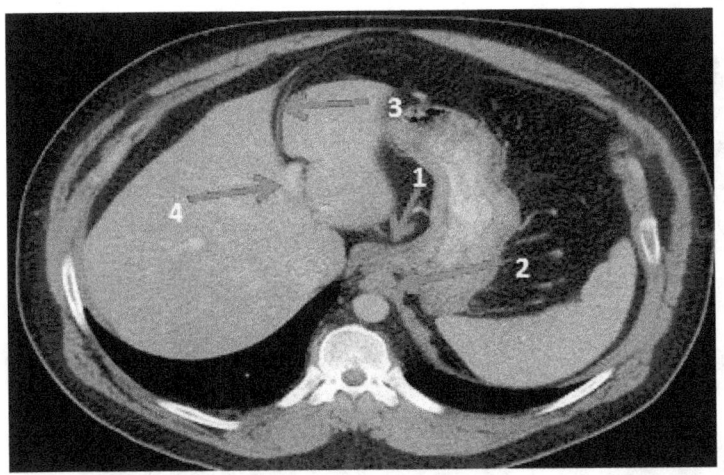

CT SCANNING OF THE ABDOMEN

Image 3

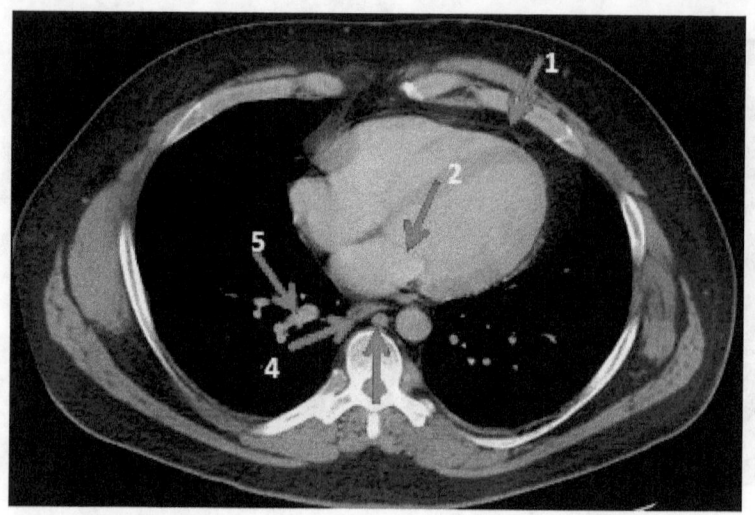

Image 4

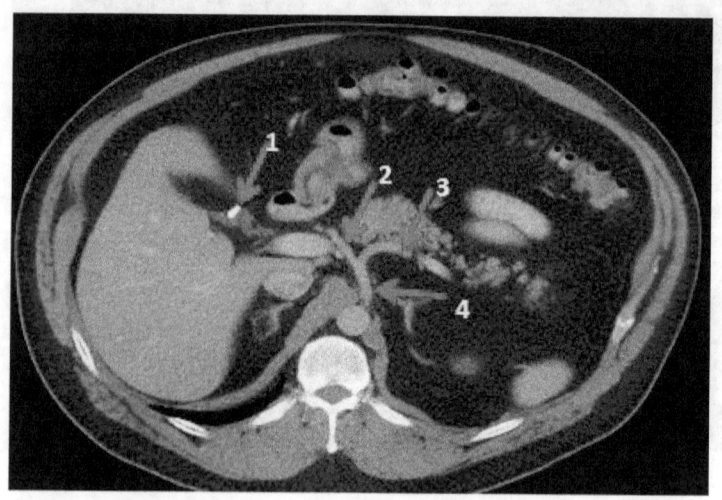

CT SCANNING OF THE ABDOMEN

Image 5

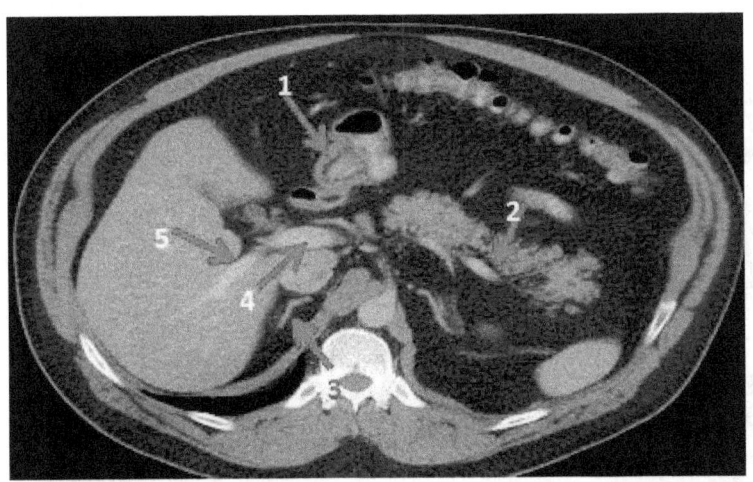

Image 6

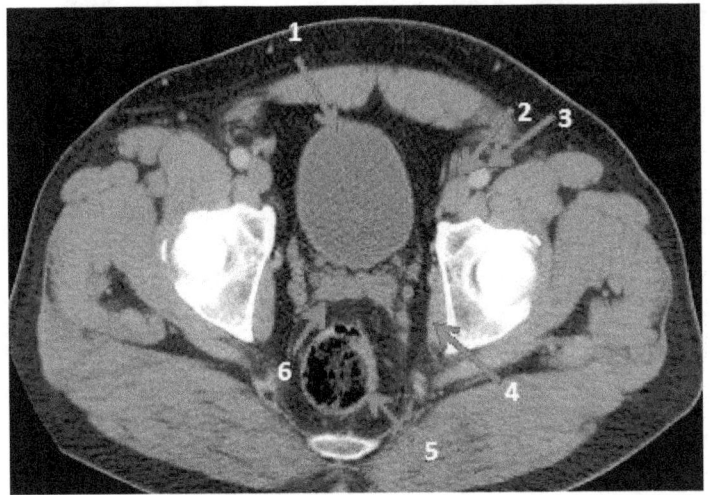

CT SCANNING OF THE ABDOMEN

Image 7

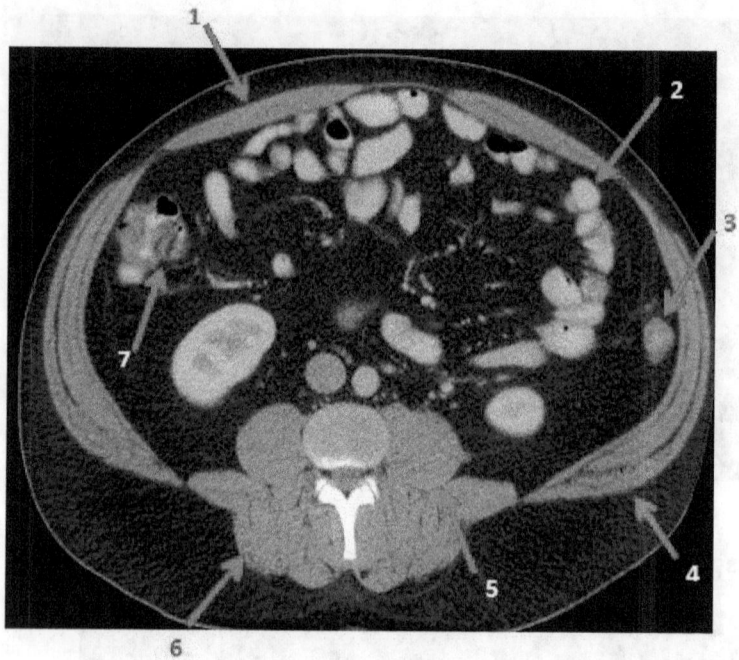

> "To give pleasure to a single heart by a single act is better than a thousand heads bowing in prayer."
>
> Mahatma Gandhi

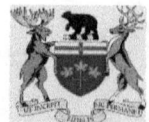

CT SCANNING OF THE ABDOMEN

Answer Sheet

The anatomical site or organ indicated by the numbered arrows in each case are given below.

Image 1
Duodenal cap
Transverse colon
Pancreas
Left hemidiaphragm
Right diaphragmatic crus
IVC
Portal vein

Image 2
GE junction
Right diaphragmatic crus
Falciform ligament
Left portal vein

Image 3
1. Pericardium
2. Mitral valve
3. Azygos vein
4. Esophagus
5. Right inferior pulmonary vein

Image 4
1. Cholecystectomy
2. Common hepatic artery
3. Splenic artery
4. Celiac axis

Image 5
1. Gastric antrum/duodenal cap
2. Splenic vein
3. Right adrenal gland
4. Main portal vein
5. Right portal vein

Image 6
1. Bladder (number cut off)
2. Left common femoral vein
3. Left common femoral artery
4. Obturator internus muscle

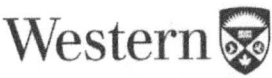

CT SCANNING OF THE ABDOMEN

5. Rectum
6. Seminal vesicle

Image 7
1. Rectus abdominus
2. Small bowel
3. Descending colon
4. External oblique muscle
5. Psoas muscle
6. Quadratus lumborum muscle
7. Cecum / ileocecal valve

MINI UPDATE

ESOPHAGUS

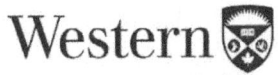

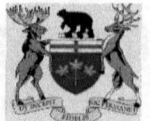

MINI UPDATE

Eosinophilic Esophagitis

Nitin Khanna

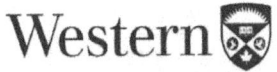

EOSINOPHILIC ESOPHAGITIS

Eosinophilic Esophagitis (EE)

- Demography
    - Increasing incidence / prevalence
    - Caucasians
    - More common in males in their 40s and 50s
    - May be associated with allergies
    - Symptoms depend on part of GI tract involved and layer of wall
        - Stomach / small bowel / colon
        - Mucosal / Muscle / Subserosa
    - Eosinophilic esophagitis (EoE) is more common among males and Caucasians.
    - Caucasians are
        - Older at diagnosis with eosinophilic esophagitis (EoE) than African Americans
        - Less likely to present with failure-to-thrive
        - More likely to have esophageal rings
    - Males were more likely to be diagnosed in childhood and more frequently report dysphagia or food impaction.
    - May mimic IBS, often diagnosed while investigating for suspected Celiac or IBD
    - May affect children
    - Symptoms present for years prior to diagnosis

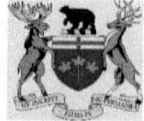

EOSINOPHILIC ESOPHAGITIS

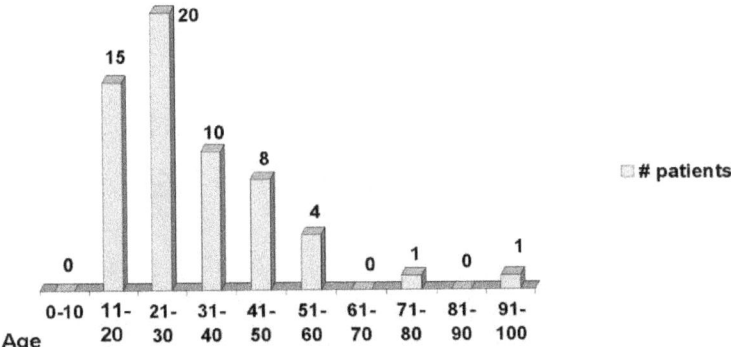

- ➢ Pathogenesis
    - o Genetically predisposed individual
        - Familial clustering
        - ? Susceptibility locus on Chromosome 5
    - o Exposed to environmental factor / antigen
    - o The immune response results in high recruitment of eosinophils to the esophagus
    - o Th2 cells involved
    - o Eotaxin (a peptide) and IL-5 are important for the recruitment of eosinophils
    - o IL-5 is also necessary for esophagitis / strictures

- ➢ Pathology
    - o Histology:
    - o > 15 eosinophils per hpf (high power field; 400x), identified in two HPFs
    - o Eosinophillic microabscesses
        - Eosinophils in aggregation
    - o Important to rule our GERD
        - Symptoms of heartburn, reflux, chest pain
        - Biopsy distal and proximal esophagus
        - Biopsy after treating with PPI

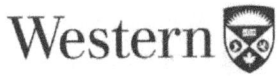

EOSINOPHILIC ESOPHAGITIS

- Consider 24 hr pH study
- \# eosinophils usually lower in GERD, and present in distal rather than proximal esophagus
  o Other histologic findings suggestive of EE:
    - Eosinophils microabscesses
      - Superficial layering
      - Sheets
      - Extracellular eosinophil granules
    - Inflammation
      - Increased number of
        - Mast cells
        - B cells
        - IgE-bearing cells
    - GERD-like histology
      - Basal cell hyperplasia
      - Papillary lengthening
      - Subepithelial and lamina propria fibrosis and inflammation

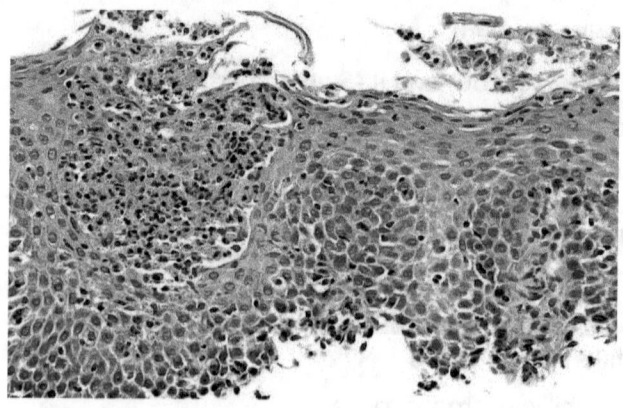

Eosinophilic Esophagitis

> Clinical Manifestations
  o Dysphagia
    - Up to 15% of patients have EE
  o Food impaction

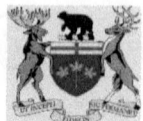

EOSINOPHILIC ESOPHAGITIS
- Up to 50% of patients
  o Chest pain
  o GERD symptom
  o Associations with other disorders
    - Food allergies
    - Environmental allergies
    - Asthma
    - Atopic dermatitis
    - Celiac disease
    - Schatzki ring

➤ Causes

- Give 8 causes/associations of eosinophilic gastrointestinal diseases (EGIDs).
  o Idiopathic
    - Eosinophilic syndromes
  o Infection
    - Fungal, parasitic and non-parasitic
  o Inflammation
    - GSE
    - IBD
    - MC
    - GERD
  o Neoplasia
    - Hodgkin's lymphoma
    - Esophageal
    - Leiomyomatosis
  o Immune
    - Autoimmune
    - GVH disease
    - Connective tissue disease (e.g. scleroderma)

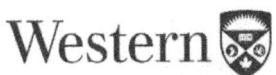

EOSINOPHILIC ESOPHAGITIS

- Hypersensitivity
- Allergy (e.g. foods)
- Allergic vasculitis
- Post-transplant

o Iatrogenic
- Drugs (e.g. gold, azathioprine)

Abbreviations: EGID, eosinophilic gastrointestinal diseases; GERD, gastroesophageal reflux disease; GSE, gluten-sensitive enteropathy; GVH, graft-versus-host disease; IBD, inflammatory bowel disease; MC, microscopic colitis

Adapted from: Mueller S. *Best Pract Res Clin Gastroenterol* 2008;22(3): pg. 427.; and Atkins D, et al. *Nat Rev Gastroentol Hepatol* 2009;6(5): 267-278.

➢ Complications
- Eosinophilic esophagitis is a high risk disease. Give 5 complications.
  o Dysphagia
  o Food impaction
  o Stricture
  o Sloughing of mucosa (mucosal eosinophils)
  o Mucosal tear
  o Perforation
    - EGD
    - Spontaneous (Boerhaave syndrome) (transmural inflammation)

Abbreviation: EGD, esophagogastroduodenoscopy

  o Intermittent, solid food dysphagia in EoE is typical
  o Basal cell hyperplasia is more common in EoE than in GERD

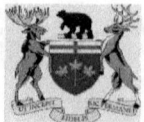

EOSINOPHILIC ESOPHAGITIS

- o Eosinophils ↑ closer to surface of esophagus in EoE than in GERD
- o It is being shown that it is safe to dilate carefully (45 F) the esophagus after mucosal biopsies have been taken.

➢ Endoscopy

- Give 5 changes on EGD in the patient with eosinophilic esophagitis (EE).
  - o Corrugation (multiple rings)
  - o Longitudinal furrows
  - o Mucosa: featureless, fragile (crepe paper)
  - o White surface vesicles (eosinophilic microabscess)
  - o Proximal or mid-esophageal stenosis/stricture
  - o Small caliber esophagus
  - o Food impaction
  - o EGD may be normal

Abbreviations: EE, eosinophilic esophagitis; EGD, esophago-gastroduodenoscopy

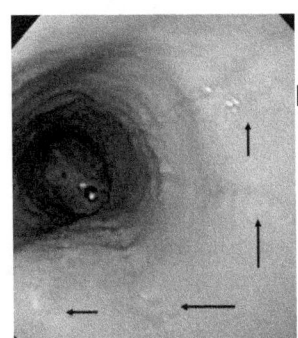

Eosinophilic Esophagitis
- Linear Furrows

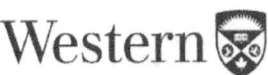

EOSINOPHILIC ESOPHAGITIS

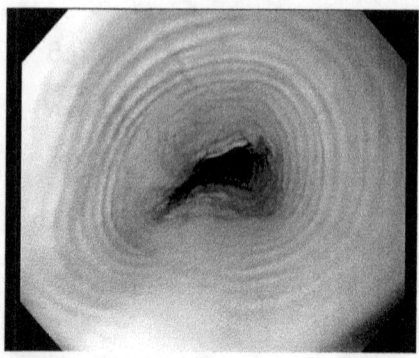

Eosinophilic Esophagitis
- Circular rings

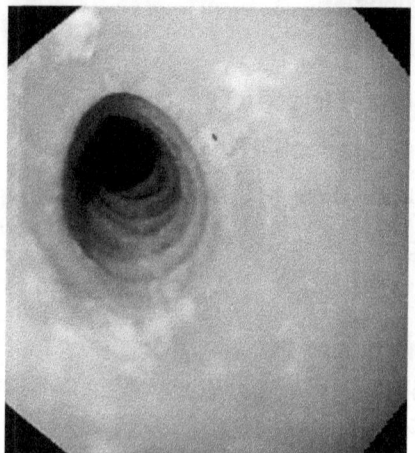

Eosinophilic Esophagitis
- Whitish papules

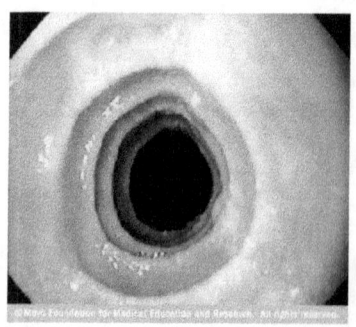

Eosinophilic Esophagitis
- Small caliber esophagus

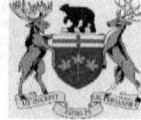

EOSINOPHILIC ESOPHAGITIS

- Differential
  - Intermittent dysphagia, sometimes severe; food impaction
  - Failed treatment with proton pump inhibitor (PPI) therapy for presumed GERD
  - Chest pain with odynophagia
  - Peripheral eosinophilia is common
  - Atopic diseases

Printed with permission: Attwood SEA, and Lamb CA. *Best Pract Res Clin Gastroenterol* 2008;22(4): 641.

- Give the diagnostic work-up for eosinophilic gastrointestinal diseases (EGIDs)
  - General without associated eosinophilia
    - Infection evaluation (stool, intestinal aspirates, and blood analyses)
    - Total and allergen-specific IgE (immunoassays and skin tests)
    - Differential blood cell count
    - Microscopic evaluation of biopsy samples from the affected and non-affected gastrointestinal parts (histological and immunohistological analysis) T-cells , mast cells
    - Granule protein and cytokine measurements (immunoassays using blood, feces, or urine)
    - Immunophenotyping of blood cells (surface marker staining and subsequent flow cytometric analysis)

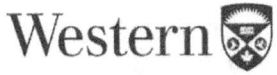

EOSINOPHILIC ESOPHAGITIS

- o With hypereosinophila, in addition to above, perform
  - Immunophenotyping of blood cells (in particular T cells and eosinophils)
  - Bone marrow analysis (cellularity, dysplastic eosinophils, spindle-shaped mast cells, cytogenetic abnormalities, etc.)
  - Measurements of vitamin B12, tryptase, IL-5, and TARC in blood
  - Genetic analysis for the presence of a FIPILI-PDGFRA gene fusion
  - Eosinophil granule protein measurements

Abbreviation: EGID, eosinophilic gastrointestinal diseases

Printed with permission: Conus S, and Simon HU. *Best Pract Res Clin Gastroenterol* 2008;22(3): pg. 443.

➢ Laboratory
  - o ↑ Serum IgE levels in 50%
  - o Peripheral eosinophilia in 50%

➢ Diagnostic imaging
  - o Helpful only to show strictures

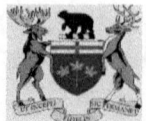

EOSINOPHILIC ESOPHAGITIS

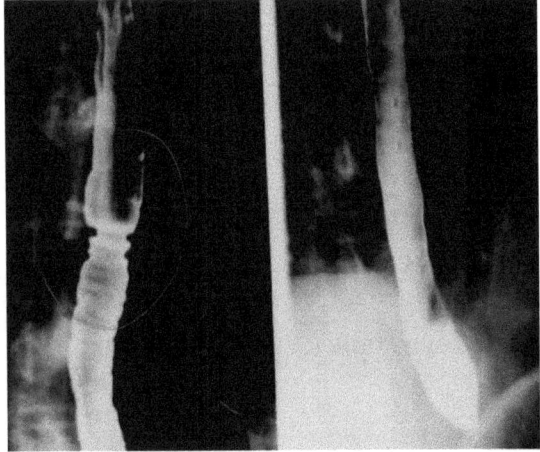

Eosinophilic Esophagitis

- o Suspect if:
  - Peripheral eosinophilia
  - ↑ serum IgE
  - Atopic person
- o Endoscopy
  - Non-specific endoscopic findings
    - Erythema
    - Erosions
    - Nodularity
- o Biopsies: > 20 eosinophils per hpf
- o 80% found within reach of EGD (esophagogastroduodenoscopy)

➢ EG: Muscle and subserosal

- o Muscle EG
  - More obstruction presentation with thickened, rigid gut
  - May have peripheral eosinophilia
  - Usually diagnosed following resection for obstruction
- o Subserosal:
  - Ascites with high eosinophils

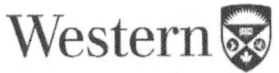

EOSINOPHILIC ESOPHAGITIS

- ➢ Other conditions to consider:
  - Intestinal parasites
  - Malignancy / lymphoma
  - IBD (typical Crohn disease architectural changes usually not seen)
  - Polyarteritis nodosa (usually have ↑↑ ESR)
  - Hypereosinophilic syndrome (usually involves several organs)

- ➢ Treatment
- Diet
  - General
    - Low residue / soft diet for strictures
    - Eat slowly, chew food well
    - Drink fluids with meal
  - Elimination diet
    - Peanuts
    - Eggs
    - Soy
    - Cow's milk
    - Wheat
    - Tree nuts
  - Elemental diet
    - Protein source is synthetic amino acids
    - Unpalatable / expensive
  - Consider possible referral allergist

- A 30 year old patient with solid food dysphagia presents for an upper endoscopy. There is no history of heartburn or regurgitation, and no family history of esophageal disease. A benign appearing stricture is seen. You suspect eosinophilic esophagitis (EoE). Give the steps in management.

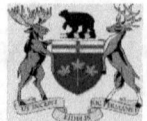

EOSINOPHILIC ESOPHAGITIS

- Exclude eosinophilic esophagitis (EoE) by biopsy of mid esophagus, >15 eosinophils
- If positive for EoE, treat for 4 weeks with PPI, before specific Rx for EoE.
- Do not do initial empiric dilation of stricture until EoE disproven, or proven by biopsy and treated
- Dilate gently and progressively only after treatment of EoE
- Use generous sedation
- If perforation occurs, try to avoid surgery, since wall does not hold sutures well; may need to do Esophagectomy
- Dietary elimination in children

Abbreviation: EoE, eosinophilic esophagitis

- Steroids
  - Topical Fluticasone
    - Swallowed fluticasone, 1-2 puffs qid for 6-8 weeks for short-term therapy, but not for maintenance
    - 70% recurrence rate after initial steroid use, and esophageal dilations may still be necessary (Helou EF, et al. *Am J Gastroenterol* 2008:2194-9).
    - Case series: 21 adults, fluticasone for 6 weeks
      - Symptoms resolved in all patients for at least 4 months
      - No patient needed endoscopic dilation
    - Case series: 19 adults, fluticasone for 4 weeks
      - Both symptomatically and histologic improvement
      - 14 (74%) of the 19 patients had a recurrence of symptoms after 3 months
    - RCT: 36 children, fluticasone vs. placebo for 3 months

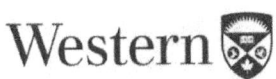

EOSINOPHILIC ESOPHAGITIS

- Histologic remission in 50% vs. 9% for fluticasone vs. placebo

Source: Arora et al. Mayo Clin Proc 2003; 78(7):830-5; Remedios et al. Gastrointest Endosc. 2006;63(1):3-12.; Konikoff et al. Gastroenterology. 2006 ;131(5):1381-91.

- Tablets, 20-40 mg prednisone po for 4-6 weeks, followed by slow taper.
- Indicated in EOE persons with acute dysphagia, high risk for esophageal perforation while undergoing repeated dilations, severe weight loss, or refractory to other symptoms.
- Topical Budesonide (BUD)
  - RCT in both adults and children show benefit
  - Both viscous and nebulized BUD
  - 36 adults with EE, 1 mg BID nebulized Bud vs. placebo for 15 days
  - Dysphagia improved in 72% vs. 22%
  - Histologic improvement seen with BUD

Source: Straumann A, et al. Gastroenterology. 2010;139(5):1526-37.

- Systemic Steroids
  - RCT in children: prednisone vs. swallowed fluticasone
  - All were symptom-free at 4 weeks
  - 45 % in both groups relapse at 24 weeks
  - Steroid adverse effects in 40% with prednisone
  - Candidal esophagitis in 15% with fluticasone

Source: Schaefer et al, Clin Gastroenterol Hepatol. 2008;6(2):165-73.Esophageal Dilation

  - Effective for improving dysphagia
  - Usually for high grade strictures or failed medical therapy

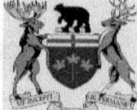

EOSINOPHILIC ESOPHAGITIS

- Dilate up 3 mm per session
- Associated with
  - Chest pain
  - Deep mucosal tears
- 2010 meta-analysis, 468 patients / 671 dilations → 1 perforation (0.1%)

Source: Jacobs et al., Dig Dis Sci 2010; 55(6):1512-5.

➢ PPI
  - Symptoms, endoscopic and histology changes may improve

➢ Esophageal Dilation
  - Improves symptoms in 75%
  - Need to be cautious due to risk of deep tears and perforation
  - Wire-guided Savary Dilation preferable
  - Risk of perforation not as high as originally thought (approx. 0.3%)
  - Free perforations require surgery

Source: Moawad et al., Aliment Pharmacol Ther 2013; 38:713 (Meta-Analysis)

➢ Alternatives
  - Antihistamines / Chromolyn: no benefit
  - Montelukast (leukotriene inhibitor)
    - Not recommended because of lack of reduction of eosinophilic infiltration in the esophageal mucosa
  - Anti-IL-5 mAb (meplizumab; humanized monoclonal IgG antibody to IL-5)
    - Poor response in placebo-controlled study

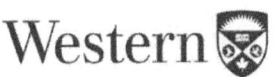

EOSINOPHILIC ESOPHAGITIS

- Anti-IgE mAb
- Azathioprine
- Infliximab

> Elimination diets (especially in children) reduce symptoms and mucosal eosinophilia

- Use skin prick testing to diagnose Type 1 IgE-mediated sensitivity, and skin patch testing for Type IV Th-2 delayed hypersensitivity reactions
- Most common food allergies are dairy, eggs, wheat, soy, peanuts, fish/shellfish
- Some recent evidence for benefit in adults, similar to benefit in children

Useful background: Limitations to medications currently used for EE

- Only one randomised, blinded, placebo-controlled trial and it was conducted with pediatric patients.
- Few trials in adults, especially those with dysphagia and anatomic narrowing of the esophagus.
- Trials only examine short-term treatment (four months or shorter); trials need to be at least one year on and off therapy.
- None of the trials address maintenance or pulse therapy, which may be critical as relapses are common.
- No validated dysphagia or quality of life questionnaires used to quantify patients symptoms resulting in patient and investigator variability.
- Diagnostic criteria and clinical endpoints vary across most studies.

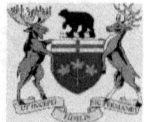

EOSINOPHILIC ESOPHAGITIS

- o Numerous confounding variables, which may affect study outcome including acid suppression, dietary restriction and allergy testing.

Printed with permission: Hait et al. *Clin Gastroenterol Hepatol* 2009;7:721-724.

- Give the comparison the advantage and disadvantages of current medical and nutritional treatment strategies for eosinophilic esophagitis

Treatment	Advantages	Disadvantages
o Oral steroids (1-2 mg/kg/day: maximum 60 mg)	- Rapid relief of symptoms	- Significant systemic side effects - Prompt recurrence when discontinued
o Swallowed fluticasone (children 440-880 µg/day; adolescents/adults, 880-1769 µg/day)	- Minimal systemic steroid absorption - Shown to relieve symptoms - Normalizes esophageal mucosa	- Risk of candidal esophagitis - Small amount systemically absorbed - Long term efficacy unknown, but prompt recurrence when discontinued - Difficult for small children and developmentally delayed patients to swallow
o Viscous budesonide (<10 y, 1 mg daily; >10 y, 2 mg daily)	- Easier to swallow - Theoretically can reach more distal areas of esophagus	- Cumbersome to mix - Theoretical risk of candidal esophagitis - Long term efficacy unknown

EOSINOPHILIC ESOPHAGITIS

Treatment	Advantages	Disadvantages
o Montelukast (20-40 mg daily)	- Shown to reduce symptoms and normalize esophageal mucosa - Symptomatic relief has been shown at high doses (100 mg) - No significant adverse effects	- Not clear whether it improve esophageal eosinophilia - Inadequate studies
o Cromolyn sodium (100 mg 4 times a day)	- No significant adverse effects	- Inadequate studies
o Mepolizumab	- Phase II trials in adults show that it is safe - Promising preliminary data in pediatric studies	- Did not induce significant histologic remission in adult study
o Elemental diet	- 92%-98% effective - Resolution of symptoms in 7-10 days - Histologic remission within 4-5 weeks	- Poor palatability - Usually requires nasogastric or gastrostomy tube - Very expensive - Socially isolating

- o Little published data, no RCTs (randomized clinical trials)

EOSINOPHILIC ESOPHAGITIS

- o Diet
  - Elimination diet (soy, wheat, corn, egg, milk, peanut, seafood)
  - Elemental diet
- o Steroids
  - Prednisone 20-40 mg / day for 2 weeks then taper
    - Most patients respond
    - Choices for relapsing EE
      - Chronic low dose prednisone
      - Repeated courses of higher dose with taper
      - Transition to Budesonide
- o No evidence of benefit for allergies.

- Give the differentiated diagnosis of the causes of food impaction / "foreign body" ingestion.
  - o Schatzki ring
  - o Peptic strictures
  - o EOE (eosinophilic esophagitis)

EOSINOPHILIC ESOPHAGITIS

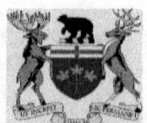

Esophageal Cancer

Mahmoud Mosli

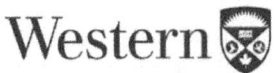

ESOPHAGEAL CANCER

- ➢ Clinical features
  - Heartburn
  - Regurgitation
  - Chest pain
  - Progressive dysphagia
  - Odynophagia
  - Hoarseness
  - Weight loss
  - Iron deficiency anemia
  - Esophago-respiratory fistula (intractable cough, or recurrent pneumonia)
  - Hematemesis
  - Symptoms of metastasis (lung, liver, bone or brain)

- Give 10 presenting symptoms for esophageal cancer.

  - Esophagus
    - Dysphagia, odynophagia
    - Back or chest pain with/without swallowing
    - Halitosis
    - Tracheoesophageal fistula
  - Nerves
    - Hoarseness from recurrent laryngeal nerve involvement
    - Horner syndrome (miosis, ptosis, absence of sweating on ipsilateral face and neck)
    - Phrenic nerve involvement from hiccups
  - Nodes
    - Supraclavicular adenopathy

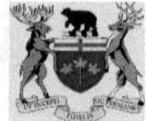

ESOPHAGEAL CANCER

- o Systemic
  - Weight loss
  - Clubbing
  - Signs/ symptoms of metastases

➢ Pathology

- Give a classification of esophageal tumors
  - o Esophageal
    - Malignant
      - Squamous cell carcinoma
      - Adenocarcinoma
      - Adenocarcinoma of the esophagogastric junction
      - Verrucous carcinoma
      - Carcinosarcoma
      - Small cell carcinoma
      - Malignant melanoma
    - Benign
      - Squamous papilloma
      - Adenoma
      - Inflammatory fibroid
      - Polyp
  - o Nonepithelial
    - Malignant
      - Lymphoma
      - Sarcoma, including malignant
      - GIST
      - Metastatic carcinoma
    - Benign
      - GIST
      - Leiomyoma
      - Granular cell tumor
      - Fibrovascular
      - Tumor
      - Hemangioma
      - Hamartoma
      - Lipoma

Abbreviation: GIST, gastrointestinal stromal cell tumor

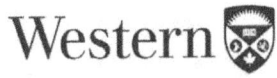

ESOPHAGEAL CANCER

➤ Risk factors

- Give 10 risk factors for squamous cell cancer
    o Demographic: "Asian esophageal cancer belt," extending from northern Iran through the central Asian republics to north-central China
    o Epidemiological factors: a African descent
    o Dietary intake:
        - Polycyclic aromatic hydrocarbons (soot extract of coal-burning stoves)
        - N-nitroso compounds (e.g. smoked pickles and a bread-like food called qocho or kocho in Ethiopia)
        - Chewing betelquid with areca nut
        - Use of gutka (pan masala, a dry powdered mixture of areca nut
        - Catecu
        - Lime
        - Flavoring agents
        - Aflatoxins
    o Dietary deficiencies
        - Selenium
        - Folate
        - Zinc
    o Tobacco use
    o Alcohol intake
        - Amount > type
    o Pre-existing esophageal diseased
        - Achalasia
        - Lye injury
        - Tylosis (autosomal dominant, hyperkeratosis of palms and soles)

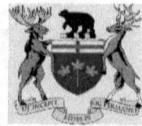

ESOPHAGEAL CANCER

- Plummer- Vinson syndrome (aka: Patterson- Kelly syndrome in the United Kingdom; iron deficiency anemia, dysphagia, and post-cricoid esophageal web)
  - History of squamous cell cancer of the upper aero-digestive tract
  - Radiation therapy following mastectomy
  - HPV infection

- Give 5 risk factors for adenocarcinoma of the esophagus.

  - Barrett esophagus
  - Dietary intake
    - High cholesterol
    - Animal protein
    - Vitamin B12
  - Dietary deficiency
    - High in fiber
    - Beta-carotene
    - Folate
    - Vitamins C, E, and B6
  - Obesity (↑BMI)

ESOPHAGEAL CANCER

- List 10 risk factors for esophageal squamous cancer and for adenocarcinoma.

	Squamous cell carcinoma	Adenocarcinoma
o Age	>60	>50
o Gender	M	M
o Alcohol	+	-
o Smoking	+	-
o GERD	-	+
o BE	-	+
o HIV	+	+

- Previous head and neck squamous cell carcinoma
- Radiation therapy
- Lye ingestion
- Plummer-Vinson (Paterson-Kelly) syndrome
- Achalasia, Tylosis palmaris
- Nutritional deficiencies– riboflavin, niacin; high-starch diet without fruits and vegetables
- Nitrosamines; "bush teas" (diterpene phorbol esters)
- Gluten sensitive enteropathy (GSE)

Abbreviations: BE, Barrett epithelium; GERD, gastroesophageal reflux disease

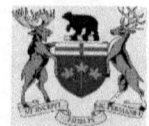

ESOPHAGEAL CANCER

- Investigations

  - Give 5 endoscopic and diagnostic imaging tests for esophageal cancer.
    - Chest x-ray
    - Contrast enhanced esophagogram
    - CT scans
    - Endoscopy and biopsy
    - Chromo-endoscopy: (Lugol's solution, methylene blue, toluidine blue, and cresyl violet and contrast stains such indigo carmine)
    - Electronic chromo-endoscopy (NBI, narrow band imaging)
    - High-resolution endoscopic imaging
    - Spectroscopic imaging

  - Give the staging of esophageal cancer : The American Joint Comitee on Cancer Staging System for Cancers of the Esophagus, and tumor node metastasis
    - Esophagus

      AJCC Stage Groupings
      - *Stage 0*
        Tis, N0, M0
      - *Stage 1*
        T1, N0, M0
      - *Stage IIA*
        T2, N0, M0
        T3, N0, M0
      - *Stage IIB*
        T1, N1, M0
        T2, N1, M0
      - *Stage III*

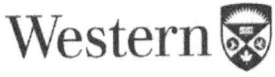

ESOPHAGEAL CANCER

　　T3, N1, M0
　　T1, any N, M0
- *Stage IV*
  　　Any T, any N, M1
- *Stage IVA*
  　　Any T, any N, M1a
- *Stage IVB*
  　　Any T, any N, M1b

Modified from American Joint Committee on Cancer (AJCC) Cancer Staging Manual. 6th ed. New York: Springer;2002: p 91.

*For tumors of the midthoracic esophagus, use only M1b because tumors with metastasis in nonregional lymph nodes have an equally poor prognosis as those with metastasis in other distant sites.

- Give 4 modalities used to stage esophageal cancer
  - Endoscopic staging
  - CT scan staging
  - PET scan staging
  - EUS staging
  - Surgical staging (laparoscopy or medianoscopy)

  - Tumor node metastasis
    - *Primary tumor (T)*
      TX: Primary tumor cannot be assessed
      T0: No evidence of primary tumor
      Tis: Carcinoma in situ (T1a or T1m)
      T1: Tumor invades lamina propria or submucosa (T1b or T1sm)
      T2: Tumor invades muscularis propria

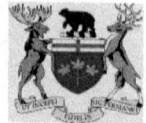

ESOPHAGEAL CANCER

T3: Tumor invades adventitia
T4: Tumor invades adjacent structures

- *Regional lymph nodes (N)*
NX: Regional lymph nodes cannot be assessed
N0: No regional lymph node metastasis
N1: Regional lymph node metastasis

- *Distant metastasis (M)*
MX: Distant metastasis cannot be assessed
M0: No distant metastasis
M1: Distant metastasis
   Tumors of the lower thoracic esophagus:
   M1a: Metastasis in celiac lymph nodes
   M1b: Other distant metastasis
   Tumors of the midthoracic esophagus*:
   M1a: Not applicable
   M1b: Nonregional lymph nodes and/ or other distant metastasis
   Tumors of the upper thoracic esophagus:
   M1a: Metastasis in cervical nodes
   M1b: Other distant metastasis

Useful background: Main classifications used in esophageal cancer

> PRE-OPERATIVE CLASSIFCATIONS

o Ultrasound (us TNM) classification for esophageal cancers

uT1   Tumour invading the mucosa and the submucosa
uT2   Tumour invading the mucosa without going beyond
uT3

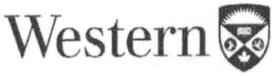

ESOPHAGEAL CANCER

uT4   Tumour invading the tunica adventitia (or the serous membrane)

Tumour invading the adjacent structures

uN0   No lymph node invasion

uN1   Lymph nodes invaded around tumour; round, same echogenicity as the tumour

uN2   Lymph nodes invaded distant from the tumour (5 cm above or below the upper or lower pole of the tumour)

- CT scan (CT) TNM classification for thoracic esophageal cancers

ctT1   Non-visibility or mass <10 mm in diameter

ctT2   Mass 10-30 mm in diameter

ctT3   Mass >30 mm in diameter with no sign of invasion t mediastinal structures

ctT4   Idem + sign of spread to mediastinal structures

- Lymph nodes (N)*

ctN0   No detectable adenopathy

ctN1   Regional adenopathy (mediastinal and/or perigastric)

- Distant metastases

ctM0   No distant metastasis

ctM1   Presence of distant metastases (including celiac and cervical adenopathies)

- *Definition of us and ct stages*

Us or ct stage
I   T1 N0 M0
IIa T2 N0 M0; T3 N0 M0

ESOPHAGEAL CANCER

IIb T1 T2 N1 M0

* lymph nodes >10 mm are considered to be high risk of being metastatic

➤ POST-OPERATIVE CLASSIFICATIONS:
- TNM classification

T-Primary tumour

T0	No sign of primary tumour
Tis	Carcinoma in situ
T1	Tumour invading the lamina propria or the submucosa
T2	
T3	Tumour invading the muscularis
T4	Tumour invading the tunica adventitia
	Tumour invading the adjacent structures

- N-Regional adenopathy

Nx	Lymph nodes not evaluated
N0	No sign of regional lymph node involvement
N1	Regional lymph node metastases

- Cervical esophagus: cervical lymph nodes, internal jugular, peri-esophageal and supraclavicular nodes

Printed with permission: Veuillez V, et al. *Best Pract Res Clin Gastroenterol* 2007;21(6): 949.

➤ Treatment

- Give the modalities for resectable and for unresectable (palliative) esophageal cancer.

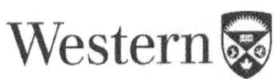

ESOPHAGEAL CANCER

- Resectable
  - Endoscopic therapy (early stage cancer; saline assisted polypectomy, lift and cut technique, cap-assisted technique, band and cut technique "EMR")
  - Surgical therapy
    - Vagal-sparing esophagectomy
  - Radiotherapy
    - External beam radiotherapy
    - High-dose
  - Chemotherapy

- Unresectable esophageal cancer
  - Compassionate care
    - Comfort, support
    - Analgesia
  - Systemic chemotherapy and radiotherapy
  - Endoscopic treatment
    - Techniques that ablate neoplastic tissue
      - Laser photo ablation using neodymium: yttrium-aluminum-garnet (Nd: YAG)
      - Potassium titanyl phosphate (KTP)
      - Argon lasers
      - APC
      - Photodynamic therapy
      - Cytotoxic injection therapy
    - Techniques that displace neoplastic tissue
      - Esophageal dilatation
      - Esophageal stent placement
  - Brachytherapy
  - Nutritional therapy

- Give 6 palliative treatments for the care of the patient with esophageal carcinoma.
  - Palliative care, including end of life care
  - Non-endoscopic techniques
    - Surgery
    - Radiation therapy

ESOPHAGEAL CANCER

- External beam radiotherapy
- Intraluminal radiotherapy (brachytherapy)
- Chemotherapy
- Endoscopic techniques
  - Laser therapy
    - Thermal (Nd:YAG)
    - Photodynamic therapy
  - Dilation
  - Electrocoagulation (BICAP probe)
  - Chemical injection therapy
  - Stent placement
- Nutritional support
  - Nasoenteric feeding tube
  - Percutaneous endoscopic gastrostomy (PEG)

Printed with permission: Siersema PD. *Nat Clin Pract Gastroenterol Hepatol* 2008;5(3): 143.

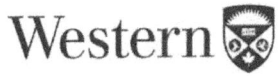

ESOPHAGEAL CANCER

References and Suggested Reading

ASGE Technology Committee. Endoscopic mucosal resection and endoscopic submucosal dissection. *Gastrointestinal Endoscopy* 2008;68:11-18.

Badreddine RJ, et al. Depth of submucosal invasion does not predict lymph node metastasis and survival of patients with esophageal carcinoma. *Clinical Gastroenterology and Hepatology*. 2010;8(3):248-53.

Curvers WL, et al. Novel imaging modalities in the detection of oesophageal neoplasia. *Best Practice & Research Clinical Gastroenterology* 2008; 22(4):687-720.

Das A, et al. Comparison of endoscopic treatment and surgery in early esophageal cancer: An analysis of surveillance epidemiology and end results data. *The American Journal of Gastroenterology* 2008;103:1340-1345

Dubecz A, et al. Modern surgery for esophageal cancer. *Gastroenterology Clinics of North America* 2008;37(4):965-987.

Greenwald BD, et al. Endoscopic spray cryotherapy for esophageal cancer: safety and efficacy. *Gastrointestinal Endoscopy*. 2010;71(4):686-93.

Hatta w., et al. Optical coherence tomography for the staging of tumor infiltration in superficial esophageal squamous cell carcinoma. *Gastrointestinal Endoscopy*. 2010;71(6):899-906.

Kendall C, et al. Evaluation of Raman probe for oesophageal cancer diagnostics. *Analyst*. 2010;135(12):3038-41.

Okines AF, et al. Epirubicin, oxaliplatin, and capecitabine with or without panitumumab for advanced esophagogastric cancer: dose-finding study for the prospective multicenter, randomized, phase II/III REAL-

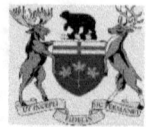

3 trial. *Journal of Clinical Oncology.* 2010;28(25):3945-50.

Pouw RE, et al. Successful balloon-based radiofrequency ablation of a widespread early squamous cell carcinoma and high-grade dysplasia of the esophagus: a case report. *Gastrointestinal Endoscopy* 2008;68(3):537-541.

Robertson E, et al. Genetics of Gastroesophageal Cancer: paradigms, Paradoxes and Prognostic Utility. *The American Journal of Gastroenterology* 2008;103:443-449.

Umar SB. Esophageal Cancer: epidemiology, pathogenesis and prevention. *Nature Clinical Practice Gastroenterology & Hepatology.* 2008;5(9):517-526.

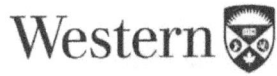

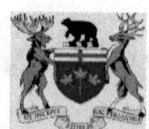

MINI UPDATE

STOMACH

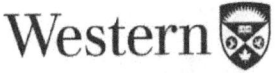

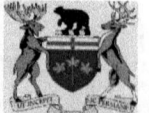

MINI UPDATE

Gastritis & Gastropathies

Melanie Beaton

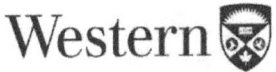

GASTRITIS & GASTROPATHIES

Gastritis

- The vocabulary
  - AMAG, autoimmune metaplastic atrophic gastritis
  - Carditis
  - DCAG ((diffuse corporal atrophic gastritis, aka autoimmune metaplastic atrophic gastritis [AMAG])
    - Diffuse corporal atrophic gastritis (aka autoimmune metaplastic atrophic gastritis, or type A gastritis)
  - EMAG (environmental multifocal atrophic gastritis)
  - GCP (gastritis cystica profunda
  - HHG (hyperplastic, hypersecretory gastropathy (Ménétrier's disease)
  - HPG (H. pylori-associated gastritis)
    - Active gastritis (aka acute gastritis)
      - Neutrophils, lymphocytes, plasma calls in mucosa and submucosa
    - Epithelial damage
      - ↓ surface mucin
      - Nuclear changes
      - Lymphoid follicles
    - May be associated with
      - EMAG (environment multifocal atrophic gastritis)
      - Lymphocytic gastritis (> 5 lymphocytes per 100 cells)
  - PG (phlegmonas gastritis)
  - MAG, multifocal atrophic gastritis, aka metaplastic atrophic gastritis)

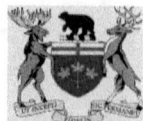

GASTRITIS & GASTROPATHIES

- Patchy
- Gastric body and antral mucosa
- Often associated with H. pylori

- When to suspect gastritis / gastropathies
    - ↑ red mucosa
    - ↑ thickness

- Causes and associations

- Give 15 causes of histologically diagnosed gastritis.

- Drugs, chemicals, radiation
    - Medications
        - Aspirin, NSAIDs, COXIBs
        - Bisphosphonates, K^+ tablets
    - Drugs, chemicals
        - Alcohol, bile, cocaine, chemotherapy, radiotherapy, red peppers, pickles

- Infection
    - Bacterial - H. pylori, Mycobacteria
    - Viral-CMV (cytomegalovirus), HSV (herpes simplex virus)
    - Fungal
    - Parasitic

- Graft-versus-host disease (GVHD)

- Autoimmune gastritis (pernicious anemia)

- Ischemia
    - Atherosclerosis

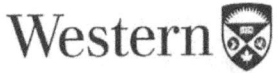

GASTRITIS & GASTROPATHIES

- o Sepsis
- o Burns
- o Shock
- o Mechanical ventilation

➢ Associated with liver disease
- o GAVE (gastric antral vascular ectasia)
- o GVE (gastric vascular ectasia)
- o PHG (portal hypertensive gastropathy)

➢ Trauma/foreign body
- o Nasogastric or gastrostomy tubes
- o Bezoar
- o Prolapse/ sliding hiatal hernia/paraesophageal hernia
- o Cameron ulcer (ulcer in hiatus hernia)

➢ Infiltration/ tumour
- o Lymphocytic/ collagenous
- o Granulomatous
- o Eosinophilic
- o Tumour

➢ Miscellaneous
- o Gastritis cystica profunda
- o Ménétrier disease (hyperplastic, hypersecretory gastropathy)

Adapted from: Lee EL, and Feldman M. *Sleisenger & Fordtran's gastrointestinal and liver disease: Pathophysiology/ Diagnosis/ Management* 2006: pg. 1068.; and Printed with permission: Francis DL. *Mayo Clinic Gastroenterology and Hepatology Board Review*; 2008:67.

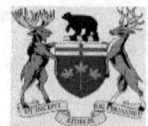

GASTRITIS & GASTROPATHIES

SO YOU WANT TO BE A GASTROENTEROLOGIST!

A patient with dyspepsia has an upper GI barium study.
- Give the gastric radiological features which help to determine if there is an infectious etiology for their dyspepsia.

  o H. pylori infection
  - Gastric folds
    - Thick
    - Polypoid
  - Area gastricae
    - Enlarged

  o Non-H. pylori causes
  - Antral erosions

- Give the classification of the causes of **Gastritis**

  o Acute
  - Hemorrhagic/ Erosive
  - Acute *H. pylori*

  o Chronic
  - Chronic *H. pylori*
    - Diffuse antral
    - Multifocal atrophic
    - Diffuse corporal
  - Autoimmune
  - Eosinophilic
  - Lymphocytic
  - CMV/GVHD

  o Chronic Nonspecific
  - ***H. pylori*** – diffuse antral predominant or multifocal atrophic pangastritis (may be w/ or w/o H.p)
  - Diffuse corporal atrophic gastritis

  o Infectious
  - Viral

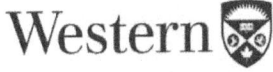

GASTRITIS & GASTROPATHIES

- Bacterial
- *H.pylori*
- Mycobacteria
- Fungal
- Parasitic

o Granulomatous
- Sarcoidosis
- TB
- Infectious
- Tumor

o Distinctive Forms
- Collagenous
- Lymphocytic
- Eosinophilic

o Miscellaneous
- Gastritis cystica profunda
- GVHD

Chronic, Nonspecific Gastritis

o Most forms are clinically silent

o Significance is that they are risk factors for other conditions (PUD, Gastric Ca)

o Three Types
- Diffuse Antral
- Corporal
- Multifocal Atrophic

Types of Gastritis

Type A	Type B
o Atrophic gastritis & hypochlorhydria	o Normal acid secretion & short segment reflux

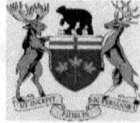

GASTRITIS & GASTROPATHIES

- Due to *H.pylori* or autoimmune gastritis
- Similar to esophageal adenocarcinoma
- Similar to non-cardia cancer
- Increasing incidence of proximal gastric cancer
  - Overall, 80% decrease in gastric cancer in NA
  - Cardia tumors now account for 50% of gastric cancer in developed world
- 80% Intestinal-type
  - Arising from metaplastic epithelium
  - GERD an important RF
  - *H.pylori*
    - Complex association, not well understood
    - Higher risk if also have atrophic gastritis (d/t Hp or autoimmune gastritis)

Diffuse Antral Gastritis

- Often *H. pylori* associated
- Most pts asymptomatic (#1 indication for EGD = Dyspepsia)
- Pathology
  - Diffuse, antral predominant
  - Chronic inflammation (lymphocytes & plasma cells) +/- PMNs (polymorphonuclear cells)
    - vs. Acute *H.pylori*: PMNs only
  - Erosions
  - Lymphoid follicles w/ germinal centres
  - *H.pylori* organisms in mucus layer on surface, usually seen best with silver stain

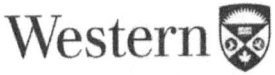

GASTRITIS & GASTROPATHIES

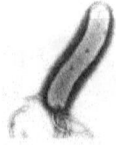

Diffuse Antral Gastritis

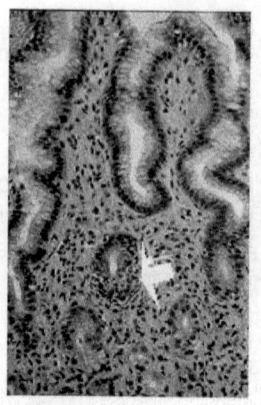

PMN's infiltrating epithelium

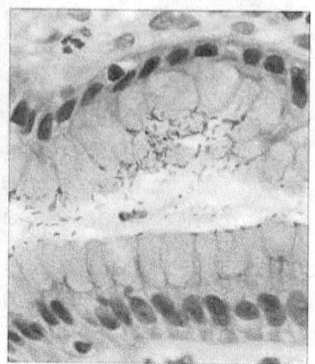

H.pylori Gastritis

- Colonizes stomachs of 50% of world
  - Greater in developing countries
  - North America
    - 10-15% of children <12years old vs. 50-60% >60 years old
    - New infection acquired by <1%/y of adults
- Virulence Factors
  - ie. cag+ & vacA
  - Both ↑ risk gastritis, PUDz & gastric cancer
  - vacA supresses inflammatory response, may contribute to longevity of colonization
- Host Factors
  - Most persons colonized are asymptomatic
  - H.pylori virulence factors cannot fully explain variable outcomes (no disease, ulcer, cancer)
  - Genetic polymorphisms influencing gastric cancer risk (IL-1β, TNFα, IL-10)

Abbreviation: PUD, peptic ulcer disease

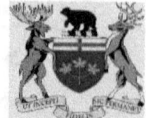

GASTRITIS & GASTROPATHIES

Disease Outcomes from H.pylori Gastric Inflammation

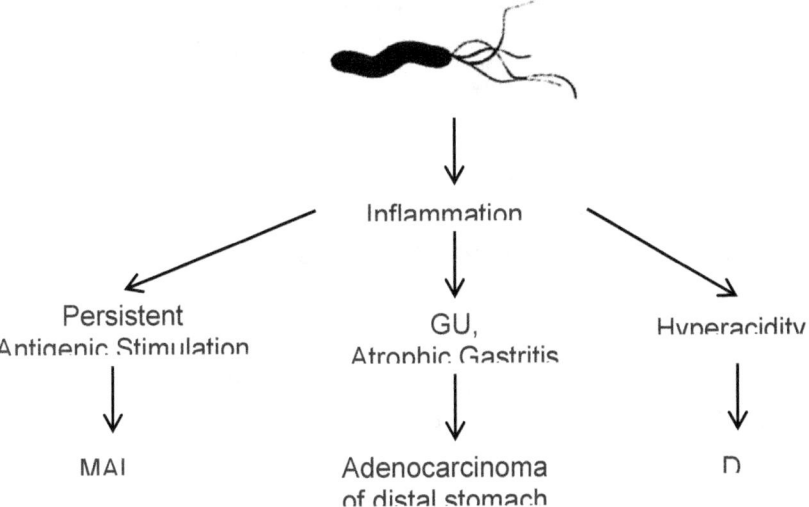

- ➢ Duodenal Ulcer
    - o Diffuse antral gastritis, minimal body/fundus involvement
    - o Gastric acid secretion normal or increased
    - o Majority of pts in developed countries
- ➢ Gastric Ulcer, Adenocarcinoma
    - o Inflammation involves body and antrum (pangastritis)
    - o Reduced acid output
    - o Gastric atrophy & intestinal metaplasia of antrum and body
    - o More common in pts from SE Asia, S America & parts of Europe

Abbreviations: Pts, patients; SE, south East; S, South

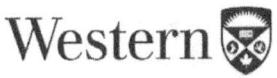

GASTRITIS & GASTROPATHIES

- o Autoimmune destruction of fundic glands
  - Anti-parietal cell & anti-intrinsic factor Ab
  - Classic pernicious anemia in small subset
- o <5% of cases of chronic gastritis
- o Achlorhydria & 2° hypergastrinemia
  - ↑ Risk gastric carcinoid tumors (2° to achlorhydria) & ↑ risk Intestinal-type G Ca
- o Mucosal changes irreversible & no standards for endoscopic surveillance

➢ AMAG / DCAG) (autoimmune metaplastic atrophic gastritis, aka diffuse corporal atrophic gastritis)
  - o Parietal cell antibodies to H^+, K^+ - ATPase
  - o Thin fundic / body mucosa
  - o Flat gastric folds
  - o ↑ gastrin
    - ↓ HCl
    - Antral G-cells (secrete antibacterial HD-5 [human defensin-5)
    - Progression of metaplasia to dysplasia / GCA: ↑ CDX_2 (type III)

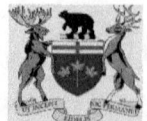

GASTRITIS & GASTROPATHIES

Atrophic Gastritis

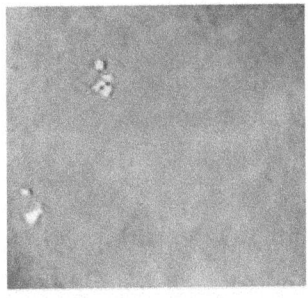

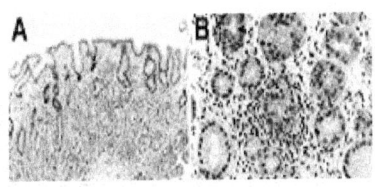

Mononuclear

Thinning of corpus mucosa: loss of folds & increased visibility of submucosal vessels

Multifocal Atrophic Gastritis

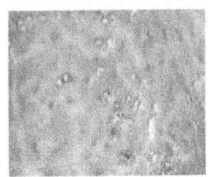

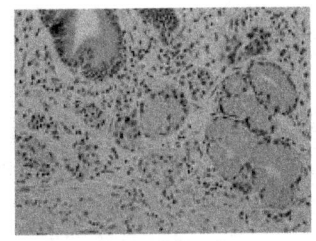

Enterochromaffin –like hyperplasia

Multifocal Atrophic Gastritis (MAG)

- EMAG (environmental multifocal atrophic gastritis)
    - 85% of EMAG caused by H. pylori
    - Body
        - Atrophic gastritis
        - Pseudopyloric metaplasia "stains positive for PG1 (pepsinogen 1)
    - Body / antrum
        - Atrophy
        - Intestinal metaplasia
    - Antrum & body
    - Mucosal atrophy & intestinal metaplasia
        - Atrophy
            - Loss of glands

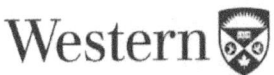

GASTRITIS & GASTROPATHIES

- Replaced by metaplastic (often intestinal) epithelium

H.pylori in 85% cases
- Genetics & environment also important
- Unclear why some *H.pylori* infected patients develop atrophy (estimated 1-3%/y)
  o Intestinal metaplasia risk factor for GCa (gastric cancer)

SO YOU WANT TO BE A GASTROENTEROLOGIST!

o AMAG / DMAG (autoimmune metaplastic atrophic gastritis) results in increased antibodies to parietal cell antigens

o The parietal cell antibodies to H^+, K^+ ATPase lead to increased CD_4^+ lymphocytes.

- Give the consequences of the increased CD_4^+ lymphocytes in AMAG/AMAG.

The increased CD_4^+ lymphocytes in the inflammation of AMAG/DMAG leads to

o ↑ Th1 cytokines → ↑ secretion of immunoglobulins by B lymphocytes

o ↑ cytotoxicity mediated by performin

o ↑ FAS ligand-mediated apoptosis

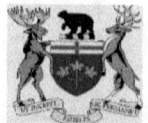

GASTRITIS & GASTROPATHIES

Hp with full thickness mucosal inflammation

Focus of intestinal metaplasia

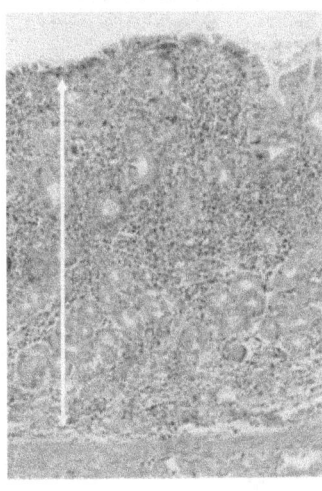
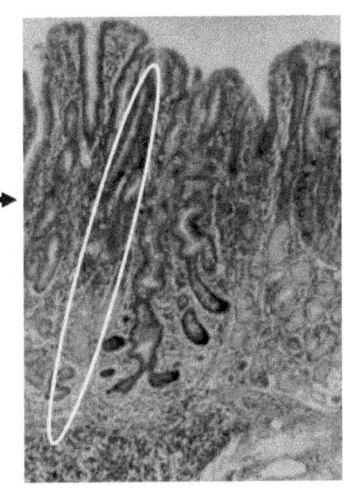

- Phlegmonous gastritis
  - Phlegmonous gastritis (PG) is also known as suppurative gastritis (SG).
  - PG/SG may progress to
    - ANG (acute necrotizing gastritis), which represents gangrene of the stomach)
    - Emphysematous gastritis, as the result of the necrotic gastric wall becoming infected with a gas-forming organism (e.g. Clostridium welchii)

- Collagenous gastritis
  - Chronic gastritis
    - Superficial
    - Patchy
  - Atrophy
    - Focal
  - Collagen
    - Focal deposits

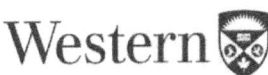

GASTRITIS & GASTROPATHIES

Subepithelial thickening of the collagen band (20 to 75 mm thick)

SO YOU WANT TO BE A GASTROENTEROLOGIST!

- Give the endoscopic and histological changes of lymphocytic gastritis.

    - Endoscopy (varioliform)
        - Thick folds
        - Nodular mucosa
        - Aphthous "ulcers" (erosions)

    - Histology
        - Antrum, body, or antrum plus body
        - ↑ lymphocytes and plasma cells in lamina
        - > 5 lymphocytes per 100 cells
        - Associated with
            - H. pylori infection
            - Celiac disease
            - Crohn disease in children

➢ Gastritis cystica profunda (GCP)
  - Rare and unknown cause
  - May be associated with
    - Gastric surgery (Bilroth II)
    - Atrophic gastritis
    - Inverted hyperplastic gastric polyp
  - Histology
    - Foveolar hyperplasia
    - Cystic glands extending into muscularis mucosae, submucosa, muscularis propria

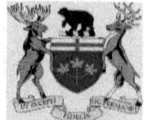

GASTRITIS & GASTROPATHIES

- For such a rare innocuous as GCP, give the reason why do we need to know about GCP?
    - GCP may be associated with
        - Synchronous or metachronous gastric adenocarcinoma (GCa)
        - GCa of postoperative gastric stump

> Reactive gastropathies (aka acute erosive gastritis)
  - Necrosis of superficial lamina propria in area of erosion
  - Foveolar hyperplasia
  - Gastric pits
    - Elongated
    - Corkscrew
  - Hemorrhage
    - From > 25% of biopsy samples
    - Atypical nuclei

"Carditis"
  - Definition: "Inflammation of the small rim of the cardiac glands at the proximal portion of the stomach" (Feldman M., et al. Sleisenger and Fordtran's Gastrointestinal and Liver Disease. 9th Edition. *Saunders/Elsevier*, Philadelphia, 2010, page 848).

- Give 3 common causes of carditis.
    - GERD
    - HPG (H. pylori-associated gastritis)

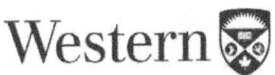

GASTRITIS & GASTROPATHIES

- o EMAG (environmental multifocal atrophic gastritis)
- o AMAG (autoimmune metaplastic atrophic gastritis)
- o Gastric Cardia
  - Most proximal part of stomach
    - Extends 10-20mm from Z-line
  - Similar to antral mucosa (columnar, mucus secreting, absent/few parietal & chief cells)
- o High incidence inflammation and metaplasia
  - 25% Asymptomatic subjects had intestinal metaplasia at GEJ
  - Due to effects of GERD & *H. pylori* infection
  - No reliable histologic markers to distinguish between gastric cardiac intestinal metaplasia and Barrett

➢ Hyperplastic Gastropathies may be confused with or miscalled Ménétrier's disease (aka [hyperplastic, hypersecretory gastropathy])

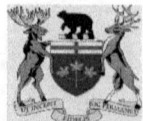

GASTRITIS & GASTROPATHIES

SO YOU WANT TO BE A GASTROENTEROLOGIST!

Even in the absence of a decrease in parietal cells in Ménétrier's disease (MD), there is reduced acid secretion (hypochlorhydria) or achlorhydria.

- Give the explanation for the change in acid secretion In MD.

Acid secretion may be reduced or absent in MD even in the absence of a reduction in parietal cells, because of

- ↑ TGF-α (transforming growth factor-alpha)
- ↑ TGF-α → ↑ EGFR (epidermal growth factor receptor)
- EGFR is a receptor for tyrosine kinase (TK)
- ↑ EGFR and ↑ TK → ↓ HCl

SO YOU WANT TO BE A GASTROENTEROLOGIST!

- Give the differences between Ménétrier's disease and HHG (hyperplastic, hypersecretory gastropathy), both of which may show foveolar hyperplasia and cystic dilation on mucosal biopsy.

	Ménétrier disease	Hyperplastic, hypersecretory gastropathy
Protein losing gastropathy	+	+/-
Acid secretion	↓	N/↑
Parietal and chief cells	N/↓	↑
Inflammation	+/-	-
Mucus secretion	N/↑	-
Associated with lymphotic gastritis	+	-
Carcinoid-like syndrome (↑ PGE_2)	+	-

Abbreviations: N, normal; PGE_2, prostaglandin E_2

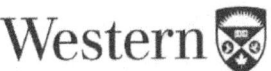

GASTRITIS & GASTROPATHIES

Compare and contrast the endoscopic findings and treatment of portal hypertensive gastropathy (PHG) and gastric antral vascular ectasia (GAVE).

➢ Feature findings	PHG	GAVE
○ Site	Fundus	Antrum
○ Mosaic pattern	Yes	No
○ Red colour signs	Yes	Yes
○ Findings on gastric mucosal biopsy		
○ Thrombi	No	+++
○ Spindle cell proliferation	Sparse	++
○ Fibrohyalinosis	No	+++
➢ Management	○ ↓ portal hypertension	○ Estrogens
	○ β adrenergic blockers	○ Antrectomy
	○ TIPS	○ (TIPS doesn't help) Argon plasma coagulation therapy
	○ Liver transplantation	○ Liver transplantation

Infectious Gastritis

- ➢ Bacterial
  - ○ Exceedingly rare (excluding *H.p*)
  - ○ Acute suppurative gastritis (aka. phlegmonous gastritis)

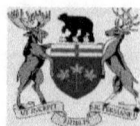

GASTRITIS & GASTROPATHIES

- Life threatening
- Submucosa & muscularis propria infected by pyogenic bacteria (α-hemolytic strep)
- Immunocompromised, elderly & alcoholics at greatest risk
- Iatrogenic causes:
    - EMR
    - Polypectomy

➢ Viral
  o CMV
    - Esophagus, stomach, small bowel, colon or anus
    - Epigastric pain, fever, lymphocytosis
    - Multi ulcers
    - "Owl-eye" intranuclear inclusion bodies
  o HSV
    - Gastric rare
    - Reactivation of dormant childhood infection
    - N/V, fever/chills, cough, weight loss
    - Multiple, small, raised ulcerated plaques or linear ulcers
    - Ground-glass nuclei & eosinophilic intranuclear inclusions
  o *Mycobacterium* TB
    - Rare, usually pulmonary TB present
    - Prepyloric ulcer(s)/mass
  o *MAC*
    - #1 in HIV
    - Gastric involvement rare
    - Chronic ulcer refractory to conventional Rx
  o Candidiasis

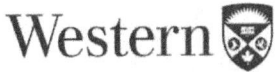

GASTRITIS & GASTROPATHIES

- Contamination from GU tract common
- May aggravate & perpetuate ulceration
- Usually Rx not necessary

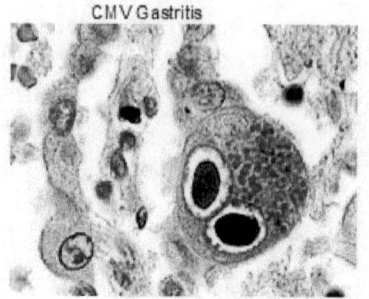

CMV Gastritis

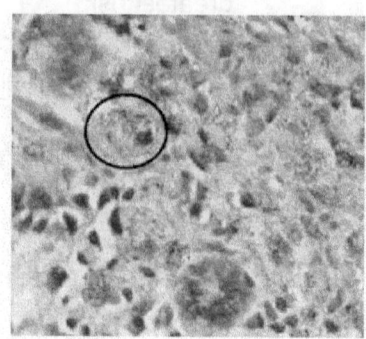

> Parasites
  - Rare in Western countries
    - *Cryptosporidium, Giardia intestinalis, Strongyloides stercoralis* in immunocompromised
  - *Anisakis*
    - Invasive cases seen in Japan
    - Consumption of raw marine fish, larvae migrate into wall
    - Multiple erosions on EGD, eosinophilic granulomas & abscesses on histology

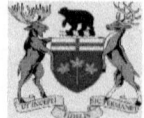

GASTRITIS & GASTROPATHIES

Granulomatous Gastritis

- o GI sarcoid rare, but stomach #1 site, usually incidental
- o Other causes:
  - Foreign Body
  - Lymphoma
  - Whipple's Disease
- o Granulomatous vasculitis
- o Infectious
  - TB
  - *Histoplasma*
  - *H.pylori*
  - *Anisakis*
- o Idiopathic

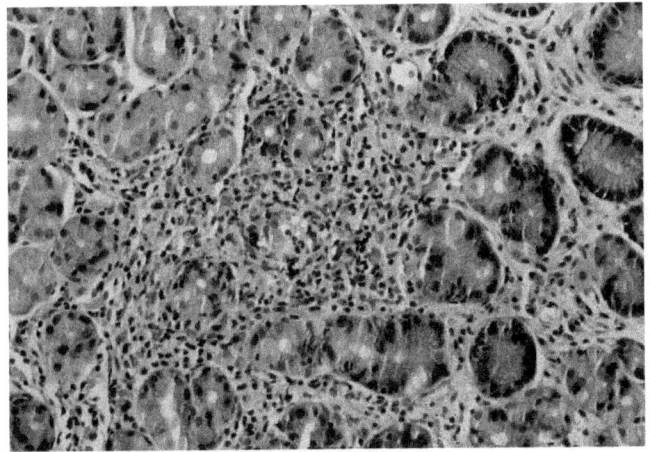

Crohn Disease of Stomach, mixed inflammatory cell infiltrate

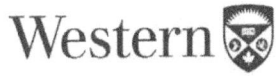

GASTRITIS & GASTROPATHIES

Lymphocytic Gastritis

- Range of endoscopic appearances
  - Normal →Thick folds → Nodular → Erosions
- Expansion of LP by lymphocytes
  - T cell origin
  - Minimum of 25 IELs/hpf
- Etiology
  - Celiac Disease (10-45%)
  - *H. pylori* (30%)
  - Crohn disease (lymphocytes most common inflammatory cell type)
  - Gastric lymphoma (MALT)
  - Lymphocytic gastritis
  - HIV

Abbreviations: IEL, interepithelial lymphocytes; LP, lamina propria; MALT, mucosa-associated lymphoid tissue

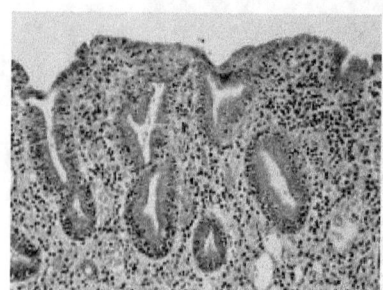

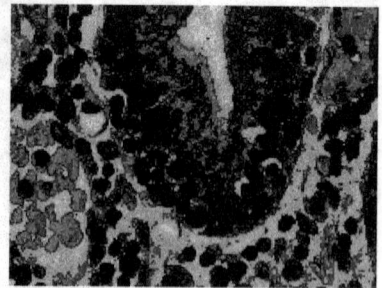

MAC within lamina propria macrophages

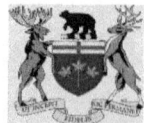

GASTRITIS & GASTROPATHIES

Eosinophilic Gastritis

- o Rare; unknown etiology
- o Classified according to layer involved
    - Mucosa (pain, nausea and vomiting, diarrhea, ↓ weight, protein losing enteropathy, perforation, iron deficiency)
    - Muscle (Obstructive symptoms)
    - Subserosal (Eosinophilic ascites)
- o Diagnosis
    - Full-thickness biopsy
    - Usually ↑ serum IgE & peripheral eosinophilia
- o Treatment
    - Symptoms
    - Corticosteroids

Gastric GVHD

- o 10-50% of Allogenic BMT pts
- o Skin > Liver > Gastrointestinal tract
    - Small & Large Bowel > Stomach, Esophagus
- o Acute
    - Post-Tx Day 21-100
    - Gastrointestinal tract commonly involved
- o Chronic
    - > Day 100
- o Gastric GVHD
    - Pain
    - N/V
    - No <u>diarrhea</u> & normal rectal biopsy
    - Biopsy
        - May be normal

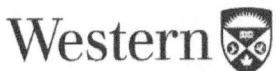

GASTRITIS & GASTROPATHIES

- Apoptotic bodies (necrosis of single cells) in mucosa

Abbreviations: BMT, bone marrow transplant; GVHD, graft versus host disease; post Tx, post-transplant; GIT, gastrointestinal tract

Gastropathy

- Disorders of the stomach with little or no associated inflammation
  - Most often caused by irritants (e.g., drugs/toxins, bile, congestion...)
  - Gastritis which results from
  - Infections,
  - Autoimmune disorders
  - Hypersensitivity reactions

- Give a classification of gastropathy
  - Reactive (erosive)
    - **NSAID/ASA,** Medication, EtOH, Cocaine
    - Stress
    - Radiation
    - Bile Reflux
    - Ischemia,
    - Congestive (PHT)
    - Prolapse, Hiatus Hernia
    - Trauma (ie. feeding tube), Bezoar
  - Hyperplastic
    - Menetrier's
    - ZES

Abbreviations: PHT, portal hypertension; ZES, Zollinger Ellison Syndrome

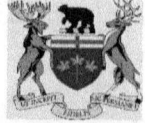

GASTRITIS & GASTROPATHIES

Reactive Gastropathy

- Aka
  - "Erosive Gastritis"
  - "Reflux Gastritis"
  - "Chemical Gastritis"
- #2 Most common diagnosis on gastric biopsy
- Erosions & ulcers
- Intervening hemorrhagic mucosa
  - Usually small & multiple
- Histology
  - Foveolar Hyperplasia
  - Reactive epithelial changes d/t regenerating mucosa
  - Often corkscrew appearance of mucosa
- ASA/NSAIDS
  - #1 cause
  - Prevalence 35-45%
- Radiation Tx
  - Usually solitary, antral
- Bile Reflux
  - Post Billroth I or II, Vagotomy & Pyloroplasty
  - ↑ed Risk GCa
- Portal Hypertensive Gastropathy
  - Vascular ectasia in mucosa w/o inflammation
  - Most prominent fundus and body

Abbreviation: w/o, without; GCa, gastric cancer

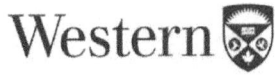

GASTRITIS & GASTROPATHIES

> **Exam Alert**
> - You are shown an example of the histopathology of the stomach taken from a person whose endoscopy is reported as showing "gastritis". First look to see if there is gastritis, and if so, can you identify the cause, such as an infectious organism.
> - Secondly, consider if there may be gastropathy, and look for a clue, including reactive changes, which might suggest NSAIDs etc.
>   - Foveolar Hyperplasia
>   - Reactive epithelial changes
>   - Regenerating mucosa
>   - Often corkscrew appearance of mucosa

CMV Inclusions

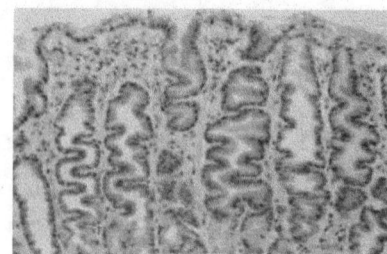

IELs in lymphocytic gastritis

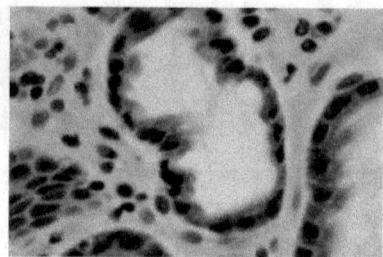

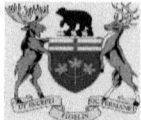

GASTRITIS & GASTROPATHIES

Portal Hypertensive Gastropathy

Reactive Gastropathy

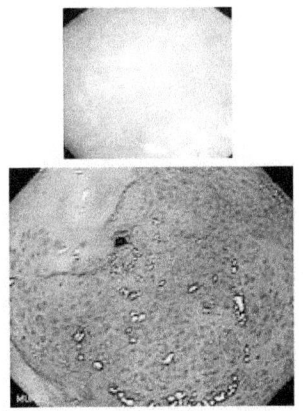
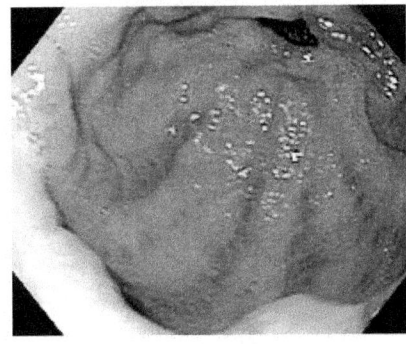

- Corkscrew appearance of foveolae
- Reactive changes in foveolar eptihelial cells
- Loss of mucus
- Enlarged nuclei

Portal Hypertensive Gastropathy

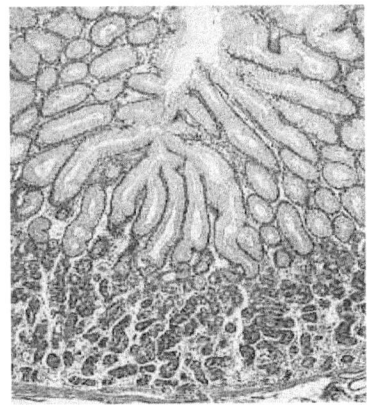

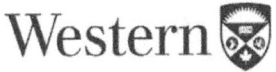

GASTRITIS & GASTROPATHIES

- Give the differential diagnosis of large thick gastric folds seen on endoscopy or diagnostic imaging.
    - Idiopathic
        - Menetrier disease
            - Protein losing enteropathy
            - Hypochlorhydria
            - Chief cells (glands replaced by mucus secreting cells)
            - Spares antrum
        - ZES (Zollinger-Ellison syndrome)
    - Infection
        - Hyperplastic, Hypersecretory Gastropathy
            - +/- Protein loss
            - ↑/N Acid secretion, parietal & chief cell hyperplasia
        - Infection:
            - *H.pylori*
            - CMV
    - Inflammation
        - Eosinophilic Gastritis
        - Lymphocytic *gastritis*
    - Infiltration
    - Neoplasm:
        - Lymphoma
        - Carcinoma
        - Amyloid
    - Vascular
        - Varices

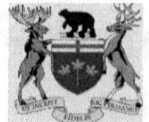

References and Suggested Reading

Abe N, et al. Long-term outcomes of combination of endoscopic submucosal dissection and laparoscopic lymph node dissection without gastrectomy for early gastric cancer patients who have a potential risk of lymph node metastasis. *Gastrointest Endosc* 2011; 74:792-797.

Agréus L, et al. Rationale in diagnosis and screening of atrophic gastritis with stomach-specific plasma biomarkers. *Scand J Gastroenterol* 2012;47(2):136-47.

Vanden Berghe P, et al Contribution of different triggers to the gastric accommodation reflex in man. *Am J Physiol Gastrointest Liver Physiol.* 2009;297(5):G902-6.

Yardley JH. Acute and chronic gastritis due to Helicobacter pylori. *UpToDate.* www.uptodate.com 2014

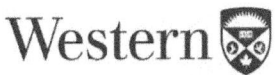

GASTRITIS & GASTROPATHIES

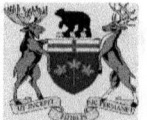

MINI UPDATE

Acid Secretion and Cytoprotection

Bandar Aljudaibi

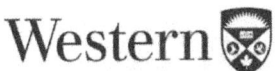

ACID SECRETION AND CYTOPROTECTION

Anatomy

- Gastric glands of different anatomic regions have different specialized epithelial cells
- Three Regions: Cardia, Oxyntic, Pyloric
- Cardia
  - Small transition zone from esophageal squamous epithelium to gastric columnar epithelium.
  - Branched and tortuous configuration
  - Secrete mainly mucus and group II pepsinogen

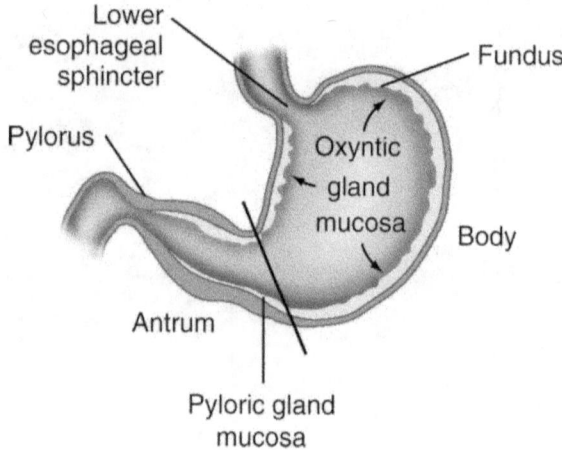

Gastric Glands

- Oxyntic (fundic or parietal) glands
  - Gastric fundus and body
  - Parietal, chief (also known as *peptic*), endocrine, mucous neck, and undifferentiated cells
- Pyloric glands
  - Antrum and pylorus

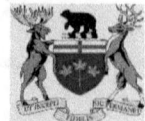

ACID SECRETION AND CYTOPROTECTION

- Composed of endocrine cells (gastrin-producing G cells) and epithelial (mucous) cells.

Oxyntic Gland (Fundic / Parietal)

- o Secretion of acid, intrinsic factor, and most gastric enzymes
- o Three areas
    - Isthmus (surface mucous cells)
    - Neck (parietal and mucous neck cells)
    - Base (mostly chief cells)
- o Endocrine cells, somatostatin-containing D cells, and histamine-secreting enterochromaffin-like (ECL) cells scattered

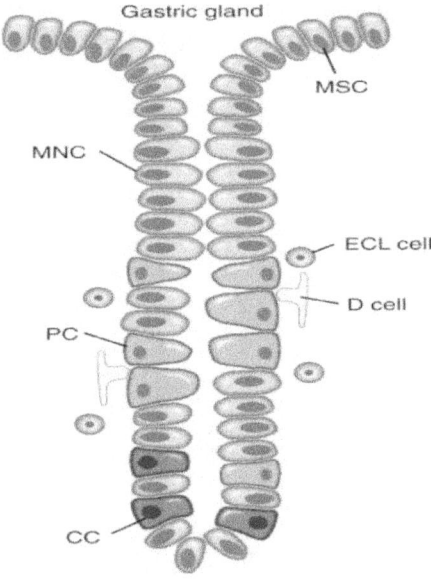

Schematic representation of an oxyntic (gastric) gland, with mucous surface cells (MSC), mucous neck cells (MNC), enterochromaffin-like (ECL) cells, somatostatin containing D cells (D cell), parietal cells (PC), and chief cells (CC).

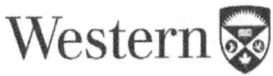

ACID SECRETION AND CYTOPROTECTION

Endocrine Cells

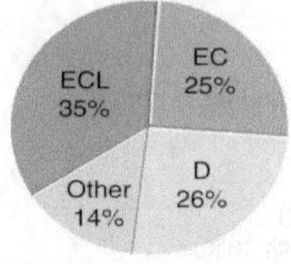
Oxyntic mucosa

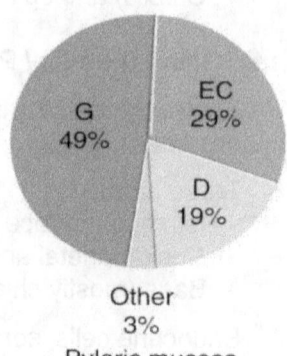
Pyloric mucosa

ECL, enterochromaffin-like (histamine); D (somatostatin); G (gastrin). Other hormones produced in the stomach include ghrelin and leptin, which play roles in food intake and satiety

Secretion

- Water
- electrolytes (H^+, K^+, Na^+, Cl^-, HCO_3^-)
- enzymes with activity at acid pH
    - Pepsins
    - Gastric
    - Lipase
- Glycoproteins (intrinsic factor, mucins)

Pepsin Secretion

The secretion of pepsinogen from gastric body chief cells is increased by
- Ach
- Gastrin / CCK
- Secretin
- VIP

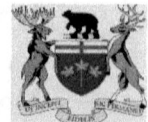

ACID SECRETION AND CYTOPROTECTION

- Give the explanation why secretion of pepsinogen is essential for normal secretion of gastric acid, and why secretion of gastric acid is essential for normal function of pepsinogens.

    o Pepsinogens are converted to pepsins, which begin the process of digestion of dietary proteins to amino acids (AA).

    o AA directly stimulate G cells to ↑ gastrin, and indirectly activated Ach neurons as well as GRP neurons.

    o This ↑ gastrin leads to ↑ histamine released from ECL cells, which in turn stimulates the H2 receptors on the parietal cell to stimulate secretion of H^+.

    o Pepsins become inactive at pH > 4, so the low intragastric pH (↑H+) maintains pepsins in an active form, which then maintains the AA-stimulation of release of gastrin from G cells, as well as release of Ach and GRP from neurons.

Gastric Acid Secretion

An understanding of gastric parietal cell secretion of HCl and G cell secretion of stimulatory gastrin as well as D cell secretion of inhibitory somatostatin, is important to understand the pathophysiology of UD, as well as the gastric effects of hypergastrinemia, including the ZES (Zollinger-Ellison Syndrome) of the sporatic or MEN- I types.

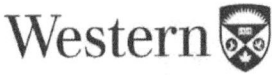

ACID SECRETION AND CYTOPROTECTION

There are redundant and overlapping pathways for acid secretion and inhibition.

- Parietal cell
  - Secretory vesicles are lined with membrane containing the H+ / K+-ATPase acid-secreting pump.
  - With food stimulation the secretory vesicles traffic to and incorporated into the luminal membrane of parietal cells, forming the secretory canaliculi.
  - The pathway for K+ to reach the H+ - K+ ATPase is in a short-circuited state in fasting state, but upon stimulation this pathway allows access of the K^+ to the H^+ - K^+ ATPase, exchange of H^+ for K^+ and thus HCl secretion.
  - The parietal cell is stimulated by the cephalic, gastric and intestinal components, with activation occurring through
    - ↑ Ca2+ (intracellular Ca2+)
    - ↑ cAMP → cAMP-dependent PK (protein kinase) cascade
  - When activation of the parietal cell causes, or inhibition increases, the H+-K+ ATPase moves back (reinternationalization) into the cytoplasmic side of the parietal cell.
  - Reinternalization of the H^+ - K^+ ATPase occurs by way of the cytoplasmic tail of the beta subunit of the enzyme.

- Gastrin and Gastrin Receptors
  - Gastrin is released from G cells in the gastric antrum as a result of amino acids (AA) in the stomach (as well as protein and peptides), and from distention of the stomach.
  - Gastrin binds to the

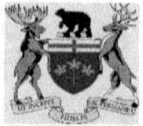

ACID SECRETION AND CYTOPROTECTION

- CCK2 (aka CCK-B, or gastrin) receptors on
    - Parietal cells
    - ECL cells in body of stomach, adjacent to parietal cells
- CCK1 (aka CCK-A) receptors on D cells, pancreas, gallbladder and brain

o Gastrin
  - Acutely
    - ↑ histamine releases from ECL cells → histamine stimulates H2 receptor of parietal cells to secrete HCl
    - Releases ↑ histamine synthesis in ECL cells
    - Releases somatostatin (more from CCK rather than gastrin) → ↓ histamine release from ECL cells
    - Stimulation of ECL cells to release histamine
      - Gastrin
      - PACAP (pituitary adenylate cyclase-activating polypeptide)
      - VIP (vasoactive intestinal peptides)

    - Antigens stimulate gastric mucosal mast cells – release of histamine
  - Chronically
    - Causes hypertrophy of parietal cells and ECL (enterochromaffin-like) cells

o Note paradoxical effect of gastrin
  - ↑ histamine release from ECL cells
    - ↑ HCl secretion
  - ↑ somatostatic release from D cells
    - ↓ G release
    - ↓ HCl secretion

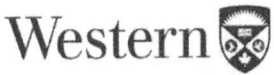

ACID SECRETION AND CYTOPROTECTION

- ➢ Somatostatin

- • Give 4 factors responsible for increasing and/or decreasing the release of somatostatin from the D cells.
    - ○ ↑ release
        - Gastric acidity (↑ H+ → somatostatin → ↓ H+ [feedback loop])
        - Minor distention of stomach, acting through VIP neurons
        - ↑ gastrin
        - ↑ VIP activation
        - ↑ gastrin → ↑ somatostatin
            - ↓ ECL secretion of histamine
            - ↓ gastrin release
        - Major inhibitory mechanism of somatostatin
            - Reduction of gastrin-stimulated release of histamine from ECL cells
    - ○ ↓ release
        - Major distention of stomach
        - Ach

- ➢ Prostaglandins
    - ○ Produced and stored in gastric macrophages and capillary endothelial cells.
    - ○ ↓ acid secretion by way of inhibiting
        - Gastrin-stimulated histamine release
        - Histamine-stimulated parietal cell acid secretion

- ➢ Other peptides which inhibit acid secretion by way of ↓ ECL histamine release from ECL histamine release
    - ○ CGRP (calcitonin gene-related peptide)

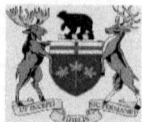

ACID SECRETION AND CYTOPROTECTION

- o PYY (peptide YY)
- o Prostaglandins
- o Galanin
- o CCK2 and CCK2 receptors are G-protein-coupled receptors
- o Signaling by way of pertussis toxin-insensitive G-proteins
- o Agonist stimulation of receptors

➢ Distention
  - o Initially, little distention
    - VIP neurons are activated to release somatostatin
    - Somatostatin inhibits antral G cells
  - o Then, more distention
    - Stimulation of release of acetylcholine (Ach; cholinergic)
      - Directly stimulates M3 receptors on parietal cell
      - ↑ gastrin
      - ↓ somatostatin

➢ AA in stomach
  - o Direct effect of AA → G cells → ↑ gastrin
  - o Indirect effect of AA
    - Activate Ach neurons
    - Activate GRP (gastrin related peptide) neurons → G cells → ↑ gastrin

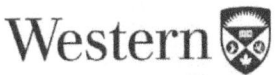

ACID SECRETION AND CYTOPROTECTION

Histamine released from ECL cells act on the H2-receptors on the basal membrane of gastric body parietal cells, increasing HCl secretion.

- Give the mechanism of action of the H3 receptors to alter gastric acid secretion.
    - Histamine stimulates H3 receptors to ↓ secretion of somatostatin from D-cells; the ↓ somatostatin leads to ↓ inhibition of parietal cell acid inhibition, and thus ↑ HCl secretion (inhibition results in stimulation).

PYY (peptide YY) is contained in ECL cells in the terminal ileum and colon. Resection of the terminal colon (R. hemicolectomy) may be associated with increased gastric acid secretion, which sometimes results in diarrhea which responds to the use of a PPI.

- Give the mechanism of this surgically induced increased acid secretion.
    - PYY inhibits gastrin-stimulated histamine release
    - This inhibition is lost with ileal resection and R. hemicolectomy

Functions of Secretion

- Hydrochloric acid
    - Provides optimal pH for pepsin and gastric lipase
    - Negative feedback of gastrin release
    - Stimulation of pancreatic HCO_3^- secretion
- Mucin/HCO_3^-
    - Protection against noxious agents including hydrochloric acid and pepsins
- Pepsins
    - Early hydrolysis of dietary proteins

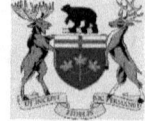

ACID SECRETION AND CYTOPROTECTION

- Gastric lipase
  - Early hydrolysis of dietary triglyceride
- Intrinsic factor
  - Binding of vitamin B_{12} for subsequent ileal absorption

Acid Secretion via the H^+, K^+-ATPase "Proton Pump" (PP)

- At rest, proton pump found in membranes (tubules, vesicles, and sacs) in cytoplasm
- When stimulated, these membranes fuse with the apical membraneparietal cell of the , transferring the activated proton pump to a position to benign to secrete HCl.
- The PP secrete protons (H^+) against a huge concentration gradient (cell interior pH 7.4 or 40 nM; acid secreted at pH 0.8 or 160 million nM)
- Chloride ions are also secreted against a gradient.
- Secretion is an active, energy-dependent process, requiring ATP provided by abundant mitochondria
- Hydrogen ions (H^+) generated by carbonic anhydrase (CA) are exchanged for K^+ by the proton pump.
- Closely associated with the proton pump is a conductance pathway for K^+ and for Cl^-. K^+ is largely recycled.
- HCO_3^- generated by CA is exchanged for Cl^- at the basolateral membrane. HCO_3^- from the parietal cell then enters the blood either to be secreted by surface epithelial cells or returned to the circulation (i.e., alkaline tide)

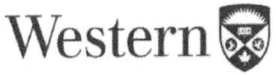

ACID SECRETION AND CYTOPROTECTION

Mechanism of action of benzimidazole proton pump inhibitors (PPIs) on parietal cell H^+, K^+-ATPase.

- PPIs are weak bases (pKa =4 to 5) and are taken up into all cells including the parietal cell (step 1).
- The PPI then crosses the apical membrane and enters the secretory canaliculus of the parietal cell, where the pH is 1 or less (step 2).
- At this point the weak base accepts a proton and ionizes to a cationic sulfonamide (PPI^+; step 3).
- Ionization to PPI^+ "traps" the drug and concentrates it. The PPI^+ then forms a covalent bond with the cystine (CYS) in position 813 of the α-chain of the proton pump, thus forming a cystinylsulfonamide (step 4).
- (PPIs bind to other cystines in the pump, but CYS 813 seems to be critical.)
- The cystinylsulfonamide blocks proton pumping until new α subunits can be synthesized and inserted into the apical membrane.

Regulation of Secretion

- Secretagogues
    - Gastrin
    - Acetylcholine and other neurotransmittor
    - Histamine
- Parietal Cell Inhibitor
    - Somatostatin
    - Cholecystokinin
    - Secretin and Related Peptides
    - Other GI peptides
    - Prostaglandin E2

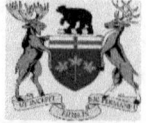

ACID SECRETION AND CYTOPROTECTION

Secretagogues: Gastrin

- Most potent endogenous stimulant of gastric acid secretion
- Not a single peptide but a family of peptides
- Major stimulant of G cells is luminal amino acids
  - Aromatic amino acids phenylalanine and tyrosine derived from peptic hydrolysis of dietary proteins
  - Amino acids turned to amines and taken up by G cells
  - Induce gastrin release into the blood
- Gastrin acts on fundic ECL cells to release histamine
  - Acts on H_2 receptors to increase H^+ secretion from the parietal cell

Negative Feedback on Gastrin

- Negative feedback occurs at lumen pH <3
- H^+ affect amino acid stimulation of G cells
  - Reduce uptake by G cells
- H^+ activate sensory nerve endings
  - Enhance somatostatin release from pyloric D cells
  - Suppress gastrin release from adjacent G cells.
- CCK also inhibit gastrin release
  - CCK released into the circulation by amino acids and fatty acids in the duodenum.
  - Stimulates CCK-1 receptor on pyloric D cell.

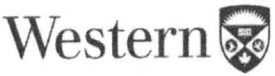

ACID SECRETION AND CYTOPROTECTION

Secretagogues: acetylcholine (Ach) and Neural Mediation
- Cholinergic neurons (postganglionic nerves with bodies in submucosal plexus) release acetylcholine
- Ach acts on muscarinic (M_3) receptors of parietal cells
- Cholinergic neurons are innervated vagal fibers and other enteric neurons
- Neuropeptide GRP may be an important neurotransmitter in the vagal-cholinergic pathway to the parietal cell.

Secretagogues: Histamine
- Secreted by ECL
- Stimulant of the oxyntic ECL cells include gastrin, CCK, and acetylcholine
- Inhibited by somatostatin from oxyntic D cells
- ECL cells can divide under the influence of gastrin
  - Hyperplasia of ECL cells occurs with hypergastrinemia (eg gastrinoma with multiple endocrine neoplasia type 1 syndrome, chronic atrophic gastritis with pernicious anemia)
  - increase in the incidence of gastric carcinoid tumors (ECLomas)

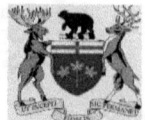

ACID SECRETION AND CYTOPROTECTION

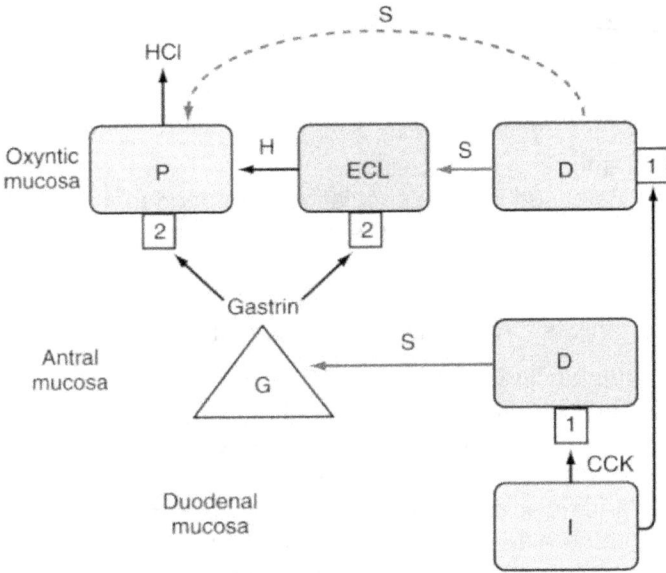

- Parietal cells located in the oxyntic gland area have stimulatory receptors for histamine (H) from oxyntic ECL cells (H_2 receptor) and for circulating gastrin and cholecystokinin (CCK) (gastrin/CCK-2 receptor, shown as 2).
- (A muscarinic receptor for the neurotransmitter acetylcholine is not shown.)
- The ECL cell also has a receptor for gastrin/CCK-2, which is more important in stimulating HCl secretion than the same receptor on the parietal cell. Oxyntic and antral D cells secrete somatostatin (S).
- D cells are stimulated by circulating CCK via CCK-1 receptors (shown as 1) that have a 1000-fold more affinity for CCK than for gastrin. Gastrin is produced by G cells in the antral mucosa.
- CCK is produced by I cells in the duodenal mucosa.

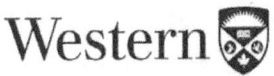

ACID SECRETION AND CYTOPROTECTION

Inhibitory Factors
- Somatostatin
- CCK
- Secretin
    - Released into the circulation from duodenal S cells in response to the entry of H^+ into the duodenum from the stomach
    - Elicit pancreatic HCO_3^- secretion
    - Inhibits further gastric H^+ secretion.
- Prostaglandin E
    - Physiologic effect of prostaglandin E_2 and others on gastric secretion is not very clear
    - Analogs such as misoprostol (Cytotec) reduce gastric acid secretion to approximately the same extent as H_2-receptor antagonists.
    - Some agents that block prostaglandin synthesis such as the cyclooxygenase inhibitor indomethacin increase basal gastric acid secretion

Measuring Gastric Acid Output
- Indications
    - Dx gastrinoma / acid hypersecretory states
    - Dx an incomplete vagotomy in postop recurrent peptic ulcer
    - Excludes achlorhydria as cause of elevated fasting gastrin level by demonstrating fasting acid secretion
- Methods
    - Gastric tube with aspirating port placed by fluoroscopy in the most dependent portion of the stomach.
    - Gastric juice is collected by suction (manual or machine).
    - The H^+ concentration determined by titration or pH measurement with electrode

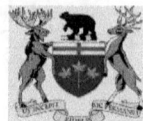

ACID SECRETION AND CYTOPROTECTION

- H^+ concentration multiplied by volume of the sample in litres to determine the *acid output* during the collection period

- Measurements
  - Basal Acid Output
    - Gastric acid secreted in the absence of intentional stimulation
      - fluctuates from hour to hour
      - Lowest between 5 and 11 am
      - Highest occurs between 2 and 11 pm
  - Maximal Acid Output / Peak Acid Output
    - Acid secretion following max IV dose of pentagastrin or histamine.
  - Post-prandial
    - In vivo intragastric titration
  - Primarily a research tool.

Cephalic – Vagal Stimulation of Gastric Acid Secretion

- Stimulation of smell, sight, and thought of nice food
  - Signals to cerebral cortex to lateral hypothalamus to medulla oblongata
  - Dorsal motor nuclei of the vagus nerves (DMN-10)
- The DMN-10 contribute long, preganglionic neurons that travel to the wall of the stomach
  - Axons terminate near short, postganglionic neurons that innervate target cells (e.g., parietal, chief, and ECL cells in oxyntic glands; G and D cells in pyloric glands).
- Cephalic-vagal stimulation a large increase in gastric acid output above the BAO, with a peak response of 50% to 60% of the PAO.

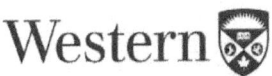

ACID SECRETION AND CYTOPROTECTION

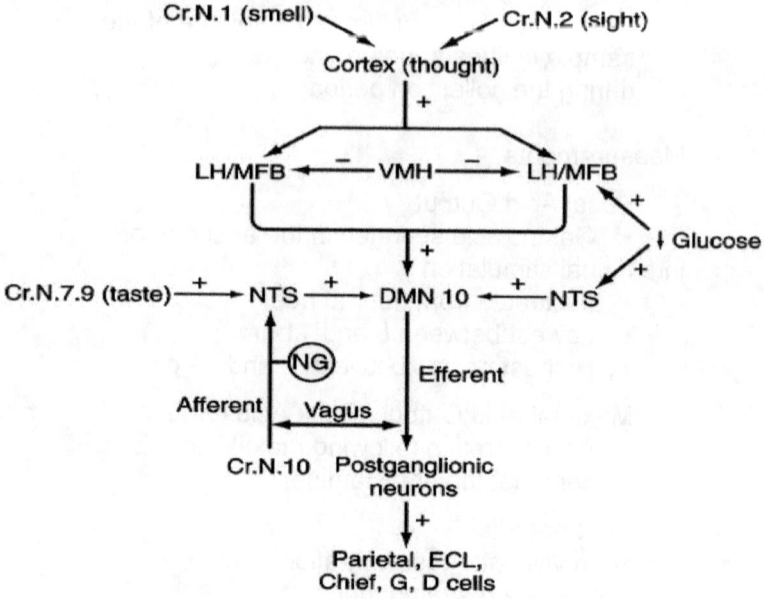

- All stimuli (i.e., smell, sight, thought, taste) ultimately activate the dorsal motor nuclei of the vagus nerves (DMN 10)
- DMN send long preganglionic efferents to the stomach, where they synapse with short postganglionic neurons near target cells.
- DMN 10 can also be activated by the nucleus tractus solitarius (NTS), either as a consequence of
  - Low blood glucose
  - Afferent vagal stimulation (e.g., induced by gastric distention)
- The lateral hypothalamus (LH) and the median forebrain bundle (MFB) are involved in stimulation of acid secretion, whereas the ventromedial hypothalamus (VMH) inhibits acid secretion.

Abbreviations: Cr.N, cranial nerve; NG, nodose ganglion of the vagus nerve.

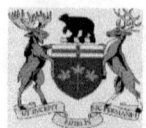

ACID SECRETION AND CYTOPROTECTION

Intraluminal Contents in Gastric Secretion

- Gastric distention releases a relatively small amount of gastrin, via local reflexes
- Proteins
  - Potent stimulants of acid secretion
- Carbohydrates / Triglycrides
  - Inhibit gastric acid secretion
- Coffee (caffeinated or decaffeinated), tea, milk, and soft drinks, Wine and beer increase gastric acid secretion
- Mucus
  - Highly viscous gel-like layer
  - Covers the gastric epithelium (surface and glands).
  - 95% water and 5% solids, mostly mucins
- Mucin
  - Glycoproteins with four subunits
  - In two forms.
- HCO_3
  - Surface cells
    - Rich in carbonic anhydrase II and secrete HCO_3
    - Also secrete mucin
    - Mucus gel with a high pH blankets the gastric epithelium.
    - Mucus gel slows H^+ diffusion
    - HCO_3 neutralizes H^+
    - Increased pH also decreases activity of pepsin
    - Therefore cells protected
  - Gastric HCO_3^- secretion
    - Energy-dependent metabolic process
    - The exact mechanism of gastric HCO_3^- secretion is unclear.

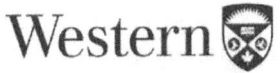

ACID SECRETION AND CYTOPROTECTION

- Vagal stimulation increases gastric HCO_3^- secretion
  - Cholinergically mediated mechanism.
- Prostaglandin E_2 analogs also stimulate gastric HCO_3^- and mucus secretion
  - Blockade of endogenous prostaglandin synthesis reduces gastric HCO_3^- secretion

- Give 10 **Diseases Associated with Increased Gastric Secretion.**
  - Duodenal ulcer
    - Gastric acid secretion is increased 30% to 50%
    - H.P. implicated
  - Zollinger-Ellison Syndrome
    - Gastrin producing tumor of pancrease / duodenum
    - serum gastrin concentrations and basal gastric acid secretion are elevated
    - BAO is >15 mmol/hr
    - BAO/PAO ratio is >= 0.6
  - Retained Antrum Syndrome
    - Rare condition
    - After an antrectomy and Billroth II gastrojejunostomy if the most distal antral and pyloric glands are not resected
    - Retained pyloric glands are bathed continuously in alkaline secretions
    - Gastrin released into the circulation
    - Gastrin-driven acid hypersecretion from remaining parietal cells occurs
    - Recurrent peptic ulceration.
  - Chronic Atrophic Gastritis
    - Inflammation destroys parietal and chief cells
    - Reduction in secretion of gastric acid and pepsin

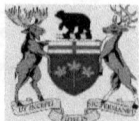

ACID SECRETION AND CYTOPROTECTION

- Autoimmune (type A) gastritis or chronic *H. pylori* gastritis
- Chronic active superficial gastritis
  - *H. pylori* infection
  - More severe in the pyloric than fundic mucosa
  - Mild hypergastrinemia
  - Cytokine mediated reduction of gastric acid secretion
- Gastric resection / vagotomy
- Antral G cell hyperplasia
- Extensive small bowel resection
- Increased intracranial pressure
- Overproduction of histamine
  - Foregut carcinoid tumors
  - Systemic mastocytosis
  - Basophilic leukemia.
- Hyperparathyroidism (increased acid secretion and peptic ulcer disease are usually caused by a coexisting gastrinoma [MEN-1 syndrome])
- AIDS
  - Not with HIV alone
- Miscellaneous
  - Gastric ulcer, gastric polyps, and gastric cancer, with associated CAG or CASG
  - Neuroendocrine tumors (VIP or somatostatin)
  - Severe hypocalcemia

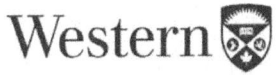

References and Suggested Reading

Madanick RD. Proton pump inhibitor side effects and drug interactions: much ado about nothing? *Cleve Clin J Med*. 2011;78(1):39-49.

Moayyedi P, et a. The risks of PPI therapy. *Nat Rev Gastroenterol Hepatol*. 2012;9(3):132-139.

Pasternak B, et al. Use of proton-pump inhibitors in early pregnancy and the risk of birth defects. *N Engl J Med*. 2010;363(22):2114-2123.

Ratuapli SK, et al. Proton pump inhibitor therapy use does not predispose to small intestinal bacterial overgrowth. *Am J Gastroenterol*. 2012;107(5):730-735.

Reimer C, et al. Proton-pump inhibitor therapy induces acid-related symptoms in healthy volunteers after withdrawal of therapy. *Gastroenterology* 2009; 137:80-87.

U.S. Food and Drug Administration. Proton Pump Inhibitor drugs (PPIs): drug safety communication—low magnesium levels can be associated with long-term use. Available from: www.fda.gov/Safety/MedWatch/SafetyInformation/SafetyAlertsforHumanMedicalProducts/ucm245275.htm.

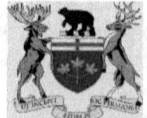

MINI UPDATE

Management of Non-Variceal Upper GI Bleeding

Jamie Gregor

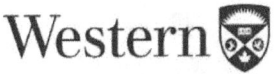

NON-VARICEAL UPPER GI BLEEDING

- ➢ Demography
  - o The overall incidence of hospitalization for UGIB was 134 per 100,000 population; incidence was higher among men than women (153 vs. 117 per 100,000)
  - o UGIB incidence, but not mortality was associated with lower socio-economic status
  - o Overall case fatality rates at 30 days after hospital admission was 10.0%; fatality rates rose with age and were higher for men than women and for those with (vs. without) comorbid illnesses.
  - o Adjusted fatality rates are 13% higher for patients admitted on weekends than on weekdays, and 41% higher for patients admitted on holidays than on weekdays (this difference in mortality could be attributed to reduced staffing and lack of availability of endoscopy on weekends and holidays in some hospitals)
  - o Patients admitted on weekends or holidays suffered higher mortality than those admitted on weekdays (13% higher on weekends, and 41% higher on holidays)
  - o Fatality rates decreased from 11.4% to 8.6% during the study period.

- ➢ Clinical
  - o A negative NG aspirate in the patient who presents with melanoma or hematoschezia reduces the likelihood of an upper GI source of the bleeding, but because of curling of the tube or duodenal bleeding which does not reflux into the stomach, 15-18% of persons with an upper GI source for bleeding will have a non-bloody aspirate.
  - o The distribution of the endoscopic type of bleeding ulcers is: clear-based, 55%; a flat pigmented spot,

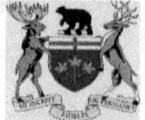

NON-VARICEAL UPPER GI BLEEDING

16%; a clot, 8%; a visible vessel, 8%; and active bleeding, 12%.

- RCTs show that adding bolus plus infusion of PPI to endoscopic hemostatic therapy (EHT) significantly decreased bleeding (NNT, 12) surgery (NNT, 28) and death (NNT, 45).

Abbreviations: NNT, number needed to treat

Learning Objectives

- Understand the role of pharmacological therapy before, during and after endoscopic evaluation for NVUGIB
- Recognize the unique characteristics of the currently available choices for the endoscopic management of NVUGIB
- Through the recognition of the advantages/disadvantages of endoscopic therapies, be able to make educated choices to optimize clinical outcomes

Case

- A 63 year old male presents to the ER with a two week history of increasing fatigue and SOBOE
- On review, he describes a four day of history of tarry black stools, the last one 12 hours previously
- Past history is remarkable for a non-ST elevation myocardial infarction three months previously
- Current medications include only atenolol 100 mg od, atorvastatin 20 mg od and ASA 81 mg od
- Hb- 69 MCV- 86
- Physical exam is unremarkable except for mild postural hypotension

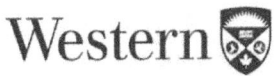

NON-VARICEAL UPPER GI BLEEDING

- Give a clinical method to estimate volume depletion

Clinical	Class I	Class II	Class III	Class IV
○ Blood loss (mL)	<750	750-1500	1500-2000	>2000
○ % blood volume	<15	15-30	30-40	>40
○ Heart rate (beats/min)	<100 Normal	>100	>120	>140
○ Blood pressure	Normal or ↑	Normal ↓ 20-30	↓	↓
○ Pulse pressure	14-20		30-40	>35
○ Ventilatory rate (breaths/min)				
○ Urine output (mL/h)	>30	20-30	5-15	Negligible
○ Mental status	Slightly anxious	Mildly anxious	Anxious and confused	Confused and lethargic
○ Fluid replacement	Crystalloid	Crystalloid	Crystalloid and blood	Crystalloid and blood

Printed with permission: Atkinson RJ and Hurlston DP.
Best Pract Res Clin Gastroenterol 2008; 22(2): pg. 234.

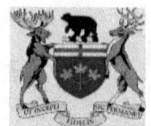

NON-VARICEAL UPPER GI BLEEDING

- Give the performance characteristics of the vital signs and acute blood loss

Physical Finding	Sensitivity (%)		Specificity (%)
	Moderate Blood Loss	Large Blood Loss	
o Postural pulse increment ≥30/min or severe postural dizziness	7-57	98	99
o Postural hypotension (≥ 20 mm Hg decrease in SBP)	9	...	90-98
o Supine tachycardia (pulse >100/min)	1	10	99
o Supine hypotension (SBP <95 mm Hg)	13	31	98

Adapted from: McGee S. R. Evidence Based Physical Diagnosis. 2nd Edition. *Saunders/Elsevier,* St.Louis, Missouri, 2007, Table 15.2 pg. 167

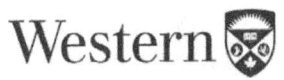

NON-VARICEAL UPPER GI BLEEDING

Useful background: Performance characteristics of hypotension and its prognosis

Finding	PLR
o Systolic blood pressure <90 mm Hg	
– Predicting mortality in intensive care unit	4.0
– Predicting mortality in patients with bacteremia	4.9
o Predicting mortality in patients with pneumonia	10.0
o Systolic blood pressure ≤ 80 mm Hg	
– Predicting mortality in patients with acute myocardial infarction	15.5

Abbreviation: PLR, positive likelihood ratio

Source: McGee S. R. Evidence Based Physical Diagnosis. 2nd Edition. *Saunders/Elsevier*, St.Louis, Missouri, 2007, Box 15.1 page 161.

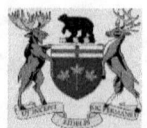

NON-VARICEAL UPPER GI BLEEDING

- Give 15 risk factors for persistent or recurrent gastrointestinal tract bleeding, as well as their approximate odds ratio (OR) for ↑ risk.

Risk Factor	OR
o Clinical Factor	
- Age ≥ 70 yr	2.2
- Age > 65	1.3
- Health status (ASA class 1 vs 2-5)	1.9-7.6
- Comorbid illness	1.6-7.6
- Erratic mental status	3.2
- Shock (systolic blood pressure < 100 mm Hg)	1.2-3.7
o Presentation of Bleeding	
- Hematemesis	1.2-5.7
- Red blood on rectal examination	3.8
- Melena	1.6
- Transfusion requirement	NA

- There are other scoring systems for risk, and the following are additional factors which increase the patient's risk for persistent or recurrent NVUGIB.
    o Rochwall score at index EGD
    o Active bleeding (Forrest Ia, Ib)
    o DU, lesser curve of stomach
    o Large GU / DU > 1 to 2 cm
    o CRF (end-stage renal disease) on dialysis, OR – 3.

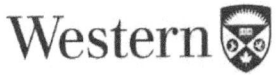

NON-VARICEAL UPPER GI BLEEDING

Risk Factor	OR
o Laboratory Factors	
- Coagulopathy	2.0
- Initial hemoglobin ≤ 10 g/dL	0.8-3.0
o Endoscopic Factors	
- Ulcer location high on lesser curve	2.8
- Diagnosis of gastric or duodenal ulcer	2.7
- Ulcer location on superior wall of duodenum	13.9
- Ulcer location on posterior wall of duodenum	9.2
- Active bleeding	2.5-6.5
- High-risk stigma	1.9-4.8
- Clot over ulcer	1.7-1.9
- Ulcer size ≥ 2 cm	2.3-3.5

Printed with permission: Barkun A, Bardou M, Marshall JK. Consensus recommendations for managing patients with non-variceal upper gastrointestinal bleed. *Ann Intern Med* 2003; 139: 843-57, Table 19-5.

- Give the **Forrest endoscopic classification** of bleeding gastroduodenal ulcers.
  - 1a, spurting
  - 1b, ouzing
  - IIa, no bleeding visible vessel
  - IIb, adherent clot
  - IIc, flat pigment spot
  - III, clean ulcer base
  - Note

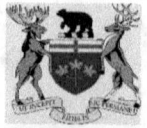

NON-VARICEAL UPPER GI BLEEDING

- No scoring system has been validated to use to predict when rebleeding will occur after endoscopic hemostatic therapy (El munzer et al., 2008).
- Thus, it is not recommended to routinely undertake a second-look EGD.
- Individualize such practice based on the unproven endpoints of clinically apparent recurrent bleeding, unexplained low level of hemoglobin concentration after appropriate transfusion, hemodynamic instability, multiple patient morbidities, or a high risk bleeding lesion seen at the index of EGD.

- Give 6 factors which are predictive of a poor prognosis after hemorrhage from peptic ulcer.

➤ Clinical
- Age > 60 years
- Bleeding onset in hospital
- Comorbid medical illness
- Shock or orthostatic hypotension
- Multiple transfusions required

➤ Laboratory
- Coagulopathy
- Multiple transfusions required

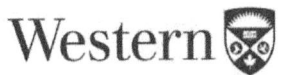

NON-VARICEAL UPPER GI BLEEDING

- Endoscopy
  - Higher lesser curve gastric ulcer (adjacent to left gastric artery)
  - Posterior duodenal bulb ulcer (adjacent to gastroduodenal artery)
  - Endoscopic finding of arterial bleeding or visible vessel

Printed with permission: Barkun A, Bardou M, Marshall JK. Consensus recommendations for managing patients with non-variceal upper gastrointestinal bleed. *Ann Intern Med* 2003; 139: 843-57, Table 19-4.

Issue 1

- How would you initiate PPI therapy?

PPI Therapy in NVUGIB prior to Endoscopy

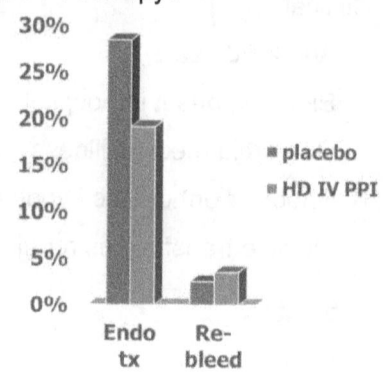

- Convincing evidence from RCT's that high dose IV PPI's given after endoscopic hemostatic therapy ↓ risk of rebleeding by as much as 75% (24% vs. 6%)
- Cohort data (i.e. RUGBE) suggests benefit in all patients

Adapted from: Lau JY, et al. *New Engl J Med* 2007; 356:1631-40.

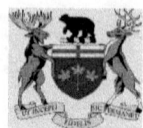

Prognostic Factors: Endoscopic

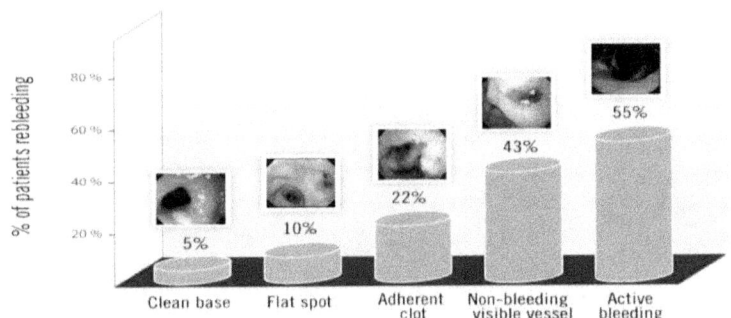

Incidence of Rebleeding by Appearance of Ulcer at Endoscopy

Adapted from: Laine L, et al. N Engl Med 1994; 331: 717-27.

Endoscopic Findings

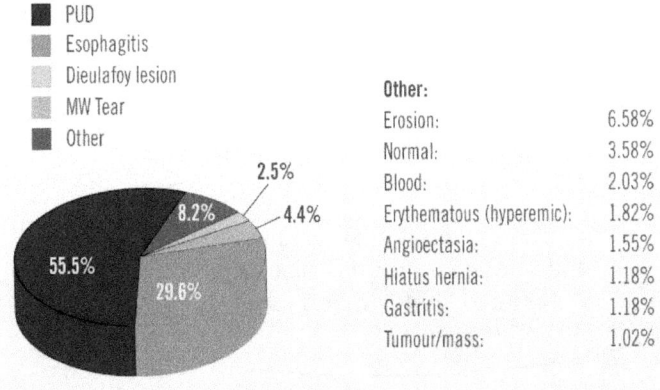

Other:
Erosion:	6.58%
Normal:	3.58%
Blood:	2.03%
Erythematous (hyperemic):	1.82%
Angioectasia:	1.55%
Hiatus hernia:	1.18%
Gastritis:	1.18%
Tumour/mass:	1.02%

Adapted from: Barkun A, et al. Am J Gastroenterol 2004; 99: 1238-46.

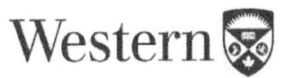

Predictors of rebleeding therapies – RUGBE registry

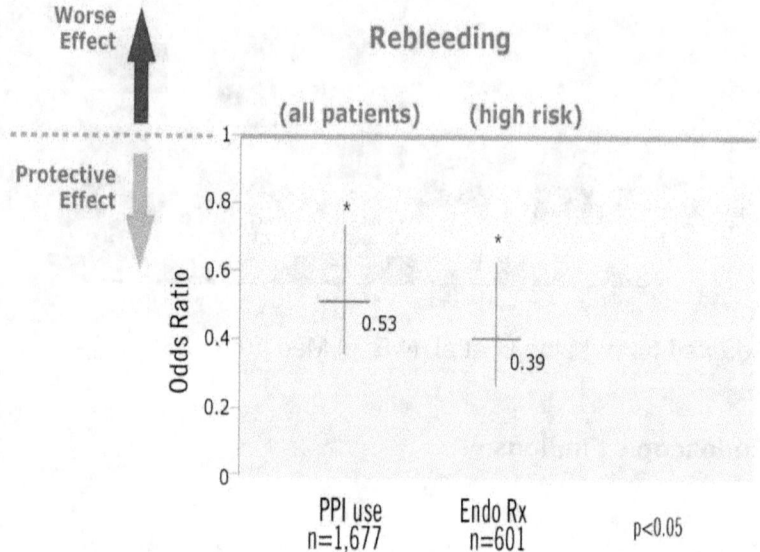

Adapted from: Barkun A, et al. Am J Gastroenterol 2004; 99: 1238-46.

> "Courage is what it takes to stand up and speak; courage is also what it takes to sit down and listen."

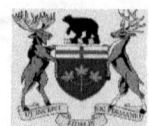

NON-VARICEAL UPPER GI BLEEDING

Effects of PPIs on outcomes in patients with PUD bleeding

o PPIs should be seen as adjuvant to endoscopic hemostasis

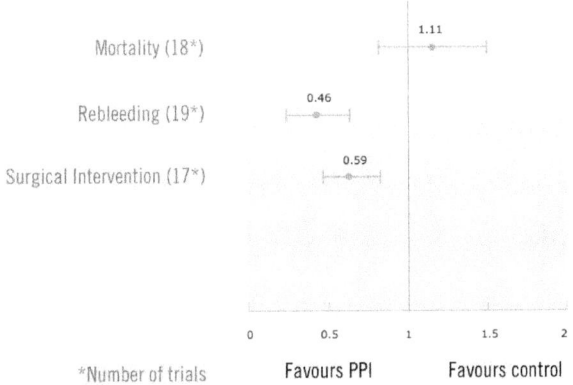

Adapted from: Leontiadis GI, et al. BMJ 2005; 330: 568.

PPI and UGI bleeding in patients with high-risk stigma and treated endoscopically: effect on mortality

Study	PPI n/N	Control n/N	Odds Ratio (fixed) 95% CI	Weight (%)	Odds Ratio (fixed) 95% CI
01 Initial EHT					
Barkun 2004	8/618	14/626		36.6	0.57 (0.24–1.38)
Javid 2001	1/50	2/54		5.0	0.53 (0.05–6.04)
Kaviani 2003	0/71	1/78		3.8	0.36 (0.01–9.01)
Lau 2000	5/120	12/120		30.6	0.39 (0.13–1.15)
Lin 1998	0/50	2/50		6.6	0.19 (0.01–4.10)
Villanueva 1995	3/45	1/41		2.6	2.86 (0.29–28.62)
Subtotal (95% CI)	954	969		85.2	0.54 (0.30–0.96)
02 Without Initial EHT					
Brunner 1990	1/19	1/20		2.5	1.06 (0.06–18.17)
Cardi 1997	0/21	0/24		0.0	Not estimable
Khuroo 1997	2/46	5/49		12.3	0.40 (0.07–2.17)
Subtotal (95% CI)	86	93		14.8	0.51 (0.12–2.12)
Total (95% CI)	1040	1062		100.0	0.53 (0.31–0.91)

Printed with permission: Leontiadis GI, et al. Cochrane Database Syst Rev 2006; CD002094

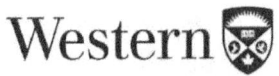

NON-VARICEAL UPPER GI BLEEDING

Treatment Options

- Injection
  - Saline, epinephrine, sclerosant
  - Fibrin
  - Thrombin
- Coagulation
  - Heater probe
  - Bicap cautery
  - APC
  - Laser (rarely required to acute hemorrhage)
- Mechanical
  - Clips

Meta-analysis

Study	Combined therapy n/N	Epinephrine alone n/N	Peto OR (95% CI)	Weight %	Peto OR (95% CI)
Balanzo 1990	5/32	6/32		4.5	0.81(0.22,2.92)
Loizou 1991	3/21	5/21		3.2	0.55(0.12,2.51)
Sollano 1991	0/29	2/32		1.0	0.14(0.01,2.35)
Chung 1993	14/98	17/98		12.8	0.80(0.37,1.71)
Villanueva 1993	8/33	4/30		4.8	2.01(0.58,7.00)
Lin 1993	5/32	12/32		6.2	0.33(0.11,1.00)
Choudari 1994	7/52	8/55		6.3	0.91(0.31,2.71)
Kubba 1996	3/70	14/70		7.3	0.23(0.08,0.64)
Chung 1996	10/79	11/81		9.0	0.92(0.37,2.30)
Villanueva 1996	2/42	7/37		3.9	0.25(0.06,1.00)
Lee 1997	4/30	10/30		5.3	0.33(0.10,1.09)
Chung 1997	6/136	15/134		9.5	0.39(0.16,0.95)
Lin 1999	4/32	12/32		5.9	0.27(0.09,0.83)
Chung 1999	5/42	8/41		5.4	0.57(0.17,1.84)
Garrido 2002	3/40	12/45		6.1	0.27(0.09,0.82)
Pescatore 2002	9/65	12/70		8.7	0.78(0.31,1.97)
Total (95% CI)	88/833	155/840		100.0	0.53(0.40,0.69)

Test for heterogeneity chi-square 17.89 df=15 p=0.26
Test for overall effect z=-4.61 p<0.00001

0.01 0.1 1 10 100
Favours combined therapy   Favours epinephrine alone

- Further bleeding rates for endoscopic treatment with epinephrine injection vs. combined therapy.
- Combination therapy beneficial over therapy in further bleeding

Printed with permission: Calvet X, et al. *GI* 2004; 441-50.

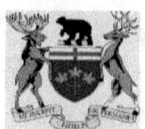

NON-VARICEAL UPPER GI BLEEDING

Study	Combined therapy n/N	Epinephrine alone n/N	Peto OR (95% CI)	Weight %	Peto OR (95% CI)
Balanzo 1990	5/32	6/32		4.5	0.81(0.22,2.92)
Loizou 1991	3/21	5/21		3.2	0.55(0.12,2.51)
Sollano 1991	0/29	2/32		1.0	0.14(0.01,2.35)
Chung 1993	14/98	17/98		12.8	0.80(0.37,1.71)
Villanueva 1993	8/33	4/30		4.8	2.01(0.58,7.00)
Lin 1993	5/32	12/32		6.2	0.33(0.11,1.00)
Choudari 1994	7/52	8/55		6.3	0.91(0.31,2.71)
Kubba 1996	3/70	14/70		7.3	0.23(0.08,0.64)
Chung 1996	10/79	11/81		9.0	0.92(0.37,2.30)
Villanueva 1996	2/42	7/37		3.9	0.25(0.06,1.00)
Lee 1997	4/30	10/30		5.3	0.33(0.10,1.09)
Chung 1997	6/136	15/134		9.5	0.39(0.16,0.95)
Lin 1999	4/32	12/32		5.9	0.27(0.09,0.83)
Chung 1999	5/42	8/41		5.4	0.57(0.17,1.84)
Garrido 2002	3/40	12/45		6.1	0.27(0.09,0.82)
Pescatore 2002	9/65	12/70		8.7	0.78(0.31,1.97)
Total (95% CI)	88/833	155/840		100.0	0.53(0.40,0.69)

Test for heterogeneity chi-square 17.89 df=15 p=0.26
Test for overall effect z=-4.61 p<0.00001

0.01 0.1 1 10 100
Favours combined therapy   Favours epinephrine alone

- Further bleeding rates for endospic treatment with epinephrine injection vs. combined therapy.
- Combination therapy beneficial over therapy in further bleeding

Printed with permission: Calvet X, et al. Gastroenterology 2004; 441-50.

"In everything, the ends well defined are the secret of durable success."

Victor Cousin

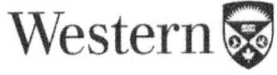

NON-VARICEAL UPPER GI BLEEDING

Study	Combined therapy n/N	Epinephrine alone n/N	Peto OR (95% CI)	Weight %	Peto OR (95% CI)
Balanzo 1990	5/32	4/32		5.8	1.29(0.32,5.22)
Loizou 1991	0/21	3/21		2.1	0.12(0.01,1.24)
Sollano 1991	0/29	1/32		0.7	0.15(0.00,7.53)
Chung 1993	14/98	16/98		18.9	0.86(0.39,1.86)
Villanueva 1993	5/33	4/30		5.8	1.16(0.28,4.70)
Lin 1993	2/32	4/32		4.1	0.48(0.09,2.57)
Choudari 1994	4/52	4/55		5.5	1.06(0.25,4.46)
Chung 1996	9/79	12/81		13.6	0.74(0.30,1.85)
Villanueva 1996	1/42	3/37		2.8	0.31(0.04,2.29)
Kubba 1996	3/70	5/70		5.6	0.59(0.14,2.45)
Lee 1997	3/30	2/30		3.5	1.54(0.25,9.44)
Chung 1997	8/136	14/134		15.0	0.54(0.23,1.30)
Chung 1999	1/42	6/41		4.8	0.21(0.04,0.97)
Lin 1999	1/32	5/32		4.1	0.23(0.04,1.25)
Pescatore 2002	4/65	7/70		7.5	0.60(0.18,2.05)
Total (95% CI)	60/793	90/795		100.0	0.64(0.64,0.90)

Test for heterogeneity chi-square 10.34 df=14 p=0.74   Favours combined therapy   Favours epinephrine alone
Test for overall effect z=2.58 p=0.010

- Surgical rates for endoscopic treatment with epinephrine injection vs. combined therapy.
- Combination therapy beneficial over single therapy in emergency surgical rates.

Printed with permission: Calvet X, et al. Gastroenterology 2004; 441-50.

Clip vs. combination therapy

- 113 patients with high-risk ulcer stigmata
- Heat probe in 57 or hemoclip in 56
- Surgical rates, mortality, initial hemostasis, length of stay and transfusion requirement similar

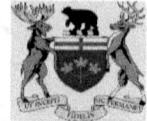

NON-VARICEAL UPPER GI BLEEDING

- Recurrent bleeding 21% vs. 1.8% (p< 0.05)

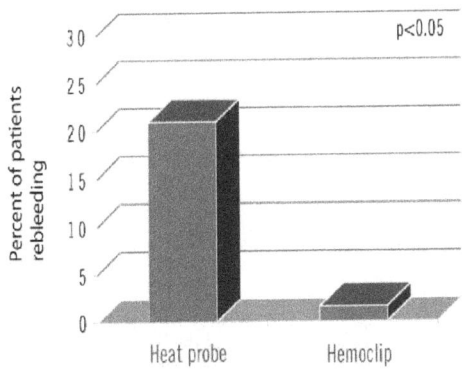

- Conclusion: Hemoclip is safe and effective

Printed with permission: Cipolletta L, et al. Gastrointest Endosc 2001; 53: 147-51.

Endoscopy
- Gastroscopy in the ER does not reveal any fresh blood
- A 1.5 cm duodenal ulcer with hematin spots is noted in the duodenal cap along with a dozen antral erosions
- An antral biopsy for rapid urease testing is negative for Helicobacter pylori

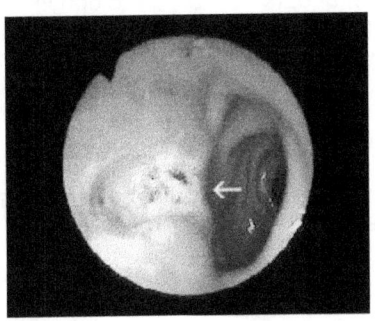

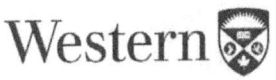

NON-VARICEAL UPPER GI BLEEDING

Useful background: The Rockall Risk Score Scheme for assessing prognosis in patients with NVUGIB (PUD), using clinical and endoscopic considerations

Variable	0	1	2	3
Age (years)	< 60	60-79	≥ 80	≥ 80
Shock	SBP $\geq$ 100, PR < 100/min	SBP $\geq$ 100, PR $\geq$ 100	SBP < 100 mm, PR $\geq$ 100	SBP < 100, PR $\geq$ 100
Comorbidity	None	None	Cardiac failure, ischemic heart disease, any major comorbidity	Renal failure, liver failure, disseminated malignancy
Diagnosis at time of endoscopy	Mallory-Weiss tear, or no lesion identified and no stigmata of recent hemorrhage	All diagnoses except malignancy	Malignancy of the upper GI tract	-

Variable	0	1	2	3
Stigmata of recent hemorrhage	None, or dark spot only		-Blood in upper GI tract -Adherent clot -Visible or spurting vessel	-

Maximum score prior to endoscopic diagnosis=7, maximum score following diagnosis=11

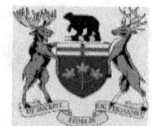

NON-VARICEAL UPPER GI BLEEDING

Abbreviations: GI, gastrointestinal; NVUGIB, non-variceal upper GI bleeding; PUD, peptic ulcer disease; PR, pulse rate

- Give 5 risk factors for peptic ulcer rebleeding after successful endoscopic hemodynamic therapy
    - Hemodynamic instability
    - Active bleeding at endoscopy (spurting more than oozing).
    - The large ulcers (either > 1 cm or > 2cm as the threshold).
    - Posterior duodenal ulcer or high lesser curve gastric ulcer.
    - Need for red blood transfusion.

- Give 6 patient-related adverse prognostic variables in persons with acute NVUGIB.
    - Increasing age
    - Increasing number of comorbid conditions (especially renal failure, liver failure, heart failure, cardiovascular disease, disseminated malignancy)
    - Shock – hypotension, tachycardia, tachypnea, oliguria on presentation
    - Red blood in the emesis or stool
    - Increasing number of units of blood transfused
    - Onset of bleeding in the hospital
    - Need for emergency surgery
    - Anticoagulant use, glucocorticosteroids

Abbreviations: NVUGIB, non-variceal upper GI bleeding

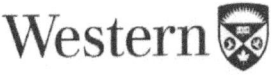

NON-VARICEAL UPPER GI BLEEDING

- Give 3 clinical endpoints which suggest recurrent NVUGIB.
  - If you see blood: NG tube bloody, hematemesis, melena
  - Blood counts ↓ hemoglobin ≥ 2 g/dL after 2 consecutive stable hemoglobins taken 3 hrs apart
  - Vital signs
    - 1 hr of hemodynamic stability: HR ≥ 110 bpm, SB ≤ 90 mm Hg (in the absence of sepsis, cardiogenic shock) or ↑ HR / ↓ SBP within 8 hr post index EGD despite
      - No other explanation e.g. sepsis, cardiogenic shock
      - Continued melena, hematochezia

In the patient with UGIB (upper GI bleeding) and with signs of chronic liver disease, give the patient

- Octreotide sc
- Antibiotics (fluoroquinolone) before and 7 days after UGIB if EV is found
- In fact, while recurrent EV bleeding is common, EGD must be performed with each presentation since just because EV are present does not mean they have bled.
- Characteristic signs on the varices and seen on EGD will establish whether the acute UBIB in the patient with liver disease or known EV arose from bleeding EV, from PUD, from a Mallory-Weiss tear of the gastroesophageal junction, from portal hypertensive gastropathy, GAVE (gastric antral vascular ectasia), or a Dieulafoy vascular disease

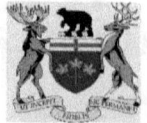

NON-VARICEAL UPPER GI BLEEDING

A patient has iron deficiency anemia, FOB-positive melena stools, a normal EGD with normal duodenal biopsies (exclude celiac disease), and normal colonoscopy with intubation of the terminal ileum. You are asked to give the "best test" from a long list of diagnostic options for obscure GI bleeding, such as

- o Diagnostic imaging
  - Small bowel follow through
  - Enteroclysis
  - CT or MR enteroscopy
  - RBC scan
  - Meckel scan
  - Angiopathy
- o Endoscopy
  - Capsule endoscopy
  - Push enteroscopy
  - Double balloon enteroscopy

And the right answer is……..None of these. Repeat the EGD / colonoscopy, perhaps by a more experienced operator

PPI infusion before EGD is recommended in the care of patients with non-variceal UGIB. Give the benefits of this empiric therapy.

- o Down grade the severity of the lesion and the risk of it rebleeding or requiring surgery (i.e., changing Forrest Ib → IIa)
- o Activation of platelets
- o Reduced peptic digestion of clot ↑ cost effectiveness

- Give the reason why a person with isolated IgA deficiency should not be given a blood transfusion.
  - o The patient would have IgG and IgE antibodies (anti-IgA antibodies), which would react against the

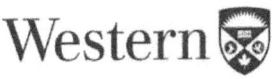

NON-VARICEAL UPPER GI BLEEDING

IgA in the transfused blood, just as would happen with IV immunoglobulins.

If a blood transfusion is contraindicated in a person with isolated IgA deficiency, give what is done if an urgent situation is faced and a blood transfusion would be life-saving.
- The RBCs may be washed, removing most of the serum containing the IgA in the blood to be transfused. The washed and packed RBC may then be given safely.

➢ Management
- Stabilize ABC's
- IV fluids
- O_2 by nasal probes / mask, as indicated
- Routine blood work, including CBC, electrolytes, Cr / BUN, Les and INR
- Monitor renal function and adequacy of fluid replacement
- Risk stratification
    - Without / before EGD   Blatchford score
    - With / after EGD   Rockall score
- Acid inhibition
    - Continuous IV PPI IV infusion may be given after EGD, to determine duration of PPI infusion
    - May given before EGD to "down grade" Rockall risk score: 80 mg IV bolus over 30 min, then 8 mg/hr
        - High stigma lesion, continuous 72 hr IV infusion, followed by PPI po, duration depending upon lesion
    - Low risk lesion o/c IV infusion after EGD; switch to PPI o, for duration dependent upon diagnosis of cause

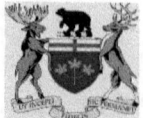

NON-VARICEAL UPPER GI BLEEDING

- o Downgrading of Forrest score when giving IV PIs prior to EGD /EHT

	IV PPI infusion	Placebo
Active bleeding on EGDs	6%	15%
Need for EHT	19%	28%

- o Oral PPIs
  - Use high dose oral PPI to approximate IV PPI infusion e.g. lansoprazole 30 mg tabs 4, then 30 mg (tabs 1) p q 30 min
- o Octreotide and somatostatin
  - Potential explanation for clinical benefit
    - ↓ splanchnic blood flow
    - ↓ gastric acid secretion
    - ↑ gastric cytoprotection
  - When to use
    - When EGD / EHT is not available, and PPI infusion or high-dose po has not been effective
    - For NVUGIB (non-variceal upper GI bleeding)
      - Octreotide 50 mcg to 100 mcg bolus, then 25 mcg per hour for up to 3 days
    - For EVB (esophageal variceal bleed)
      - 50 mcg bolus, followed by 50 mcg per hr
    - If somatostatin to be used for NVUGIB
      - 250 mcg by bolus, then 250 mcg/hr, for 3 to 7 days
- o Co-morbidities to be treated
- o Endoscopy
  - Diagnosis
    - Exclude EVB / GVB (esophageal or gastric variceal blood) if liver disease and varices

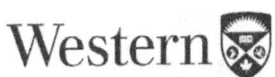

NON-VARICEAL UPPER GI BLEEDING

- Prophylactic antibiotics
- If EVB or GVB → EBL

- Give the rates (%) of rebleeding, surgery and mortality, without and with **endoscopic hemostatic therapy** (ET), using the Forrest classification of bleeding peptic ulcers.

EGD appearance	Prevalence	Rebleeding Rate (%)		Surgery Rate (%)		Mortality rate (%)	
		No EHT		No EHT		No EHT	
		EHT(~70%↓)		EHT (~80%↓)		EHT (~50%↓)	
		EHT	EHT⁺	EHT°	EHT⁺	EHT	EHT⁺
Active Bleeding (Ib, ouzing)*	18	55	20	35	7	11	<5
Visible vessel (IIa); not bleeding	17	43	15	34	6	11	<5
Adherent clot (IIb)	15	22	5	10	2	7	<3
Flat pigmented spot (IIc)	15	10	<1	6	<1	3	<1
Clean ulcer base (III)	35	<5	<1	<1	<1	<1	<1

*Forrest 1a, active bleeding (spurting)

Abbreviation: EHT, endoscopic hemostatic therapy

Printed with permission: Atkinson RJ and Hurlstone DP. *Best Pract Res Clin Gastroenterol* 2008; 22(2): pg. 235.

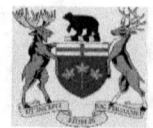

NON-VARICEAL UPPER GI BLEEDING

- o Exclude risks for future rebleeding
  - ASA / NSAIDs
    - Use preventive maintenance co-therapy
  - H. pylori
    - Test and treat, then repeat UBT ± EGD biopsies when off PPI for > 7 days
  - H. pylori-negative, NSAID-negative ulcer
    - Maintenance PPI po, in standard dose, ½ hr before breakfast

Abbreviations: ABC's, airway breathing circulation; EVB, esophageal variceal bleed; GVB, gastric variceal bleed; UBT, urea breath test (for H. pylori infection); EHT, endoscopic hemostatic therapy

- o Overall benefit of EHT, 2/3 ↓ in risk of rebleeding, surgery, death
  - OR for use of EHT in high-risk lesions
    - Recurrent bleeding, 0.46
    - Need for surgery, 0.59
- o Overall benefit of PPI infusion after EHT, ~ ½ further ↓ in risk of rebleeding, surgery, death
- o Timing
  - Usually with 24 hrs of index bleed
  - Earlier may be necessary in some patients
  - Best done with full GI bleeding term of experience endoscopy nurses, staff, trainees, and available anaesthesiologists and general surgeons
- o Adherent clots
  - Gently wash to visualize nature of underlying lesion
- o Use two modalities of endoscopic hemostatic treatment, e.g. injection of epinephrine plus thermal coagulation or hemostatic clips

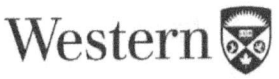

NON-VARICEAL UPPER GI BLEEDING

- Epinephrine 1:10,000 dilution, 0.5 to 2.0 mL aliquots given into 4 quadrants, within 3 mm of bleeding site

> **Clinical Heads-Ups**
>
> Hemospray®, a nanopowder which promotes hemostasis, has been shown in preliminary studies to be 95% effective in achieving acute hemostasis in persons with ouzing peptic ulcers.

- Planned and unplanned
  - A planned second-look EGD within 24 hrs of the index EGD may be justified, if there is
    - Poor visualization in the initial EGD
    - Possible poor EHT in the initial EGD
  - An unplanned second-look EGD or recurrent bleeding
    - Persistent

- Interventional Angiography: TAE (transarterial embolization)
  - Success of TAE for index bleed 52% to 88%
  - Risk of rebleeding 10% to 20%
  - After failure EHT – consider TAE for high surgical risk
    Hematobilia or bleeding into pancreatic duct

NON-VARICEAL UPPER GI BLEEDING

- ➢ Surgery in NVUGIB
  - o Mortality rate
    - Urgent ~25%
    - Elective ~5%
  - o Recurrent (post-op) bleeding ~5%

- Give 15 differential diagnoses of bleeding from the upper and from the lower GI tract in persons suffering from HIV/AIDS, excluding non-AIDS-related diagnoses.

Infection	Esophagus	Stomach	Small bowel	Colon
o Candida	+			
o Cytomegalovirus	+	+	+	+
o Herpes simplex	+			
o Idiopathic ulcer	+			+
o Cryptosporidiosis			+	+
o Salmonella sp.			+	
o Entamoeba histolytica				+
o Campylbacter				+
o Clostridium difficile				+
o Shigella sp				+
o Kaposi's sarcoma		+	+	+
o Lymphoma		+	+	+

Adapted from: Wilcox, C. Mel. *Sleisenger & Fordtran's gastrointestinal and liver disease: Pathophysiology/Diagnosis/Management* 2006: pg. 676.

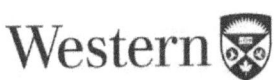

NON-VARICEAL UPPER GI BLEEDING

- What are the clinical features of upper gastrointestinal bleeding elderly versus younger patients?

  ➢ Similarities
    o Presenting manifestations of bleeding: hematemesis (50%); melena (30%); hematemesis and melena (20%)
    o Peptic ulcer disease most common etiology
    o Safety and efficacy of endoscopic therapy

  ➢ Differences (elderly vs. younger patients)
    o Fewer antecedent symptoms (abdominal pain, dyspepsia, heartburn)
    o Prior aspirin and NSAID use
    o Presence of comorbid conditions
    o Higher rates of hospitalization
    o Higher rates of rebleeding Higher mortality rate

Adapted from: Farrell JJ, and Friedman LS. *Gastroenterol Clin North Am.* 2001;30(2):377-407, viii.

- Compare and contrast the endoscopic findings and treatment of portal hypertensive gastropathy (PHG) and gastric antral vascular ectasia (GAVE).

  ➢ Feature findings

	PHG	GAVE
o Site	Fundus	Antrum
o Mosaic pattern	Yes	No
o Red colour signs	Yes	Yes
o Findings on gastric mucosal biopsy		

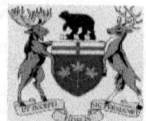

NON-VARICEAL UPPER GI BLEEDING

- Thrombi	No	+++
- Spindle cell proliferation	Sparse	++
- Fibrohyalinosis	No	+++

- Management
  - ↓ portal hypertension
  - β adrenergic blockers
  - TIPS
  - Liver transplantation
  - Estrogens
  - Antrectomy
  - (TIPS doesn't help) Endoscopic laser therapy
  - Liver transplantation

- **Case discussion**
- **Case 1**

  - The patient is treated with pantoprazole 40 mg po bid, transfused overnight and discharge is planned for the following morning
  - What are benefits of antiplatelet therapy in this patient?

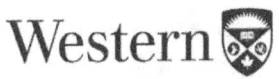

Benefits of antiplatelet therapy in high risk patients

- Meta-analysis 287 studies (135,000 patients) [1]
- 1/4 reduction in serious vascular events
- 1/6 reduction in vascular mortality
- clopidogrel 10% more effective than ASA 75-150 mg / day

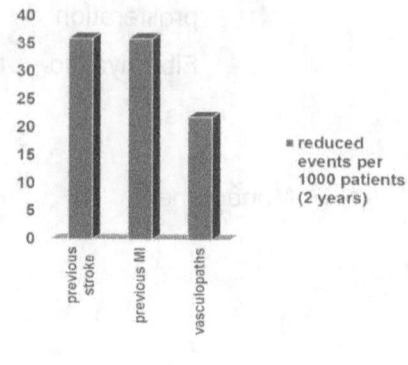

Printed with permission: Antithrombotic Trialists' Collaboration. *BMJ* 2002;324:71-86.

- **Case 2**
  - Overnight he is noted to have an incidental rise in his troponin level
  - Consideration is given to switching the patient's antiplatelet therapy to clopidogrel
  - Might there be any benefits to be expected from such a strategy?

NON-VARICEAL UPPER GI BLEEDING

ASA vs. clopidogrel and ticlopidine in patients at high risk for vascular events

- Meta-analysis four studies (22,000 high risk patients) [2]
- Clopidogrel and ticlopidine associated with a 1% statistically significant reduction in serious vascular events
- Comparable rates of GI hemorrhage
- Not patients with recent GI bleeding

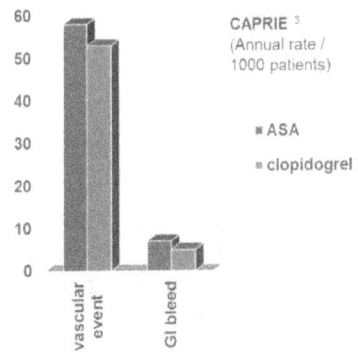

Adapted from: [2]*Cochrane Database Syst Rev 2000;* CD001246; [3]*Lancet 1996; 348:1329-39.*

- **Case 3**
  - The cardiologist caring for the patient would be more comfortable if the duration of antiplatelet withdrawal could be minimized
  - Would it be possible to treat this ulcer without withdrawing ASA?

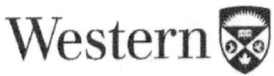

PPI's and ASA-induced ulcer healing

- Patients medically treated for bleeding PUD have a risk of recurrence of approximately 10% over the next 2-3 years [4]
- Risk of recurrent bleeding can be significantly lowered by the use of cytoprotective agents
- Ulcers can be effectively treated and bleeding risk reduced by PPI therapy even if anti-platelet therapy held for as little as one day [5]

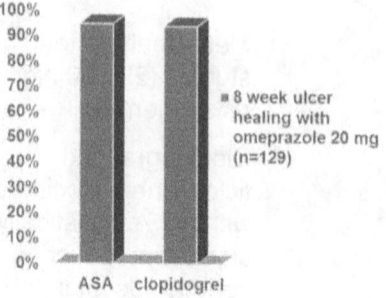

Adapted from: [4]*Epidemiology 1999;10:228-32*; [5]*Aliment Pharmacol Ther 2004;19:359-65*

NON-VARICEAL UPPER GI BLEEDING
Early ASA reintroduction after endoscopic therapy

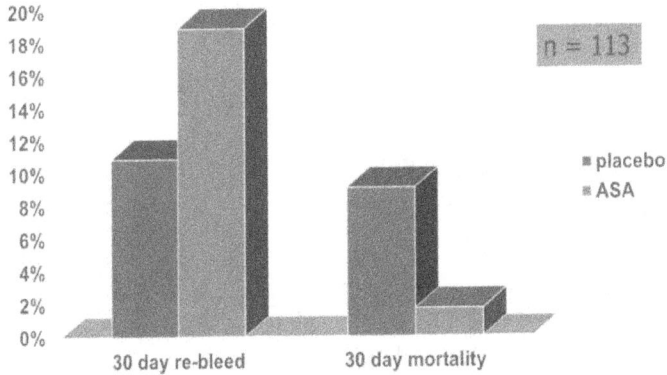

Adapted from: Shanahan F, et al. *Gastroenterology 2006;130 Suppl 2:A-44.*

- **Case 4**
  - The patient was negative for Helicobacter pylori
  - Would your long term management strategy be different if the rapid urease test had been positive?

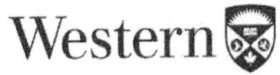

Helicobacter and ASA-induced ulcers

- Helicobacter eradication is a highly effective strategy to treat peptic ulcers and prevent recurrence and complications
- Does not appear to be as effective as chronic PPI therapy for NSAID ulcers but may be for ulcers associated with low dose ASA [6]

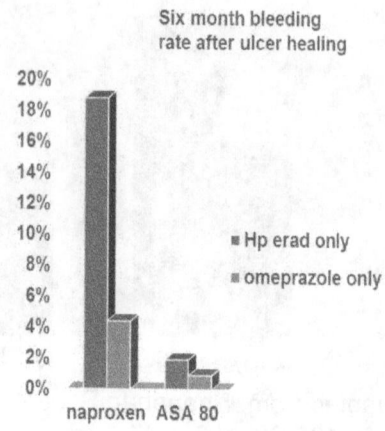

Adapted from: Chan FK, et al. *N Engl J Med* 2001;344:967-73.

NON-VARICEAL UPPER GI BLEEDING

- **Case 5**
  - A decision is made to hold antiplatetet therapy for 4 weeks, continue pantoprazole 40 mg daily and repeat the endoscopy
  - At endoscopy, the ulcer is found to be completely healed
  - What antiplatelet therapy and/or cytoprotective strategy if any would you now recommend?

Post-bleed antiplatelet strategies

- Re-introduction of ASA or NSAIDs after ulcer complications without cytoprotection puts patients at significant risk of recurrence
- Numerous studies have demonstrated that PPI therapy can reduce the risk of endoscopic recurrence [7]

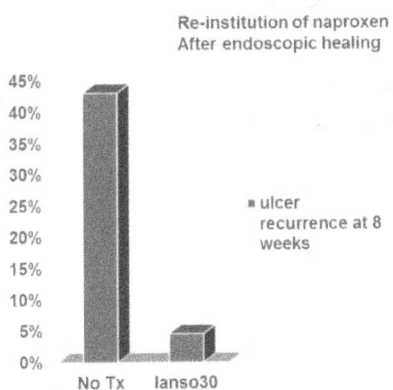

Adapted from: [7] Lai KC, et al. *Aliment Pharmaco Ther* 2003;18:829-36

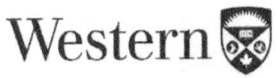

NON-VARICEAL UPPER GI BLEEDING

- Studies have also shown that PPI's reduce the rate of ulcer complications in patients using low dose ASA chronically, particularly after post-bleed Helicobacter eradication therapy [8]

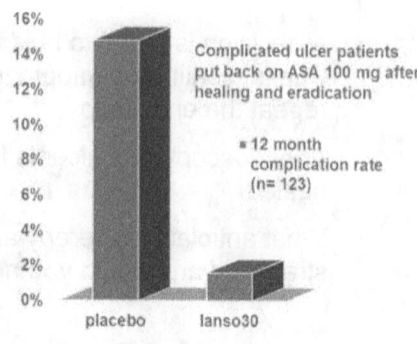

Adapted from: [8] Lai KC, et al. N Engl J Med 2002;346:2033-8.

"The things you do for yourself are gone when you are gone, but the things you do for others remain as your legacy."

Kalu Ndukwe Kalu

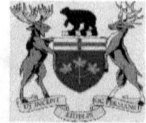

NON-VARICEAL UPPER GI BLEEDING
Post-Bleed Cytoprotection

- Once an ulcer is healed US guidelines had been to use clopidogrel instead of ASA as the preferred antiplatelet agent
- Two studies have compared clopidgrel to ASA/PPI combination after an ASA-induced ulcer bleed in Hp-negative or Hp-eradicated patients [9,10]
- Both have demonstrated clear superiority of the ASA/PPI strategy in preventing recurrent bleeding at one year

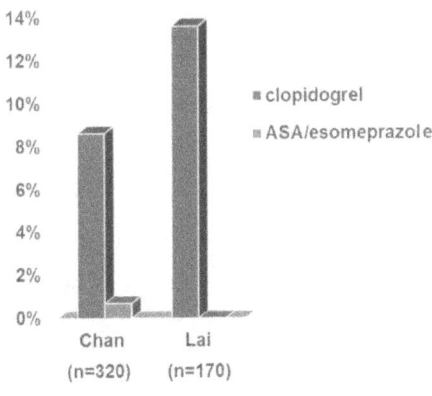

Adapted from: [9] Chan FK, et al. *N Eng J Med* 2005;352:238-44; [10] Lai KC, et al. *Clin Gastroenterol Hepatol* 2006; 4:860-5

- Give 3 clinical endpoints which suggest recurrent NVUGIB.
    - If you see blood: NG tube bloody, hematemesis, melena
    - Blood counts ↓ hemoglobin ≥ 2 g/dL after 2 consecutive stable hemoglobins taken 3 hrs apart
    - Vital signs
        - 1 hr of hemodynamic stability: HR ≥ 110 bpm, SB ≤ 90 mm Hg (in the absence of sepsis, cardiogenic shock) or ↑ HR / ↓ SBP within 8 hr post index EGD despite

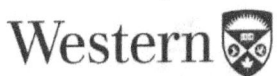

NON-VARICEAL UPPER GI BLEEDING

> No other explanation e.g. sepsis, cardiogenic shock
> - Continued melena, hematochezia

- Give 5 factors which increase the patient's risk for persistent or recurrent NVUGIB.
  - Rochwall score (R) at index EGD
  - Active bleeding (R Ia, Ib)
  - DU, lessor curve of stomach
  - Large GU / DU > 1 to 2 cm
  - CRF (end-stage renal disease) on dialysis or (odds ration) of 3.8 versus CRF not on dialysis, or non-CRF patients with NVUGIB

➤ Interventional Angiography: TAE (transarterial embolization)
  - Success of TAE for index bleed 52% to 88%
  - Risk of rebleeding 10% to 20%
  - After failure EHT – consider TAE for high surgical risk
    - Hematobilia or bleeding into pancreatic duct

➤ Surgery in NVUGIB
  - Mortality rate
    - Urgent ~25%
    - Elective ~5%
  - Recurrent (post-op) bleeding ~5%

- Give 6 patient-related adverse prognostic variables in persons with acute NVUGIB.
  - Increasing age

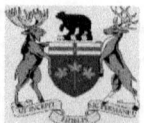

NON-VARICEAL UPPER GI BLEEDING

- Increasing number of comorbid conditions (especially renal failure, liver failure, heart failure, cardiovascular disease, disseminated malignancy)
- Shock – hypotension, tachycardia, tachypnea, oliguria on presentation
- Red blood in the emesis or stool
- Increasing number of units of blood transfused
- Onset of bleeding in the hospital
- Need for emergency surgery
- Anticoagulant use, glucocorticosteroids

Abbreviations: NVUGIB, non-variceal upper GI bleeding

Conclusions

- Anti-platelet agents are important in the prevention of vascular morbidity and mortality
- Re-institution of anti-platelet therapy in vasculopaths at the earliest possible time after a GI bleed should be a priority
- Both Helicobacter eradication and maintenance PPI therapy play an important role in anti-platelet therapy associated ulcer prevention
- Low dose ASA and a PPI is a safer cytoprotective strategy than clopidogrel alone

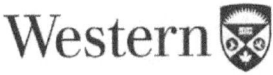

References and Suggested Reading

Atkinson RJ, et al. Usefulness of prognostic indices in upper gastrointestinal bleeding. *Best Pract Res Clin Gastroenterol* 2008;22(2):233-242.

Bardou M, et al. Diagnosis and management of nonvariceal upper gastrointestinal bleeding. *Nat Rev Gastroenterol Hepatol.* 2012;9(2):97-104.

Bardou M, et al. Diagnosis and management of nonvariceal upper gastrointestinal bleeding. *Nat Rev Gastroenterol Hepatol* 2012;9(2):97-104.

Barkun A, et al. A one-year economic evaluation of six alternative strategies in the management of uninvestigated upper gastrointestinal symptoms in Canadian primary care. *Can J Gastroenterol* 2010;24(8):489-498.

Barkun AN, et al. International consensus recommendations on the management of patients with nonvariceal upper gastrointestinal bleeding. *Ann Intern Med.* 2010;152(2):101-113.

Barkun AN, et al. Proton pump inhibitors vs. histamine 2 receptor antagonists for stress-related mucosal bleeding prophylaxis in critically ill patients: a meta-analysis. *Am J Gastroenterol* 2012;107(4):507-520.

Barkun AN, et al. Upper Gastrointestinal Bleeding Conference Group. International consensus recommendations on the management of patients with nonvariceal upper gastrointestinal bleeding. *Ann Intern Med* 2010;152(2):101-113.

Bhatt DL. ACCF/ACG/AHA 2008 expert consensus document on reducing the Gastrointestinal risks of antiplatelet therapy and NSAID use. *Am J Gastroenterol* 2008;103:2890-2907.

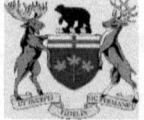

NON-VARICEAL UPPER GI BLEEDING

Blatchford O, et al. A risk score to predict need for treatment for upper-gastrointestinal haemorrhage. *Lancet* 2000;356(9238):1318-1321.

Button LA, et al. Hospitalized incidence and case fatality for upper gastrointestinal bleeding from 1999 to 2007: a record linkage study. *Aliment Pharmacol Ther* 2011;33:64-76.

Calvet X, et al. High-dose vs non-high-dose PPIs after endoscopic treatment in patients with bleeding peptic ulcer: current evidence is insufficient to claim equivalence. *Arch Intern Med* 2010; 170:1698-1699.

Cheung J, et al. Peptic ulcer bleeding outcomes adversely affected by end-stage renal disease. *Gastrointestinal Endoscopy* 2010;71:44.

Dall M, et al. An association between selective serotonin reuptake inhibitor use and serious upper gastrointestinal bleeding. *Clin Gastroenterol Hepatol* 2009;7:1314-1321.

Dall M, et al. Helicobacter pylori and risk of upper gastrointestinal bleeding among users of selective serotonin reuptake inhibitors. *Scand J Gastroenterol* 2011;46(9):1039-1044.

Dall M, et al. There is an association between selective serotonin reuptake inhibitor use and uncomplicated peptic ulcers: a population-based case-control study. *Aliment Pharmacol Ther* 2010;32:1383-1391.

Elmunzer BJ, et al. Systematic review of the predictors of recurrent hemorrhage after endoscopic hemostatic therapy for bleeding peptic ulcers. *Am J Gastroenterol* 2008; 103:2625-2632.

Enestvedt BK, et al. An evaluation of endoscopic indications and findings related to nonvariceal upper GI hemorrhage in a large mulitcenter consortium. *Gastrointestinal Endoscopy* 2008;67:422-429.

García-Iglesias P, et al. Meta-analysis: predictors of rebleeding after endoscopic treatment for bleeding

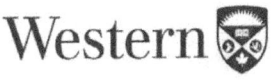

peptic ulcer. *Aliment Pharmacol Ther* 2011;34(8):888-900.

Gralnek IM. Will surgery be a thing of the past in peptic ulcer bleeding? Gastrointest Endosc 2011; 73:909-910.

Greenspoon J, et al. Upper Gastrointestinal Bleeding Conference Group. Management of patients with nonvariceal upper gastrointestinal bleeding. *Clin Gastroenterol Hepatol* 2012;10(3):234-239.

Jairath V, et al. Mortality from acute upper gastrointestinal bleeding in the United kingdom: does it display a "weekend effect"? *Am J Gastroenterol* 2011;106(9):1621-1628.

Kafes AJ, et al. Clinical outcomes after double-balloon enteroscopy in patients with obscure GI bleeding and a positive capsule endoscopy. *Gastrointestinal Endoscopy* 2007;66(2):304-309.

Kobilica N, et al. Major complication after Histoacryl injection for endoscopic treatment of bleeding peptic ulcer. *Endoscopy* 2012; 44 Suppl 2:E204-205.

Laine L, et al. Management of patients with ulcer bleeding. *Am J Gastroenterol*. 2012;107(3):345-360.

Laine L and McQuaid KR. Endoscopic therapy for bleeding ulcers: an evidence-based approach based on meta-analyses of randomized controlled trials. *Clin Gastroenterol Hepatol* 2009; 7:33-47.

Lanas A, et al. Clinical predictors of poor outcomes among patients with nonvariceal upper gastrointestinal bleeding in Europe. *Aliment Pharmacol Ther* 2011;33(11):1225-1233.

Lanas A, et al. Low doses of acetylsalicylic acid increase risk of gastrointestinal bleeding in a meta-analysis. *Clin Gastroenterol Hepatol* 2011;9(9):762-768.

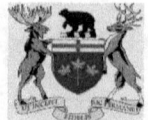

NON-VARICEAL UPPER GI BLEEDING

Lanas A, et al. Time trends and impact of upper and lower gastrointestinal bleeding and perforation in clinical practice. *Am J Gastroenterol* 2009: 104(7):1633-41.

Laursen SB, et al. The Glasgow Blatchford score is the most accurate assessment of patients with upper gastrointestinal hemorrhage. *Clin Gastroenterol Hepatol.* 2012;10(10):1130-1135.

Lin KJ, et al. Acid suppressants reduce risk of gastrointestinal bleeding in patients on antithrombotic or anti-inflammatory therapy. *Gastroenterology.* 2011;141(1):71-9.

Marmo R, et al. Mortality from nonulcer bleeding is similar to that of ulcer bleeding in high-risk patients with nonvariceal hemorrhage: a prospective database study in Italy. *Gastrointest Endosc.* 2012;75(2):263-272.

Ng FH, et al. Esomeprazole compared with famotidine in the prevention of upper gastrointestinal bleeding in patients with acute coronary syndrome or myocardial infarction. *Am J Gastroenterol* 2012;107(3):389-396.

Raju GS. American Gastroenterological Association (AGA) Institute Technical Review on Obscure Gastrointestinal Bleeding. *Gastroenterology* 2007;133:1697-1717.

Saltzman JR, et al. A simple risk score accurately predicts in-hospital mortality, length of stay, and cost in acute upper GI bleeding. Gastrointest Endosc 2011;74(6):1215-1224.

Schrier SL. Approach to the adult patient with anemia. *UpToDate*; www.uptodate.com

Schrier SL. Causes and diagnosis of anemia due to iron deficiency. *UpToDate*; www.uptodate.com 2014

Sreedharan A, et al. Proton pump inhibitor treatment initiated prior to endoscopic diagnosis in upper gastrointestinal bleeding. *Cochrane Database Syst Rev.* 2010;(7):CD005415.

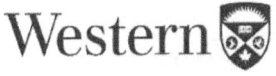

Straube S, et al. Mortality with upper gastrointestinal bleeding and perforation: effects of time and NSAID use. *BMC Gastroenterology* 2009;9:41.

Sung JJ, et al. Asia-Pacific Working Group consensus on non-variceal upper gastrointestinal bleeding. *Gut* 2011;60(9):1170-1177.

Sung JJ, et al. Early clinical experience of the safety and effectiveness of Hemospray in achieving hemostasis in patients with acute peptic ulcer bleeding. *Endoscopy* 2011; 43:291-295.

Targownik LE, et al. Selective serotonin reuptake inhibitors are associated with a modest increase in the risk of upper gastrointestinal bleeding. *The American J Gastroenterol* 2009; 104(6):1475-1482.

Tsoi KK, et al. Second-look endoscopy with thermal coagulation or injections for peptic ulcer bleeding: a meta-analysis. *J Gastroenterol Hepatol* 2010; 25:8-13.

Van Rensburg C. Clinical trial: intravenous pantoprazole vs. ranitidine for the prevention of peptic ulcer rebleeding: a multicentre, multinational, randomized trial. *Aliment Pharmacol Ther* 2009;29:497-507.

Veitch AM. Guidelines for the management of anticoagulant and antiplatelet therapy in patients undergoing endoscopic procedures. *Gut* 2008;57:1322-1329.

Wang CH, et al. High-dose vs non-high-dose proton pump inhibitors after endoscopic treatment in patients with bleeding peptic ulcer: a systematic review and meta-analysis of randomized controlled trials. Arch Intern Med 2010; 170:751-758.

Wong GL, et al. Gastroprotective therapy does not improve outcomes of patients with Helicobacter pylori-negative idiopathic bleeding ulcers. *Clin Gastroenterol Hepatol*. 2012;10(10):1124-1129.

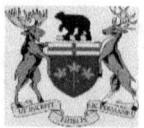

Wong RCK. Nonvariceal upper gastrointestinal hemorrhage: Probing beneath the surface. *Gastroenterology* 2009;137:1897-1911.

Wu CY, et al. Histamine$_2$ receptor antagonists are an alternative to proton pump inhibitor in patients receiving clopidogrel. *Gastroenterology* 2010;139:1165-1171.

Wu CY, et al. Long-term peptic ulcer rebleeding risk estimation in patients undergoing haemodialysis: a 10-year nationwide cohort study. *Gut* 2011;60(8):1038-1042.

Yachimski PS. Gastrointestinal Bleeding in the Elderly. *Nat Clin Pract Gastroenterol Hepatol* 2008;5(2):80-93.

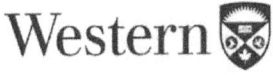

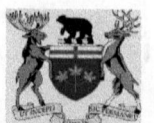

MINI UPDATE

Bariatric Surgery for the Gastroenterologist

Michael Sey

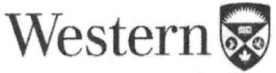

BARIATRIC SURGERY

Reasons Why We Need to Know About Bariatric Surgery

- Pre-operative reasons
  - Cardiovascular benefits from an internal medicine perspective
  - Potential treatment for NAFLD and diabetes

- Post-operative reasons
  - Bariatric surgery predisposes to a large number of UGI symptoms
  - Knowledge of anatomy crucial prior to upper endoscopic procedures
  - Management of long term complications

Reasons for Rise of Bariatric Surgery

- Difficulty and limited efficacy of lifestyle measures

- Limited pharmacologic options

- Reduced mortality and morbidity with laparoscopic surgical approaches

- Give the **indications for bariatric surgery.**

Criteria	NIH (1991)	NICE (2006)	IDF (2011)
Based on BMI only	>40	>40	>35
BMI + co-morbid condition	35-40 + 1 serious weight loss responsive co-morbidity	35-40 + 1 serious weight loss responsive co-morbidity	>30 + 1 serious weight loss responsive co-morbidity

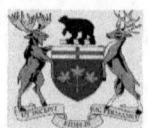

BARIATRIC SURGERY

**All guidelines require prior failure of non-surgical treatment plus motivated patient who is committed to life-long diet and follow-up

NIH: National Institute of Health (US)

NICE: National Institute for Health and Clinical Excellence (UK)

IDF: International Diabetes Federation

- Give the benefits of bariatric surgery.
    - ↓ appetite (related to altered GI peptides)
    - ↓ BMI / waist curcumference
    - ↓ all cause mortality rate (CV, CRC), as well as and other obesity-related cancers
    - ↓ diabetes (↓ insulin resistance, ↓ insulin requirements)
    - ↓ NAFLD histology score in > 80% (↓ fibrosis in 60%)
    - ↑ quality of life for patien

Gems & Pearls

URSO ↓ risk of gallstones by 40% after R-en-Y gastric bypass

VBG (vertical banded gastroscopy) → pseudoachalasia

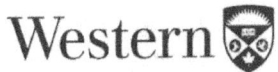

Bariatric Surgery is Effective at Reducing Weight

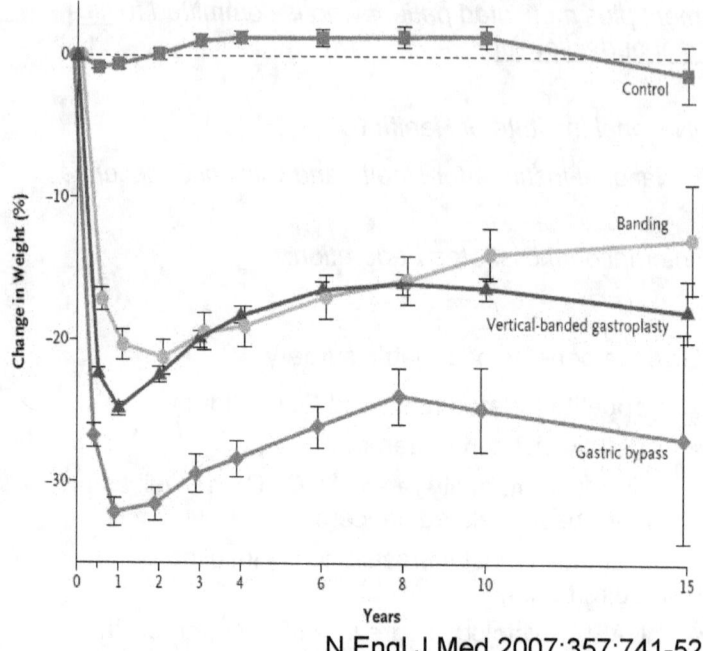

N Engl J Med 2007;357:741-52

Bariatric Surgery Reduces Obesity-Associated Mortality

➢ Swedish Obese Subjects study
  - Prospective case-control study of bariatric surgery vs. conventional therapy in 4047 obese patients
  - Follow up of 10 years
  - Mean starting BMI 40
  - Outcome: ↓ mortality

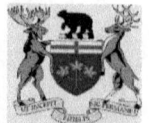

BARIATRIC SURGERY

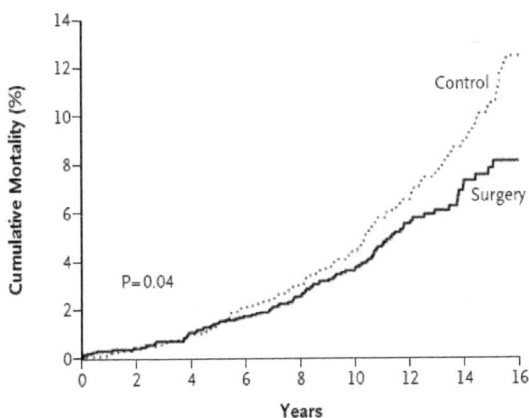

N Engl J Med 2007;357:741-52.

Bariatric Surgery Reduces Obesity-Associated Morbidity Diabetes

- Meta-analysis of resolution of diabetes after bariatric surgery (various techniques)
- 621 studies with 135,246 patients included

Table 8 Overview of Weight Loss, Surgical Procedure, and Diabetes Resolution

	Total	Gastric Banding	Gastroplasty	Gastric Bypass	BPD/DS
% EBWL	55.9	46.2	55.5	59.7	63.6
% Resolved overall	78.1	56.7	79.7	80.3	95.1
% Resolved <2 y	80.3	55.0	81.4	81.6	94.0
% Resolved ≥2 y	74.6	58.3	77.5	70.9	95.9

%EBWL = percent excess body weight loss; BPD/DS = biliopancreatic diversion/duodenal switch.

Am J Med 2009;122:248-56.

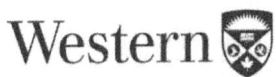

BARIATRIC SURGERY

Types of Bariatric Surgery

- Give the major **types of bariatric surgery,** and be prepared to draw the post-operative analog.

    o Restrictive
    - Laparoscopic adjustable gastric band
    - Sleeve gastrectomy
    - Vertical banded gastroplasty ("stomach stapling")*

    o Mixed
    - Roux-en-Y gastric bypass

    o Malabsorptive
    - Biliopancreatic diversion +/- duodenal switch*
    - Ileo-jejunal bypass*

No longer routinely performed

    o Mixed procedure

BARIATRIC SURGERY

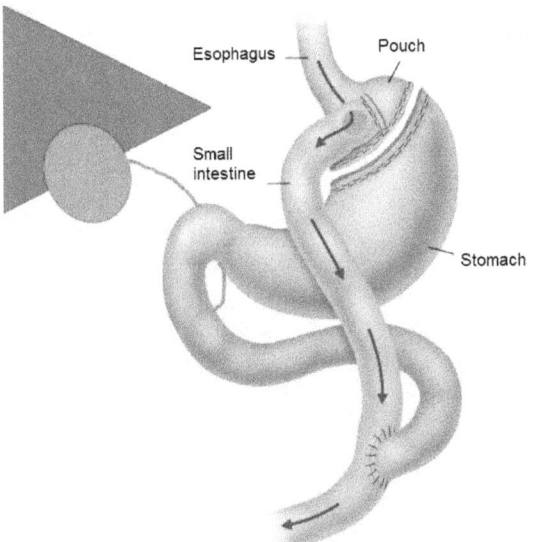

Roux-en-Y gastric bypass

Source: UpToDate

> Restrictive procedures

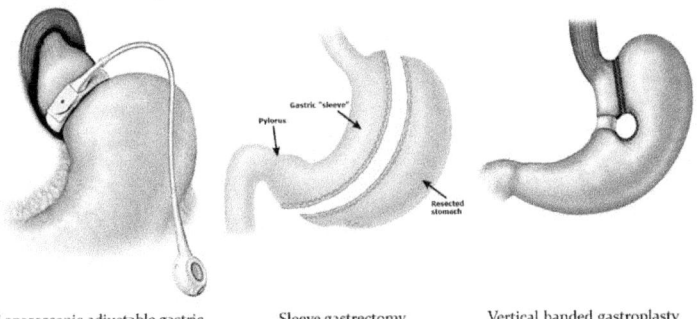

Laparoscopic adjustable gastric band   Sleeve gastrectomy   Vertical banded gastroplasty

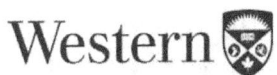

BARIATRIC SURGERY

> Malabsorptive procedures

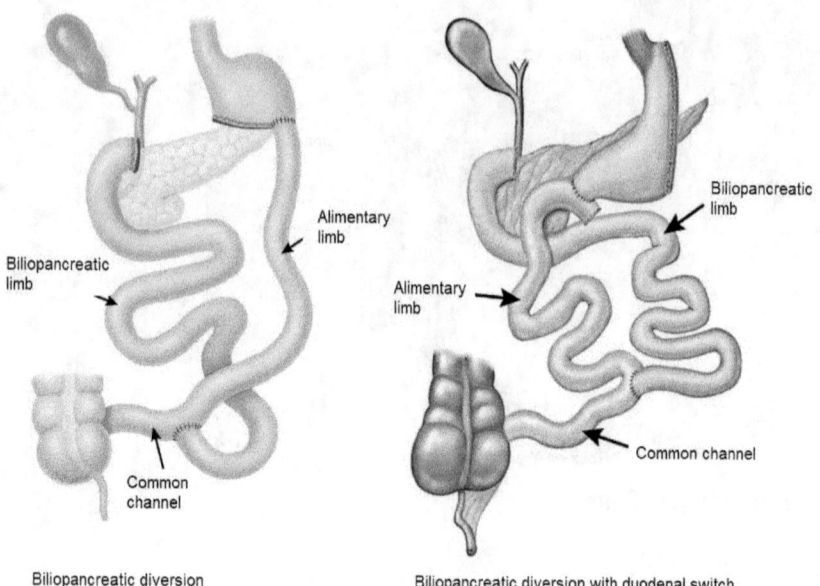

Biliopancreatic diversion

Biliopancreatic diversion with duodenal switch

Source: UpToDate

BARIATRIC SURGERY

Choice of Bariatric Surgery

	Laparoscopic adjustable gastric band	RYGB	Sleeve gastrectomy
o Excess weight loss at 3-5 years	54%	60%	50-60%
o Pattern of weight loss	Gradual, maximal at 2-3 years	Rapid, maximal at 1-2 years	Rapid, maximal at 1-2 years
o Long term data available	Y	Y	N
o Mortality reduction	Y	Y	N
o 30-day post-op mortality	0.05-0.1%	0.3-0.5%	0.4%

Nat Rev Gastroenterol Hepatol 2011;8:429-37.

- NAFLD
    - Meta-analysis: bariatric surgery improve NAFLD histology
    - 15 studies (766 patients with liver biopsy pre and post-surgery)
    - Duration between biopsies ranged from 2 to 111 months
    - % reduction in BMI ranged from 20-40%

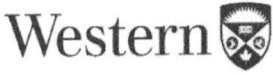

BARIATRIC SURGERY

Bariatric Surgery Improves NAFLD Histology

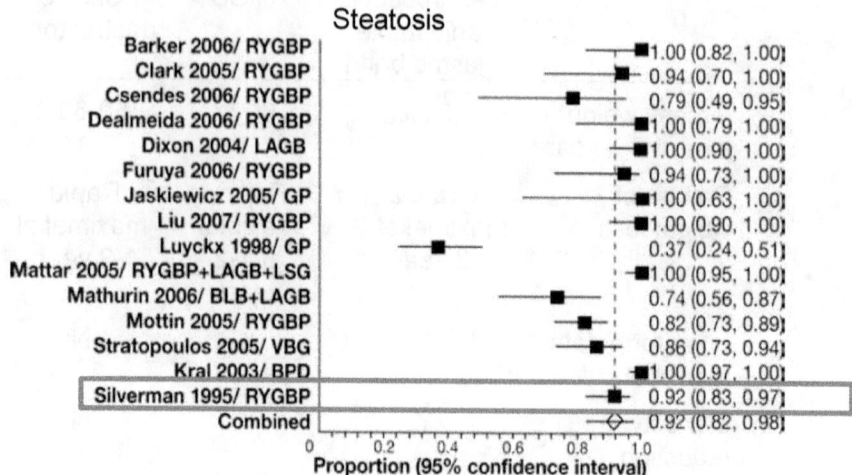

Steatosis

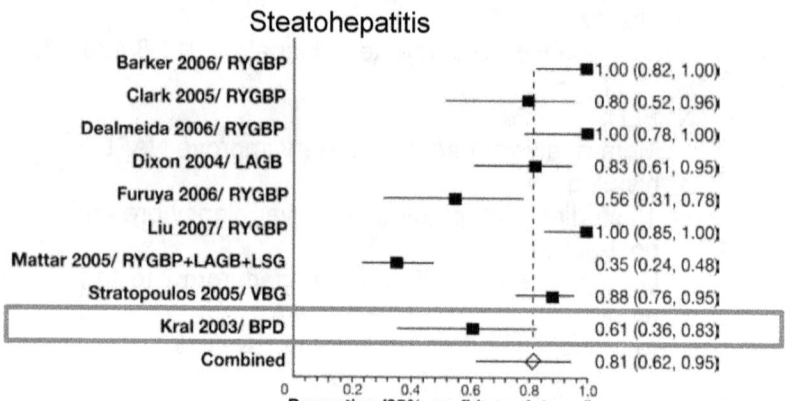

Steatohepatitis

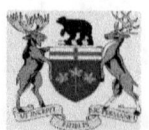

BARIATRIC SURGERY

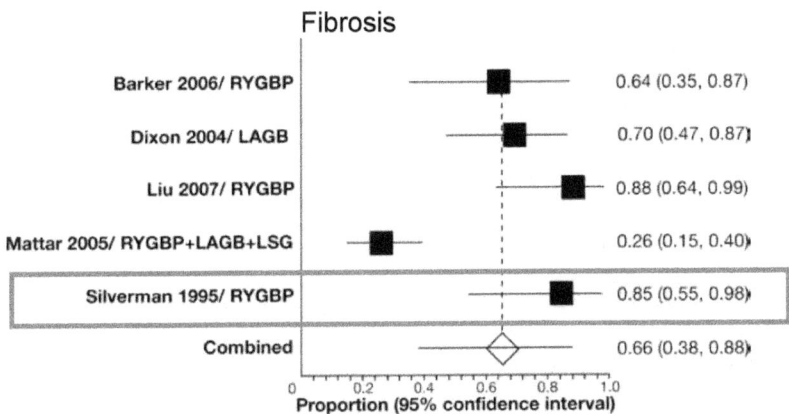

- o Limitations of studies
  - None are RCTs
  - Small studies (20-100 patients)
  - No long-term follow up
  - Magnitude of histologic improvement unclear
  - Rare cases of liver deterioration with rapid weight loss

  Clin Gastroenterol Hepatol 2008;6:1396-02.

Complications

- o All procedures are prone to complications
- o Lifelong commitment to diet and medical follow up needed for patients after their surgery
  - Bariatric surgery is not a cure for obesity
  - Maladaptive eating behaviour #1 cause of weight regain (grazing throughout the day or, soft foods like ice cream can overcome restriction of bariatric surgery)
- o Complications are often unique to the type of surgery performed
  - Understand the anatomy and physiology is crucial in caring for these patients

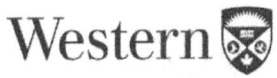

BARIATRIC SURGERY

- LAGB
  - Band related
    - Band erosion
    - Band slippage and gastric prolapse
    - Dysphagia
  - Port related
    - Infection
    - Port malfunction
  - Nutritional deficiency risk (low)

Band Slippage and Gastric Prolapse

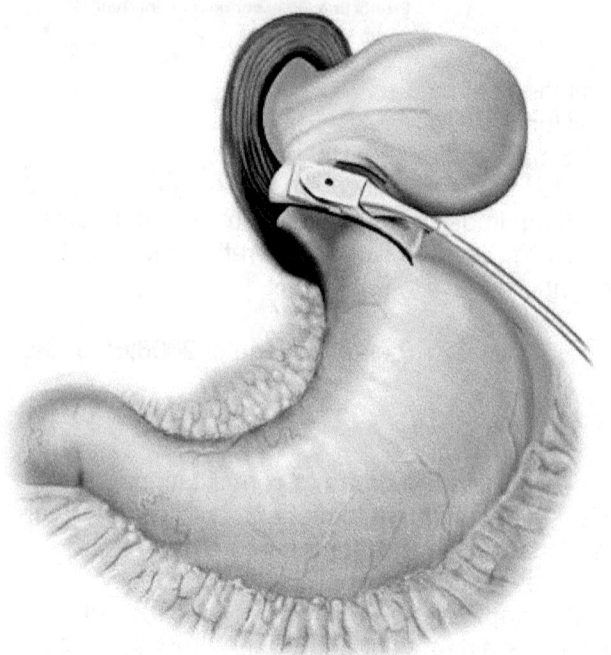

Source: UpToDate

BARIATRIC SURGERY

- Sleeve gastrectomy
  - Stenosis
    - Commonly occurs at GE junction or incisura angularis
    - Due to over-sewing or using a bougie that is too small when creating the "sleeve"
    - Presents as nausea and vomiting, pain, dysphagia
    - Treatment is endoscopic dilation
  - Nutritional deficiency risk (moderate)
    - Fe, B12, folate, Ca, vitamin D

- Vertical banded gastroplasty
  - Staple line disruption
    - Weight regain due to loss of restrictive capability of pouch
  - Stomal stenosis/band erosion
    - Fibrosis around band
    - Presents as GERD, gastric outlet obstruction
    - Endoscopic dilation or surgical removal of band
  - Nutritional deficiency risk (low)

- Roux-en-Y gastric bypass

- Give 5 late complications of Roux-en-Y gastric bypass.

  - Anastomotic ulcer
    - Ischemia
    - Presence of FB (foreign body)
    - Excessive acid exposure
    - Smoking
    - H. pylori infection
  - Stomal stenosis
    - Ischemia
    - Treat by endoscopic dilation
  - Gastric remnant distension
    - Consequence of distal bowel obstruction or ileus
    - Gastric blow-out may occur due to inability to vent gastric remnant

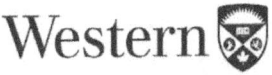

BARIATRIC SURGERY

- Dumping syndrome
  - Not seen with restrictive procedures due to preservation of pylorus
  - Early dumping
    - <15 min
    - Hyperosmolar large simple CHO load → fluid shift in SI hypotension + adrenergic response
  - Late dumping
    - 2-3 hours post prandial
    - Hyperinsulinemia due to large simple CHO load reactive hypoglycemia
  - Tx:
    - Complex CHO and protein rich meals
    - Smaller, more frequent feeds
- Nutritional deficiency risk (moderate)
  - Fe, folate, Ca, vitamin D due to proximal SI diversion
  - B12 deficiency (hypochlorhydria, fat maldigestion, trypsinogen)
- Oxalate nephrolithiasis
  - Fat maldigestion → excess luminal free fatty acids (FFA) bind to dietary oxalate (OXA)
  - FFA – OXA is absorbed in colon, excreted in kidney, where stones form
- Cholelithiasis
  - Not unique to RYGB
  - Rapid weight loss increases lithogenicity of bile
  - Difficult access to papilla for ERCP
  - Prevention:
    - URSO x 6 months post op
    - Prophylactic cholecystectomy at time of bariatric surgery

Abbreviations: CBD, common bile duct; URSO, ursodeoxycholic acid; CHO, carbohydrate

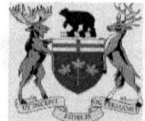

BARIATRIC SURGERY

- Biliopancreatic diversion

  - Nutritional deficiency risk (high)
    - Protein calorie malnutrition
      - Very short common limb severely restricts CHO and protein digestion and absorption
    - Fe, folate, Ca malabsorption
      - Bypass proximal SI
    - Fat soluble vitamin deficiency and oxalate nephrolithiasis
      - Steatorrhea due to pancreatic diversion
    - B12 deficiency

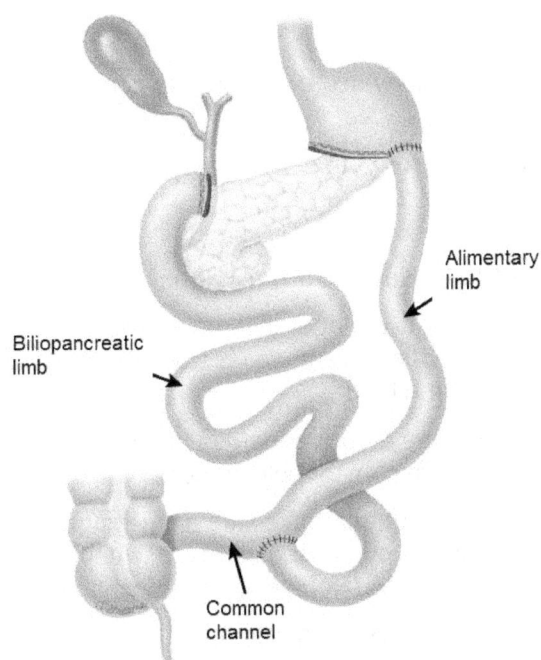

Source: UpToDate

BARIATRIC SURGERY

> **Remember**
>
> In a sentence, state the indications for bariatric surgery
>
> - BMI > 40 kg/m², or
> - BMI > 35 kg/m² plus comorbid complications

- Give the benefits of bariatric surgery
    - ↓ all cause mortality rate (CV, CRC), as well as and other obesity-related cancers
    - ↓ diabetes
    - ↓ NAFLD histology score in > 80% (↓ fibrosis in 60%)
    - ↑ quality of life for patient

Endoscopy in the Bariatric Surgery Patient
- Be smart: review the operative notes and any relevant post-operative imaging studies to be aware of the "lay of the land".
- Visualization may require the use of a narrower pediatric gastroscopy or colonoscopy.
- ERCP of the biliopancreatic limb and retrograde evaluation of the by passed stomach is especially difficult after RYGB (Roux-en-Y gastric bypass).
- This difficult is increasing with more use of "distal bypass", with anastomosis of the biliopancreatic limb only 150 cm proximal to the ileocecal value.
- Retrograde evaluation may be made easier with use of

BARIATRIC SURGERY

- Shapelock™ enteroscopy guide
- Deep small bowel enteroscope
  - Ballon assited enteroscopy

Common Endoscopic Findings after Bariatric Surgery

- RYGB
  - "gastritis" is common, but clinical significance is unclear
  - ~1/3 of symptomatic RYGB have a normal EGD
  - ~1/4 will have stenosis of stoma, usually 1 month after surgery

Endoscopic treatment of complications after bariatric surgery

- Stoma
  - Narrowing
    - Symptomatic stomal stenosis
    - Bougie dilators or balloons, using guide wire TTS (through-the-scope placement)
    - Optimal aperture diameter 10 mm to 15 mm
    - If multiple dilators needed, dilate slowly (up to 3 mm [3 French sizes] at each session, every 1 to 2 weeks until symptoms resolve
  - Reduction in size of enlarged stomas and pouches
    - Aim for stomal diameter ~ 12 mm
    - Objective is to reduce / eliminate symptoms e.g. slowing of expected weight loss from surgery; during syndrome)
    - Use sclerosants endoluminal, suturing device (Overstitch)

- Leaks
  - Fistulae, dehiscence of stale line, gastric leaks
    - Tissue apposition
      - Fibrin glue
      - Biomaterial (from pig intestine)

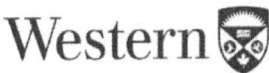

BARIATRIC SURGERY

- Stents
  - SEPS (self-expanding plastic stents)
  - SEMS (self-expanding esophageal metal stents)
- Endoluminal suturing (Overstitch)

➢ Band erosion
  - Removal of band with endoscopic scissors, YAG laser, APC

➢ Marginal ulcer (MU) bleeding
  - Usually on jejunal side of gastrojejunal anastomosis
  - Early MU in 10%, late in 1%
  - Risk of MU associated with smoking, H. pylori infection, NSAIDs use
  - If bleeding occurs early after surgery, perform EGD in OR
  - The post-operative complications of bariatric surgery are often subdivided into 3 phases
    1. 1 to 6 weeks
    2. 7 to 12 weeks
    3. 13 to 52 weeks

The gastroenterologist is often involved in the Phase 2 and Phrase 3 medical problems.

- Give the Phase 2 and 3 post-operative medical care of the patient with bariatric surgery.

  - Nutrition
    - Eat slowly (< 1 oz per 10 minutes)
    - Eat solids, wait 30 min, then take beverage
    - Be aware of possible new food intolerance, e.g. red meat

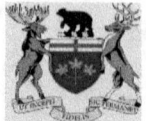

BARIATRIC SURGERY

- Avoid snacks and high calorie fluid drinks, e.g. "pop"
- Identify and correct any vitamin D deficiency
- Beware alcohol use disorder (10% in second post-op year)
- Anticipate, possible deficiencies of
  - Thiamine
  - Copper 2 mg / day
  - Zinc 8 mg / day
  - Calcium (use calcium citrate po, which does not need gastric acidity for dissolution)

o Medications
- Medicals need to be crushable, or liquid
- If anti-diabetic therapy, use metformin po (only small changes in blood sugar)
- Reassess need for treatment of GERD (GERD symptoms may improve with weight loss)
- Reassess need for contraception
  - ↑ fertility as weight is lost
  - Menses may return
  - Consider use of non-oral hormonal
- Reassess need for drugs for obesity-associated arthralgias
  - ↓ need or NSAIDs is possible
  - Use acetaminophen if arthralgias persist
  - Return of post psychiatric issues

o Be on lookout for
- Psychiatric disorders
  - Emotional liability
  - Self-destructive behaviour
  - Bulimia
  - Somatization (nausea, vomiting)
- GI disorders

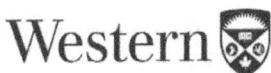

BARIATRIC SURGERY

- - Dyspepsia from development of stomal (aka marginal)
  - Nausea / vomiting
- Cholelithiasis
  - 22% at 6 months post-op
  - Consider UCDA (ursodeoxycholic acid, ursodiol) 300 mg bid for 6 months
- Dumping syndrome
  - Avoid foods which are associated with causing symptoms (e.g. sugar, pop)
  - Eat slowly, "by the clock"
  - Take liquids at end of rather than during a meal
  - Focus on complex CHO and proteins
- Prolonged vomiting
  - Only slowly advance intake to solid foods
  - Stomal stricture
  - Marginal ulcers
  - Small bowel obstruction, such as from internal hernia
  - Food intolerances
  - Somatization
- New onset of heartburn, regurgitation, dysphagia
  - Gastric band slippage
  - Gastric outlet obstruction (especially in VBG and RYGB)
- Hematemesis
  - Marginal ulcer
  - Mallory Weiss tear from vomiting
  - Severe esophagitis from partial gastric outlet obstruction
  - Band erosion through the wall of the stomach

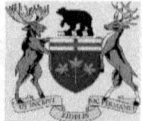

BARIATRIC SURGERY

- Slowing of initially satisfactory weight loss
  - Recidivism
  - Development of new and poor eating habits
  - Development of gastrogastric fistula in RYGB
- Expected weight loss
  - RYGB
    - First 6 months 10 lbs to 15 lbs per month
    - 2 years
      - 65% of excess body weight, or
      - 35% of initial body weight
  - LAGB
    - 2 years
      - 45% of excess body weight, or
      - 25% of initial body weight

➤ Cosmetic and body image issue

Weight loss after RYGB may be partially from the restriction of food intake, and partially from the associated malabsorption.

- Give the changes in GI peptides which occur after RYGB and which may contribute to the improved insulin secretion, glucose tolerance, and weight loss.

    o Malabsorption in the jejunum leads to ↑ delivery of nutrients to the ileum
    o ↑ nutrients in the ileum lead to
      - ↑ PYY (peptide YY)
        - ↑ GLP-1 (glucagon-like petide-1)
        - ↑ GIP (glucose dependent insulin otropic polypeptide)

With rapid weight loss after bariatric surgery, a woman's menses may stop. In any situation when menses stop, you

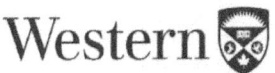

BARIATRIC SURGERY

would suspect pregnancy and you would arrange pregnancy testing.

- Give the reason why this index of suspicion should be high in the post-bariatric surgery female patient.
    - Fertility improves with the post-surgical weight loss
- Give 6 mechanisms or causes of iron- and B12-deficiency associated anemia, diarrhea, metabolic bone disease, and recurrent gastric ulceration in a patient having had a Billroth II partial gastrectomy for peptic ulcer disease (PUD), gastric cancer (GCA) or morbid obesity (bariatric surgery) and Roux-en-Y.

➤ Iron
  - Pre-surgery iron deficiency
  - Decreased intake from post-op symptoms (anorexia, early satiety)
  - Decreased acid leads to decreased pepsin and decreased meat (iron) digestion
  - Decreased acid: inhibits the acid-mediated solubilizing and reducing of inorganic dietary iron (Fe^{3+} .[ferric] .. Fe^{2+})ferrous])
  - Decreased absorption of Fe^{2+}, Ca^{2+}, BII, bypassing site of maximal absorption (duodenum)
  - Can be slow bleeding at surgical site
  - Bile gastritis
  - Gastric stump cancer

➤ B12
  - Pre-surgery deficiency
  - Decreased intake

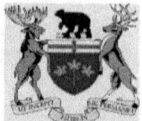

BARIATRIC SURGERY

- o Loss of stimulated and co-ordinated release of "R" factor
- o Decreased intrinsic factor
- o Loss of HCl/pepsinogen to liberate food B12
- o Bacterial overgrowth syndrome

➢ Metabolic bone disease
- o Pre-existing osteoporosis ↓ Ca^{2+} solubilization
- o ↓ vitamin D or Ca^{2+} intake
- o Bypass of site of maximal absorption of Ca^{2+} (duodenum)
- o Binding Ca^{+2} (unabsorbed fatty acids)

➢ Diarrhea
- o Magnesium-containing antacids, PPI's
- o Early dumping syndrome
- o Retained antrum (↑ gastrin)
- o Hypergastrinemia → HCL hypersecretion (↑ volume, mucosal damage); loss of PPY from ileum, loss of inhibition of gastrin → ↑s. gastrin
- o Bypassed duodenum
- o Unmasked celiac disease
- o Unmasked lactose intolerance
- o Unmasked bile acid wastage
- o Primary or secondary (unmasked) pancreatic insufficiency
- o Bacterial overgrowth syndrome (BOS)

➢ Peptic ulceration (previous peptic ulcer disease [PUD])

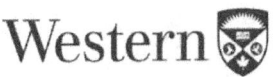

- ↑ gastrin – ZES, incomplete vagotomy, gastric retention, afferent loop syndrome
- H. pylori infection
- NSAIDs, ASA use
- "Stump" Cancer
- Ischemia at anastomosis
- Bile gastritis

➤ Presentations of ZES (Zollinger Ellison Syndrome) (see Question #16)
- PUD – severe, multiple, unusual sites; GERD-like symptoms
- Diarrhea
- Recurrent ulceration (with or without gastric surgery)
- Associated MEN I syndrome
- Thick gastric folds
- Fundic gland polyps

Abbreviations: BOM, bacterial overgrowth syndrome; GCa, gastric cancer; MEN, multiple endocrine neoplasia; PPIs, proton pump inhibitor; PUD, peptic ulcer disease; ZES, Zollinger-Ellison syndrome

Summary

- Bariatric surgery is an effective treatment for obesity in well selected, motivated patients.
- Patients require lifelong follow up to preserve weight loss and avoid nutritional deficiencies.
- A knowledge of the anatomy and physiology of the changes to the UGI tract is crucial prior to

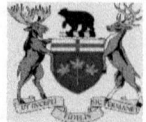

endoscopy and provides a framework for understanding the potential complications of bariatric surgery.

"Life doesn't require that we be the best, only that we try our best."

H. Jackson Brown Jr.

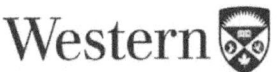

References and Suggested Reading

Azagury DE, et al. Marginal ulceration after Roux-en-Y gastric bypass surgery: characteristics, risk factors, treatment, and outcomes. *Endoscopy* 2011;43(11):950-4.

Bueter M, et al. Why patients lose weight after bariatric operations. *Zentralbl Chir* 2010;135(1):28-33.

Decker GA. Gastrointestinal and Nutrition complications after bariatric surgery. *Am J Gastroenterol* 2007; 102:2571-2580.

DeVault KR, et al. Insights into the future of gastric acid suppression. *Nat. Rev. Gastroenterol Hepatol* 2009;6:524.

Gertler R, et al. Pouch vs. No pouch following total gastrectomy: meta-analysis and systematic review. *The American Journal of Gastroenterology 2010;*105(5):1208.

Jeffrey D, et al. Increased Perioperative Mortality Following Bariatric Surgery Among Patients With Cirrhosis. *Clinical Gastroenterology and Hepatology* 2011;9:897-901.

Lau DC. Canadian clinical practice guidelines on the management and prevention of obesity in adults and children. *Canadian Medical Association Journal* 2007;176(8 Suppl):S1-13.

Laville M, Disse E. Bariatric surgery for diabetes treatment: why should we go rapidly to surgery. *Diabetes & Metabolism.* 2009;35(6 Pt 2):562-563.

Mathus-Vliegen E.M, et al. The role of endoscopy in bariatric surgery. *Best Practice and Research Clinical Gastroenterology* 2008; 22 (5): 839-864.

Mosko JD, et al. Increased perioperative mortality following bariatric surgery among patients with cirrhosis. *Clin Gastroenterol Hepatol* 2011;9(10):897-901.

Nguyen NT. Complications of antiobesity surgery. *Nat Clin Pract Gastroenterol Hepatol* 2007; 4(3): 138-147

O'Brien PE, et al. Laparoscopic adjustable gastric banding in severely obese adolescents: a randomized trial. *Journal of American Medical Association* 2010;303(6):519-526.

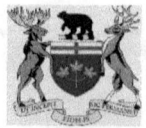

Rugge M, et al. Operative link for gastritis assessment vs operative link on intestinal metaplasia assessment. *World J Gastroenterol* 2011;17(41):4596-601.

Talley NJ. Is there an increased risk of hip fracture in patients on long-term PPI therapy? *Nature Clinical Practice Gastroenterology & Hepatology* 2007;4(8):420-421.

Tsesmeli N, et al. The future of bariatrics: endoscopy, endoluminal surgery, and natural orifice transluminal endoscopic surgery. *Endoscopy.* 2010;42(2):155-162.

Vetter ML, et al. Narrative Review: Effect of Bariatric Surgery on Type 2 Diabetes Mellitus. *Annals of Internal Medicine* 2009;150:94-103.

Wolfe BM. Bariatric Surgery: A review of Procedures and Outcomes. *Gastroenterology* 2007;132:2253-2271.

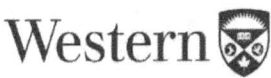

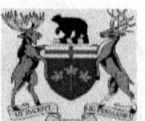

MINI UPDATE

Management and Risk of Interruption of Anti-Thrombotics for Endoscopic Procedure

Mohammed Aljawad

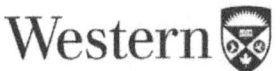

Overview

- Procedure risk for bleeding
- Risk factors for thromboembolism
  - Atrial fibrillation (AF)
  - Cerebrovascular event (CVA)
  - Deep venous thrombosis
  - Acute coronary syndrome
- Guidelines for management
  - Anticoagulants
  - Anti-platelet drugs
  - Vascular stents
  - Mechanical valves

Procedure Risk for Bleeding

Procedure	Risk of bleeding
Low risk of bleeding (< 1%): proceed without interruption of warfarin or anti-platelet agents	
o Diagnostic endoscopy with or without biopsy	
– EGD	0.01-0.13%
– Double-balloon enteroscopy	0.1%
– Colonoscopy	0-0.02%
o Biliary / pancreatic stent without sphincterotomy	0.26%
o Endosonography without FNA	-
o Wireless capsule endoscopy	-
High risk of bleeding (≥ 1%)	
o Polypectomy	
– Gastric	7.2%
– Duodenal / ampullary	
▪ 1-3 cm	4.5%
▪ > 3 cm	10.3%
▪ Colonic	0.7-3.3%
o Endoscopic mucosal resection	22%

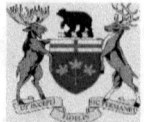

MINI UPDATE

- Biliary sphincterotomy — 2.0-3.2%
- Pneumatic / balloon dilation in achalasia — 1.7%
- Esophageal stenting — 0.5-5.3%
- PEG placement — 2.5%
- Endosonography with FNA — 1.3-6%
- Laser ablation and coagulation — 1.1%
- Variceal sclerotherapy — 4-25.4%
- Variceal band ligation — 2.4-5.7%
- Thermal ablation and coagulation — 5%

Printed with permission: ACG - Am J Gastroenterol 2009; 104:3085–3097.

Diagnostic Endoscopy

- Risk of bleeding with ASA/NSAIDs use

- Incidence of major and minor bleeding after endoscopic biopsy or polyectomy

Group*	UGI endoscopy		Colonoscopy	
	Minor bleeding (%)	Major bleeding (%)	Minor bleeding (%)	Major bleeding (%)
- NSAIDs	0	8.8	8.8	0.9
- Control	1.4	0	2.5	0.9

*Total number of patients evaluated = 694; Significant different from control (p = .006)

Minor self limited bleeding was higher in the NSAIDs group
Major bleeding occurred only after polypectomy with no difference between the two groups

Source: Shiffman ML, et al. Gastrointest Endosc. 1994; 40(4): 458-62.

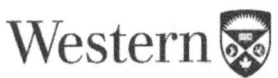

Colonscopic Polypectomy

Use of antiplatelet agents, NSAIDs / ASA, and anticoagulants in patients with and without bleeding

Drug use	No bleeding	Bleeding
o Antiplatelet agents	13.2%	16%
o Aspirin	7.5%	13.5%
o NSAIDs	5.2%	2.7%
o Aspirin plus NSAIDs	0.4%	0%
o Warfarin	0.8%	10.8%

Total number of patients evaluated, 1657; Significant different from patients with bleeding

- o Polypectomy-associated bleeding, 2.2%
- o Warfarin usage was an independent risk factor for bleeding, odds ratio (OR) 13.4
- o Univariant analysis showed no ↑ risk of bleeding (p = 0.62) for anti-platelet agents, NSAIDs, or aspirin plus NSAIDs
- o Median INR 1.4 in both groups
- o Unknown what is "ideal" INR for safe mucosal biopsy (i.e. not post-biopsy bleeding)

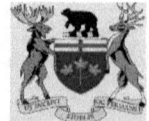

MINI UPDATE

Colonoscopic Polypectomy: clopidogrel

	On clopidogrel Group A	Not on clopidogrel Group B
○ Overall PPB	5.6%	3.0%
○ Immediate PPB (intraprocedural)	2.1%	2.1%
○ Delayed PPB (postprocedural)	3.5%	1%
○ Significant PPB (all delayed)	2.1%	0.4%

Abbreviation: PPB, postpolypectomy bleeding

Eight of PPB patients in group A and 16 of 38 PPB patents in group B taking aspirin (P = .002)

Clopidogrel alone was not an independent risk factor for PPB.
Concomitant use of clopidogrel and ASA/NSAIDs significantly increased PPB.

Definition of Significant PPB patients requiring transfusions, other interventions, or hospitalization

"With the new day comes new strength and new thoughts."

Eleanor Roosevelt

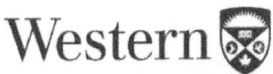

Conditions Associated with Postpolypectomy Bleeding (PPB)

	PPB	No PPB
o Age, (mean ± SD)	67.8 ± 11.0[†]	64.12 ± 10.0
o Hypertension, %	78	66
o Diabetes mellitus, %	24	28
o CAD, %	35	30
o COPD, %	28	20
o CrCl, mL/min	85 + 35	92 + 33
o Platelets	208 + 67	225 + 71
o INR	1.07 + 0.3	1.08 + 0.2
o Clopidogrel,	17.4	10
– ASA / NSAIDs, % [†]	44	34
– Clopidogrel and ASA / NSAIDs, % [†]	17.4	2.7
o Polyps per patient	5.3 + 4.0	2.5 + 2.0

[†] significantly different from no PPB, p < .05

Significant risk factors for PPB are:
1- concomitant use of clopidogrel and ASA/NSAIDs
2- Number of polyps removed

Source: Singh M, et al. Gatrointest Endosc 2010; 71: 998-1005.

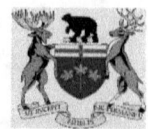

MINI UPDATE
Risk Factors for Hemorrhage after ERCP Sphincterotomy

- Give 4 factors shown on multivariant analysis to be significant to contribute to hemorrhage after sphincterotomy.

Risk factor	Patient with hemorrhage (N=48)	All patients (N=2347)	Univariate P value	Adjusted Odd Ratio (95% CI)†
➢ Significant in the univariate analysis				
o Cirrhosis – no. (%)	5 (10)	73 (3)	0.003	
o Stone as indication for procedure – no. (%)	41 (85)	1600 (68)	0.01	
o Periampullary diverticulum – no. (%)	14 (29)	382 (16)	0.02	
o Distal bile-duct diameter – mm	10.7 + 5.5	9.3 + 4.4	3.3	
➢ Significant in the multivariate analysis				
o Coagulopathy before procedure – no. (%)	10 (21)	120 (5)	< 0.001	3.32 (1.54 – 7.18)
o Anticoagulation within 3 days after procedure – no. (%)	4 (8)	37 (2)	< 0.001	5.11 (1.57 – 16.68)
o Cholangitis before procedure – no. (%)	17 (35)	339 (14)	< 0.001	2.59 (1.38 – 4.86)
o Mean case volume of endoscopist	35 (73)	1189 (51)	0.002	2.17 (1.12 – 4.17)
o Bleeding during procedure – no. (%)	23 (48)	678 (29)	0.04	(1.15 – 2.65)

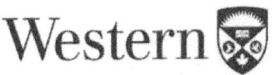

- Not significant
    - Extension of previous sphincterotomy – no. (%)   3 (6)   101 (4)   0.50
    - Ampullary tumor – no. (%)   1 (2)   36 (2)   0.75
    - Length of incision – mm   10.0 + 3.0   9.9 + 3.7   0.82
    - Aspirin or NSAID use within 3 days – no. (%)   6 (12)   292 (12)   0.99

Source: Freeman ML, et al. N Engl J Med 1996;335; 909-18.

Sphincterotomy

- Withholding Aspirin or NSAIDs up to 7 days before sphincterotomy
    - No reduction in risk of bleeding [1]
- Anticoagulation within 3 days after procedure
    - Increase risk of bleeding [2]

[1] Aliment Pharmacol Ther 2002; 16: 929-36
[2] Aliment Oharmacol Ther 2007; 25: 579-84

Risk of Venous Thromboembolic Events
- Low risk patients
    - Uncomplicated or paroxysmal novalvular atrial fibrillation
    - Bioprosthetic valve (> 3 months)
    - Mechanical valve in the aortic position
    - Deep vein thrombosis (> 3 months)

Source: ASGE Standards of Practice Committee. Gastrointest Endosc 2009; 70(6):1060-70).

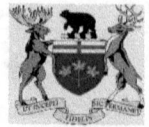

MINI UPDATE

- o High risk patients

- Give 3 conditions which predispose to a high risk of venous thromboembolic events after endoscopic.
  - o Atrial fibrillation
    - Previous stroke / transient ischemic attack
    - $CHADS_2 \geq 3$
    - Associated valvular heart disease
  - o Prosthetic valve
    - Discontinuing antiplatelet / anticoagulant in bioprosthetic valve < 3 months
    - Mechanical valve in mitral position
    - Mechanical valve with previous thromboembolic event
  - o Coronary disease and stents
    - Recent acute coronary event < 4- weeks
    - Discontinuing dual antiplatelet therapy in
      - Drug-eluting stent < 1 yr
      - Bare metal stent < 1 month
  - o DVT / PE
    - Discontinuing anticoagulation in event < 3 months
    - Recurrent DVT / PE
    - Severe hypercoagulable states
      - Active cancer
      - Myeloproliferative syndromes

Source: Kwok A and Faigel DO. Am J Gastroenterol 2009; 104: 3085-97.

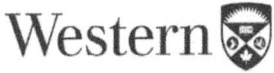

Atrial Fibrillation and Stroke risk

Patient category	Risk, % (95% CI)	
	Per-patient	Per-procedure
○ Total population (No 165,554)	0.02 (0.016-0.031)	-
○ Patient with AF		
− Anticoagulation not adjusted	-	-
− Anticoagulation adjusted		
▪ Heart valves	1.32 (0.27-3.8)	1.15 (0.24-3.33)
▪ Mechanical	0.60 (0.02-3.3)	0.52 (0.01-2.87)
▪ Other	3.28 (0.40-11.4)	2.94 (0.36-10.2)
▪ Normal valves		
− Routine	0.38 (0.05-1.35)	0.31 (0.04-1.13)
− Complex	3.10 (1.26-6.28)	2.93 (1.19-5.94)
○ AF total	1.22 (0.63-2.11)	1.06 (0.55-1.84)

Risk Factors for stroke in patients with A. Fib. after interruption of anticoagulation:

Age >80, history of stroke, hypertension, hyperlipidemia, and family history of vascular disease

Source: Blacker DJ, et al. Neurology 2003; 61(7): 964-8.

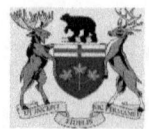

MINI UPDATE

Prosthetic Cardiac Valves (risk of thromboembolism)

- o Mechanical valves
  - No anticoagulation: 4% per patient-yr
  - Aspirin: 2.2% per patient-yr
  - Warfarin: 0.7%-1% per patient-yr
- o Bioprosthetic Valves
  - 0.2 – 0.7 % per yr in sinus rhythm
  - Mitral valve prostheses has twice the risk of aortic valve
  - Risk of thrombosis is higher in the first 90 days

Source: Cannegieter SC, et al. Circulation 1994; 89: 635-41.

Deep Vein Thrombosis

- o Within the first month after an acute episode of VTE
  - Risk of recurrence without anticoagulation is 1% per day
- o By two to three months after an acute episode
  - The risk of recurrence is significantly reduced

Source: Levine MN, et al. Thromb Haemost 1995; 74: 74: 606-611.

> "Model the traits you have observed in your best and favourite teachers."
>
> Madam Justice Elained Adair

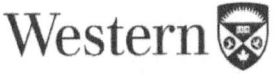

Risk of thromboembolism with/without interruption of anticoagulation

Indication	Rate without therapy (%)	Risk reduction with therapy (%)
o Acute venous thromboembolism*		
– Month 1	40	80
– Month 2 and 3	10	80
o Recurrent venous thromboembolism	15†	80
o Nonvalvular atrial fibrillation	4.5†	66
o Nonvalvular atrial fibrillation and previous embolism	12†	66
o Mechanical heart valve	8†	75
o Acute arterial embolism		
– Month 1	15	66

† statistically significant, $p < 0.05$

Source: Kearon C and Hirsh J. N ENgl Med 1997; 336: 1506-11.

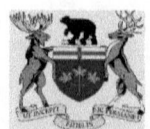

MINI UPDATE
Management of Anticoagulants

Procedure risk	Condition risk	ASGE Guidlines
o Low	– LOW/HIGH	- Continue warfarin
o High	– LOW	- D/C warfarin 3-5 d prior - Restart same night
o High	– HIGH	- Postpone if possible - Same as above - Consider bridging therapy

Note: administration of vitamin K to reverse anticoagulation for elective procedures should be avoided

Source: ASGE Standards of Practice Committee. Gastrointest Endos 2009; 70(6): 1060-70.

Management of Anti-Platelet Medication

- Give the management of anti-coagulants and anti-platelet medication prior to endoscopic procedures.

Procedure risk	Condition risk	ASGE Guidelines
o Low	– Low/High	- Continue Anti platelet drug
o High	– Low	- Continue ASA - D/C Plavix 7-10 days prior - If not on ASA, consider ASA while off plavix - Restart once hemostasis achieved

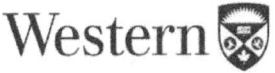

- o High   – High   - Consider postponing procedure until risk is low if possible
                             - Same as above

Source: ASGE Standards of Practice Committee. Gastrointest Endos 2009; 70(6): 1060-70.

Dabigatran

- o Cr Cl ≥ 50 mL/min
  - Half-life : 12 to 14 hours
  - D/C Dabigtran 1 to 2 days before the procedure
- o Cr Cl <50 mL/min
  - Half life : 28 hours
  - D/C Dabigtran 3 to 5 days before the procedure

Source: Stangier J, et al. Clin Pharmacokinet 2010; 49(4): 259-68.

LateStent Thrombosis

- o 161 patients with late DES thrombosis
- o 48 patients stopped both agents >>> 36 cases (75%) of stent thrombosis occurred within 10 day
- o 94 patients discontinued a thienopyridine but continued ASA, only 6 cases (6%) occurred within 10 days.
- o Median time to event
  - 7 days : both agents were stopped
  - 122 days : still on ASA but other anti-platelet agent was stopped

Conclusion: It is safe to discontinue dual therapy for short period in patients with DES while maintained on ASA

Source: Eisenberg MJ, et al. Circulation 2009;119(12):1634-42.

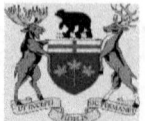

MINI UPDATE

Liver Cirrhosis

- Patients are not at increased risk for procedure-related bleeding
- Correcting the INR to 1.4 - 1.7 before carrying out high-risk procedures
- INR less than 2.5 is generally adequate for mucosal biopsies

Source: ASGE management recommendation of patients with disorders of hemostasis. *Gastrointest Endosc* 1999; 50:536.

Post-EVL Bleeding

- Give the risk of post-EVL bleeding in persons with cirrhosis, as related to their Child-Pugh class and to selected laboratory factors.

Parameter	Post-EVL	No post-EVL
Child-Pugh class †		
- A/B	5 (45%)	111 (80%)
- C	6 (55%)	28 (20%)
Platelet count		
- $< 50 \times 10^3$	1 (8%)	17 (12%)
- $\geq 50 \times 10^3$	10 (91%)	122 (88%)
INR		
- > 1.5	3 (27%)	25 (18%)
- ≤ 1.5	8 (73%)	114 (82%)
PTT		
- ≥ 1.2	4 (36%)	24 (17%)
- < 1.2	7 (64%)	115 (83%)

† Only Child-Pugh class was statistically significant, $p = 0.0174$

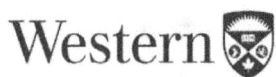

Source: Vieira da Rocha EC, et al. Clin Gastroenterol Hepatol 2009; 7(9): 988-93.

Does the patient with supratherpeutic INR need EGD for their NVUGIB

- Retrospective study of 55 patients
- High INR > 4
- Finding (%)
  - Normal (19)
  - Peptic ulcer disease (19)
  - Gastritis (35)
  - Angiodysplasia (16)
  - Esophagitis (16)
  - Duodenitis (12)
- Answer to question above – Yes!

Abbreviations: EGD, esophagogastroduodenoscopy; NVUGIB, non-variceal upper GI bleeding

Source: Rubin TA, et al. Gastrointest Endosc 2003; 58: 369-73.

Target INR for Endoscopic Therapy in patients with non varcieal bleeding

- 233 patients
- 44 % of the patients had an INR ≥1.3
- 95 % of the anticoagulated patients had an INR 1.3 to 2.7
- The rebleeding rate was 23% in the anticoagulated patients (INR ≥ 1.3), and 21% in the patients with INRs<1.3.

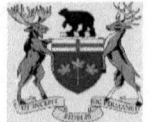

MINI UPDATE

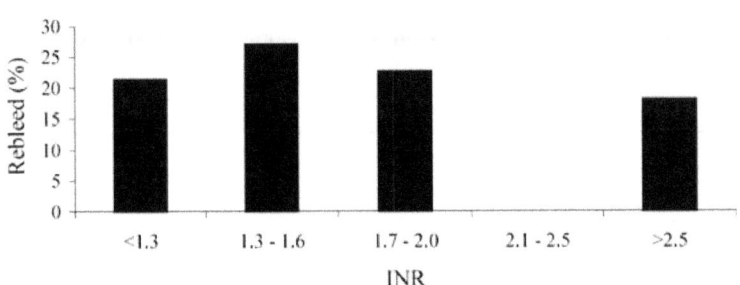

Success rate for endoscopic therapy in patients with mild to moderate anticoagulation is comparable to non anticoagulated patients.

Source: Wolf AT, et al. Am J Gastroenterol. 2007;102(2):290-6.

Acute Bleeding

Drug class	Specific agent(s)	Duration of action	Routes for reversal	
			Elective	Urgent
o Antiplatelet agents	o Aspirin	10 days	NA	Transfuse platelets
	o NSAIDs	Varies	NA	Transfuse platelets
	o Dipyridamole	2-3 days	Hold	Transfuse platelets
	o Thienpyridines (clopidrogel, ticlopidine)	3-7 days	Hold	Transfuse platelets ± desmopressin if overdose
	o GP IIb/IIIa inhibtors (tirofiban, abciximab, epifibatide)	Varies	NA	Transfuse platelets; in case of overdose, some agents can be removed with dialysis

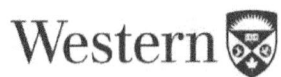

Drug class	Specific agent(s)	Duration of action	Routes for reversal	
			Elective	Urgent
o Anticoagulants	o Warfarin	3-5 days	Hold	FFP + vitamin K; consider protamine sulfate*
	o Unfractionated heparin	4-6 h	Hold	Hold, or consider protamine sulfate*
	o LMWH	12-24 h	Hold	Hold, or consider protamine sulfate*

Source: ASGE Standards of Practice Committee. Gastrointest Endos 2009; 70(6): 1060-70.

Anticoagulation and Mechanical Heart Valves

- o Low-dose vitamin K (eg, 1-2 mg) with or without FFP, is appropriate
- o FFP is preferable to high-dose vitamin K
- o High-dose (10 mg) vitamin K should NOT be given routinely to patients with mechanical valves

Source: ACC/AHA 2005 Guidelines

GI Bleeding in ACS / Recent Stent

- o 1-3 % of patients with ACS will develop GIB
- o GIB in ACS: ↑ hospital mortality by 4-7 x
- o High procedure complication
  − Up to 12 % >> if endoscopy done on Day 1 of ACS

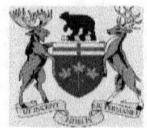

MINI UPDATE

- GIB causing ACS more likely to benefit from endoscopy

Abbreviations: ACS, acute coronary syndrome; GIB, gastrointestinal bleed

EGD vs Cath strategy

- Safety if EGD
    - EGD complication rate, recent AMI is 8%
    - EGD fatality rate, recent AMI is 5%
- EGD bleeding source identified
    - AMI with hematermesis, melena, or bloody NG aspirate
    - Any patient with occult / guaiac + stool: 24%

Source: Yachimski P and Hur C. Dig Dis Sci 2009; 54: 701-11.

"People might tell you it's impossible, or that it won't work, but I think it's rarely true."

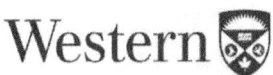

Result of the base-case analyses for safety of EGD vs cath

	EGD	CAH	Difference (%)
o Analysis 1 (OVERT)			
- Deaths	97	600	-503 (5)
- UGIB (recurrent or ongoing)	471	6,000	-5,529 (55)
- EGD complications	800	0	800
- UGIB / EGD complications combined	1,271	6,000	-4,729 (47)
o Analysis 2 (OCCULT)			
- Deaths	59	16	0.4)
- UGIB (recurrent or ongoing)	88	160	-72 (0.7)
- EGD complications	800	0	)
- UGIB / EGD complications combined	888	160	728 (7)

Source: Yachimski P and Hur C. Dig Dis Sci 2009; 54: 701-11.

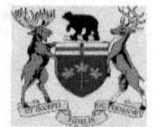

MINI UPDATE

- Give the recommended reinstitution of anticoagulant / antiplatelet therapy after gastrointestinal endoscopy.

Drug	Timing of reinstitution	Special considerations
o Warfarin	– Same night (Grade 1C)	▪ Consider recommencing ≥ 3 days in the case of – Sphincterotomy – Gastric /duodenal polypectomy – Large colonic polypectomy – EMR
o Heparin	– 2-6 h after procedure	
o LMWH	– 24 h after procedure	▪ Higher risk procedure – 48-72 h after – Lower dose (Grade 1C)
o Aspirin / NSAIDs	– Next day	
o Clopidogrel	– Next day	▪ Consider delayed reinstitution if higher risk procedure performed

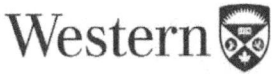

Summary

- Consider withholding elective procedures until minimum duration of antithrombotics is completed
- Low-risk procedures do not require an adjustment of anti-thrombotic agents
- Higher-risk procedures:
  – Need to balance the perceived thromboembolic risk and bleeding risks
- Decision to stop , (reverse antithrombotics) in acute bleeding should be individualized according to patient risks

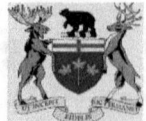

MINI UPDATE

Helicobacter Pylori Infection and Its Associated Diseases

Malcolm Wells

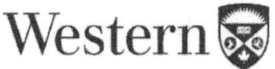

HELICOBACTER PYLORI Infection and Its Associated Diseases

What is Helicobacter pylori?

- H. pylori is a spiral shaped, microaerophilic, gram negative bacterium measuring approximately 3.5 microns in length and 0.5 microns in width
- In 1982, Marshall and Warren identified and subsequently cultured the gastric bacterium, Campylobacter pyloridis, later reclassified as Helicobacter pylori (H. pylori)
- Survives on dry inanimate surfaces for at most 90 minutes, based on 1 citation in systematic review

Source: BMC Infect Dis 2006;6:130; Lancet 1983 Jun 4;1(8336):1273.

When is it acquired?

- Infection acquired during childhood
- Most cases of Helicobacter pylori infection develop by age 10
    - 224 patients were followed from age 1-3 years until 21 years
        - 8% had H. pylori antibodies at baseline
        - 18% developed H. pylori antibodies by age 21

Source: Lancet 2002 Mar 16;359(9310):931.

> Incidence/Prevalence

- ~ 30-40% of North American population currently infected
- Up to 80-90% in rural areas
- Rates in N.A. children vary widely

Source: Pediatrics 2006;117(3):e396; BMC Public Health 2005;10;5:118.

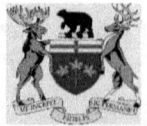

HELICOBACTER PYLORI Infection and Its Associated Diseases

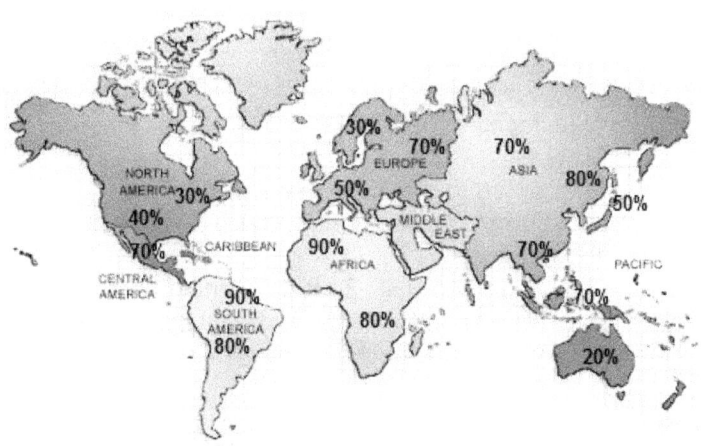

- ➢ Pathogenesis
- Give 3 virulence factors for H. *pylori* infection
    - o Urease and flagella
        - Urease production and motility essential for first step of infection.
        - Urease hydrolyzes urea into carbon dioxide and ammonia, thereby permitting
            H. *pylori* to survive in an acidic environment
    - o Adhesion
        - BabA, is a 78-kD outer-membrane protein that binds to the fucosylated Lewis B blood-group antigen.
        - BabA, BabA and SabA, is relevant in H. *pylori*-associated disease and may influence disease severity.
    - o Exotoxin
        - Most H. *pylori* strains express a cytotoxin VacA.
        - VacA is also targeted to the mitochondrial membrane, where it

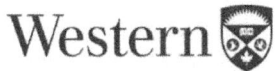

HELICOBACTER PYLORI Infection and Its Associated Diseases

- Causes release of cytochrome c, and
- Induces apoptosis.
  - VacA is not essential for colonization.

- *Cag* pathogenicity island
  - Translocates the 120-kD protein CagA into the host cell.
  - After entering the epithelial cell, CagA is phosphorylated and binds to SHP-2 tyrosine phosphatase.
  - This binding to SHP-2 tyrosine phosphatase leads to a growth factor–like cellular response and cytokine production by the host cell.

➢ Pathophysiology

SST (somatostatin) and gastrin are produced with the gastric antrum, and gastric acid is secreted by the parietal cells in the gastric body.

- Give the explanation why gastric acid secretion falls with acute or chronic H. pylori pancreatits, yet why gastric acid secretion rises with antral gastritis.

➢ Acute or chronic H. pylori pangastritis
  - H. pylori
    - Directly
      - ↓ gene expression of parietal cell H^+ / K^+-ATPase α-subunit
      - ↓ gastrin release
      - ↓ duodenal HCO_3^-

    - Indirectly
      - Produces anti-secretory cytokines IL-1β and TNF-α
      - Activates CGRP sensory neurons → ↑ SST (somatostatin) → ↓ gastrin

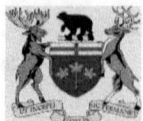

HELICOBACTER PYLORI Infection and Its Associated Diseases

- ↓ HCl secretion for body parietal cells

➢ Chronic H. pylori antral gastritis
  - ↓ somatostatin (SST)
    - Proinflammatory / prosecretory cytokines
    - Prosecretory H_3 agonist (N^3-methyl histamine)
  - ↑ gastrin (from ↑ SST, and from ↑ IL-8 and PAF)
  - ↑ gastrin → ↑ ECL cells in fundus / body → ECL hyperplasia
  - ECL hyperplasia → ↑ HCL secretion from parietal cell antibodies

- Give 10 bacterial factors and 10 host factors which are important in the H. pylori-associated development of peptic ulcer, lymphoma and gastric cancer.

➢ The H. pylori organism
  - Adhesion / colonization
    - The genetically 'distinct strains'
    - Bacterial genes encoding proteins in the motility apparatus of H. pylori (movement of organism from lumen of stomach, into the mucus layer) and genes for urease (provides for 2 pH optimum values of 3.0 and 7.2).
    - Colonization occurs only in gastric epithelium or where there is gastric metaplasia.
    - O-glycans in deeper portions of the glandular mucosa present colonization
    - SLPI (secretory leucocyte protease inhibitor) produced by H. pylori reduces colonization.
    - F3 ab A, a bacterial gene product may be liquid for the host Lewis (Le) b receptor or MUC 5AC, enhancing colonization.

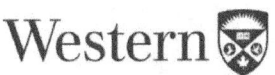

HELICOBACTER PYLORI Infection and Its Associated Diseases

- H. pylori urease binds to MHC (major histocompatibility) class II molecules to ↑ apoptosis.
- TFF_1 (trefoil protein) on gastric epithelial cells and mucus bind H. pylori
- TLRs (Toll-like receptors) in the PAMPS (pathogen-associated molecular receptors) family recognize H. pylori or their bacterial products which recognize LPS (lipopolysaccharide) or flagellin.
- Cag PAI (cag pathogenicity island) is a segment of H. pylori DNA which provides cag E (type N secretion apparatus)
- Cag PAI
    - Allow host gastric cellular membrane translocation
    - ↑ IL-8 expression
    - SRC kinase s phosphorylate tyrosine in Cag A protein
- All H. pylori have the vac A gene, and half produce the protein, Vac A (vacuolating cytotoxin)
- Vc A is a ligand for the cell membrane receptor, protein-tyrosine phosphatase.

➢ The host
- Intensity of host inflammatory response
    - OipA (outer inflammatory protein A)
    - ↑ IL-8 → ↑ neutrophil infiltration
    - Peptidoglycan, acting by type IV secretion system
    - HP-NAP (H. pylori neutrophil-activating protein)
        - ↑ chemotaxis of neutrophils, monocytes

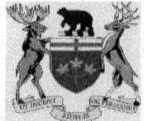

HELICOBACTER PYLORI Infection and Its Associated Diseases

- ↑ ROIs (reactive oxygen intermediates)
- ↑ recruitment of neutrophils and macrophages → ↑ iNOS (inducible nitric oxide synthase)

○ Host immune response
- Polymorphism for IL-1β → ↑ IL-1 → intense mucosal inflammation (gastritis)
- IL-8, IL-10, TNF-α (tumor necrosis factor) also ↑ gastritis
- Morphological changes in gastric epithelial cells
  - TJ (tight junctions) complexes become broken
  - ↑ epithelial cell proliferation and apoptosis
- ↑ gene expression
- Inflammatory cytokine
  - ↑ signaling mechanism for gene expression
- ↑ MAP (mitogen-activated protein) kinases
- ↑ lost cell redox factor-1
- ↑ activity of NF-kB (nuclear factor kappa B)
- ↑ activity of AP-1 (activator protein-1)
- ↑ oxidative stress
  - ↑ oxidation of DNA
- NOD_1 (nucleotide-binding oligomerization domain-1) in host

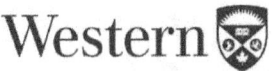

- Sense H. pylori
- ↑ NF-kB
- GI physiology
  - SST (somatostatin), gastrin effects on secretion of gastric HCl and duodenal HCO_3^-
  - Mucus - ↓ volume
  - ↓ mucosal hydrophobicity
- TNF-α and IFN-γ (interferon-gamma)
  - ↑ effects of HP-NRP
  - Prime neutrophils
- ↑ phagocytosis of H. pylori infected gastric epithelial cells
- ↑ chemokines e.g. ENA-78 GRO-α activate neutrophils
- ↑ cytokine induction
  - TNF-α
  - IL-6, IL-12, IL-17, IL-18
  - Heat shock protein 60
- T cell
  - ↓ IL-4 activation of STAT6 → ↑ Th1 and ↓ Th2 response
  - ↑ Th1 response
  - ↑ apoptosis
  - ↑ inflammation
  - ↑ atrophy
  - ↑ dysplasia
- ↑ IL-1β, IFN-α, TNF-α
  - ↑ Fas antigen expression → Fas-FasL (ligand) interactions → ↑ gastric epithelial cell death by apoptosis

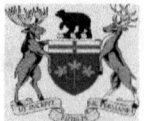

HELICOBACTER PYLORI Infection and Its Associated Diseases

- ↓ NFAT (↓ nuclear translocation of a transcription factor) → ↓ IL-2
- Dysregulation of Treg (regulatory T cells)
- ↑ IgA, IgA, IgM and complement
- ↑ monoclonal antibodies to H. pylori cross-react with gastric epithelial cells
- Innate host responses impaired by catalase, urease

o How does H. pylori cause DU?
- Antrum D cells ↓ - ↓ S - ↓ inhibition of G cells - ↑ G - ↑HCl - ↑ metaplasia – H. pylori in metaplasia H. pylori infection develops in metaplasia of the duodenum.

o Why is the rate of symptom relief with Hp-triple therapy higher for dyspepsia in functional dyspepsia with an EGD, than in uninvestigated dyspepsia.
- EGD shows an ulcer, so pretest probably for symptom relief is higher.

➤ Risk Factors for H. *pylori* infection
- Likely transmission within families
  o Maternal infection associated with risk of *Helicobacter pylori* infection in children (in Japan)
    - Based on case series of 42 patients aged 4-19 with *H. pylori* gastritis
    - Identical DNA analyses in
      - 32 (76%) patients and their family members
      - 29 (69%) of patients and their mothers
      - 7 (17%) of patients and their fathers (including 6 also identical to their mothers)

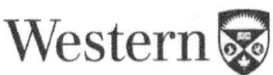

HELICOBACTER PYLORI Infection and Its Associated Diseases

Source: Konno M, et al. Pediatr Infect Dis J 2008;27(11):999.

- o H. pylori infection clusters within families

Source: Dominici P et al. BMJ 1999;319(7209):537-541.

- Possible crowded conditions
    - o Crowded conditions with poor sanitation may be risk factor for *Helicobacter pylori* infection
        - Based on seroprevalence study in 1,104 children aged 4-11 years in northeastern Brazil
- Give the modes of transmission of H. pylori (Hp), and the impact of one person in the family being positive for H. pylori on the rate of H. pylori infection by others in the family.

    - o Modes of transmission of Hp
        - Gastro-oral
        - Vomitus-oral
        - Fecal-oral

- Give the impact of an infected family member on others in the family group

    - o Hp positive parent
        - Spouse 68% Hp$^+$
        - Children 40% Hp$^+$
    - o Hp negative parent
        - Spouse 9% Hp$^+$
        - Children 3% Hp$^+$
    - o Community Risk
        - Adults - approximately 25-30% (depends on person's age)
        - Higher (30%) in older persons

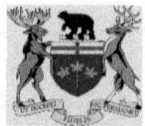

HELICOBACTER PYLORI Infection and Its Associated Diseases

- >50% First Nations Canadians, new Canadians from high Hp prevalence areas
- New Canadians from high prevalence countries

- Presence of anti-*H. pylori* IgG antibodies associated with
  - Age > 8 years
  - Larger sibling number
  - Nursery attendance
  - Location of house at unpaved street
  - Absence of flush toilet

Source: Helicobacter 2010 Aug;15(4):273 full-text.

- Gastroenterologists performing endoscopies have increased risk for obtaining *H. pylori* infection compared with general population
  - Based on case-control study
  - 92 gastroenterologists and 168 healthy control subjects underwent urea breath testing
  - 54 gastroenterologists and 103 controls were negative and had follow-up test 5-8 years later
  - 7 vs. 1 tested positive for annual conversion rate of 2.6% vs. 0.14%

Source: Hildebrand P et al. BMJ 2000; 15;321(7254):149.

- Give 8 GI and 8 non-GI conditions which may be associated with H. pylori (Hp) infection.

- Hp-associated GI diseases
  - Non-ulcer dyspepsia
  - Acute/chronic gastritis

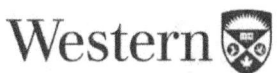

HELICOBACTER PYLORI Infection and Its Associated Diseases

- Atrophic gastritis (AG) – acceleration with PPI of AG-IM-Dys-GCa → intestinal metaplasia (IM) → dysplasia (Dys) → GCa (non-cardia gastric cancer)
- Duodenal and gastric ulcer (DU and GU) (only ~20% of Hp^+ persons develop clinical disease)
- Accentation of effect of smoking on PUD
- Accentuation of ASA/NSAID effects on peptic PUD
- Maltoma
- Fundic gland polyps
- Hypertrophic gastric folds
- Protective against GERD (possible)
- Halitosis
- Carcinoid tumours
- Colorectal cancer (possible association, due to hypergastrinemia)
- Pancreatic cancer (possible)

> Possible Hp-associated non-GI diseases
- Head –otitis media, migraines, headaches
- CNS – Parkinsonism, CVA
- Heart – atherosclerotic diseases
- Lung – chronic bronchitis, COPD, SIDS
- Blood – ITP, iron deficiency
- Skin – idiopathic chronic urticaria, acne, rosacea; Rosacea's
- Growth retardation in children
- Vomiting in pregnancy

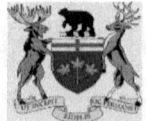

HELICOBACTER PYLORI Infection and Its Associated Diseases

Abbreviations: COPD, chronic obstructive pulmonary disease; CVA, cerebrovascular accident; DU, duodenal ulcer; GCa, gastric cancer; GERD, gastroesophgeal reflux disease; GU, gastric ulcer; ITP, idiopathic thrombocytopenic purpura; PUD, peptic ulcer disease; SIDS, sudden infant death syndrome.

Adapted from: Hunt R. *AGA Institute Post Graduate Course* 2006; pg. 333-342.; and adapted from Graham DY. and Sung JJY. *Sleisenger & Fordtran's gastrointestinal and liver disease: Pathophysiology/ Diagnosis/ Management* 2006. pg. 1054; and 2010, pg. 839.

- Peptic ulcer disease
  - About 50% of the world's population have an H. pylori infection, but only about 15% develop peptic (gastric or duodenal) when disease, and ~1% develop gastric cancer or MALT lymphoma. So, there a disconnect between H. pylori infection in the stomach, and H. pylori-associated diseases
  - H. pylori may be
    - Associated with, or causative of GU and DU
    - Worsen chance of developing ASA / NSAID-associated GU / DU
    - Worsen effect of smoking on slow healing of peptic ulcer, and higher risk of relapse of ulcer

    (Note: once associated H. Pylori infection has been cured, smoking loses these adverse on ulcer healing and relapse.

    - ↑ risk of ulcer relapse (80% for H. pylori +, 10% for H. pylori-)

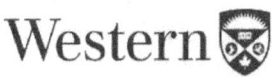

HELICOBACTER PYLORI Infection and Its Associated Diseases

- Give the way in which H. pylori can cause DU?
  - Antrum D cells ↓ - ↓ S - ↓ inhibition of G cells - ↑ G - ↑HCl - ↑ metaplasia – H. pylori in metaplasia H. pylori infection develops in metaplasia of the duodenum.
  - Why is the rate of symptom relief with Hp-triple therapy higher for dyspepsia in functional dyspepsia in functional dyspepsia with an EGD, than in uninvestigated dyspepsia.
    - EGD shows an ulcer, so pretest probably for symptom relief is higher.
  - Combine anti-H. pylori therapy with PPI to
    - ↑ anti-H. pylori effect of antibiotics
    - Accelerate improvement of ulcer healing and symptom relief
  - Optimal pH for outcomes for different upper GI disorders (18 hours per day)

≥ 3	GU, DU
4	GERD
5	H. pylori eradication
6	Non-variceal upper GI bleeding

  - With NSAIDs: *H. pylori* infection and NSAIDs independently and synergistically increase risk for peptic ulcer disease
    - based on systematic review of 25 observational studies
    - HP + NSAIDs vs NSAIDs (41.7% vs. 25.9%, OR 2.12, 95% CI 1.68-2.67)
    - HP + NSAIDs vs neither (OR 61.1; 95% CI 9.98-373)
    - risk of ulcer bleeding increased
      - 1.79 times with *H. pylori* infection

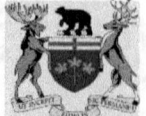

HELICOBACTER PYLORI Infection and Its Associated Diseases

- 4.85 times with NSAID use
- 6.13 times with both factors

Source: Lancet 2002;359(9300):14.

- Gastric cancer
  - Meta-analysis suggests association between *Helicobacter pylori* infection and gastric cancer
    - Review of 42 heterogeneous studies (8 cohort, 34 case-control)
    - Pooled results showed increased risk for gastric cancer (odds ratio 2.04, 95% CI 1.69-2.45)

Source: Am J Gastroenterol 1999 Sep;94(9):2373.

  - Histologic progression of gastric intestinal metaplasia associated with persistent *H. pylori* infection
    - Randomized trial of *H. pylori* eradication in 587 patients, 435 (74%) of whom were followed at 5 years

Source: Gut 2004 Sep;53(9):1244.

- Gastric lymphoma
  - *H. pylori* infection associated with increased risk for gastric lymphoma, specifically mucosa associated lymphoid tissue (MALT) lymphoma

Source: Am J Gastroenterol. 2007 Aug;102(8):1808-25.

- Growth Retardation
  - *H. pylori* infection may reduce growth velocity in children
    - Based on prospective cohort study

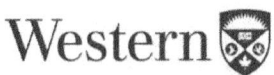

HELICOBACTER PYLORI Infection and Its Associated Diseases

- 347 healthy children aged 1-5 years who tested negative for urea breath test
- Monitored every 2 months for growth and every 4 months with urea breath test
- Followed for 2.5 years
- 105 (30%) developed *H. pylori* infection during follow-up
- *H. pylori* infection reduced growth velocity by about 0.5 cm/year starting 1-2 months after infection, irrespective of age of child
- *H. pylori* infection associated with absenteeism due to upper respiratory infection

Source: J Pediatr Gastroenterol Nutr 2003 Nov;37(5):614.

- Not clear that this difference is clinically significant
- Proportion of children with clinically significant growth retardation (if any) not reported

➤ Associations

- Give 6 associations with *H. pylori* infection, and state whether the association is positive or negative, or unclear.

- **Positive**

➤ Gastritis

  o *Helicobacter pylori* frequently found in biopsy-proven gastritis, especially if lymphoid follicle formation
    - Based on series of 185 gastric antral biopsy specimens
    - 114 (62%) had *H. pylori* detected on Giemsa stain
    - Among 51 cases with lymphoid follicle formation, 44 (86%) had *H. pylori*

Source: Siddiqui ST, et al. J Pak Med Assoc 2011;61(2):138-41.

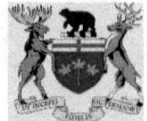

HELICOBACTER PYLORI Infection and Its Associated Diseases

- **Unclear**
  - Non-ulcer dyspepsia
    - No strong association between *Helicobacter pylori* infection and nonulcer or uninvestigated dyspepsia
      - Based on systematic literature review
      - Insufficient evidence to confirm or refute weak association

Source: Arch Intern Med 2000 Apr 24;160(8):1192.

  - H. pylori eradication has a modest benefit in patients with *H. pylori*-positive nonulcer dyspepsia (level 1 [likely reliable] evidence)
  - Adolescent recurrent abdominal pain
    - Unclear association between Helicobacter pylori infection and recurrent abdominal pain (RAP) in children
      - Based on systematic review and multiple observational studies with inconsistent findings
      - Systematic review
        - 38 studies evaluating association between gastrointestinal symptoms and *H. pylori* in 17,017 children ≤ 18 years old
        - Studies had poor methodological quality
        - No significant association observed

Source: Spee LA, et al. Pediatrics 2010;125(3):e651-6.

  - Prurigo chronica multiformis

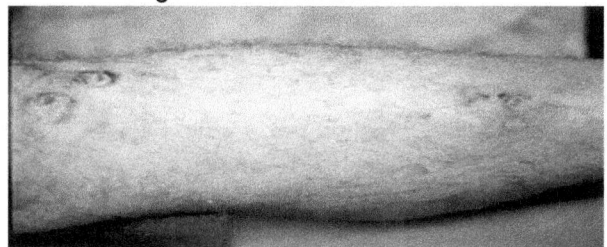

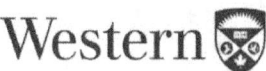

HELICOBACTER PYLORI Infection and Its Associated Diseases

- Presents with prurigo nodules, lichenification, eczematization, enlarged lymph nodes and esinophilia.
- Associated with rectal and esophageal cancer (Motoori M, et al. Surg Today. 2001;31(12):1087-90)
- Unclear association between *H. pylori* and prurigo chronica multiformis
    - 82 patients with chronic urticaria and 17 patients with prurigo chronica multiformis were tested with *H. pylori* stool antigen
    - *H. pylori* stool antigen detected in 25 (30.5%) patients with chronic urticaria and 10 (59%) patients with prurigo chronica multiformis, but results not significantly higher than rates found in healthy age-matched controls

Source: Akashi R, et al. J Dermatol 2011;38(8):761-6.

- o Hyperemesis gravidarum
    - Helicobacter pylori infection may be associated with hyperemesis gravidarum
        - Based on systematic review of studies with considerable heterogeneity
        - 14 case-control studies included 1,732 persons with hyperemesis gravidarum and controls tested for *H. pylori*
        - 10 studies showed significant association (3 with odds ratios < 1)

Source: Golberg D, et al. Obstet Gynecol 2007;110(3):695-703.

- o Vitamin B12 deficiency
    - Helicobacter pylori infection not clearly associated with vitamin B12 deficiency
        - Possible association reported in uncontrolled prospective study

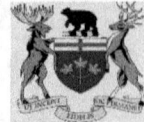

HELICOBACTER PYLORI Infection and Its Associated Diseases

- 138 patients with megaloblastic anemia and serum vitamin B12 levels < 147 pmol/L (200 pg/mL) without clear cause of cobalamin deficiency had upper gastrointestinal endoscopy with extensive testing (4 biopsies) for *H. pylori* infection
- 77 (56%) had *H. pylori* detected
- *H. pylori* eradication associated with improved hematologic parameters in 31 (40%) treated patients

Source: Kaptan K, et al. Arch Intern Med 2000;160(9):1349-53.

- Other studies
  - Adv Med Sci 2008;53(2):205
  - J Clin Gastroenterol 2003;36(2):130
  - Eur J Clin Invest 2002;32(8):549
  - Am J Gastroenterol 2001;96(1):63
- MI and atrial fibrillation
  - Weak association between *H. pylori* infection and early onset myocardial infarction (MI)
    - Based on case-control study
    - 1,122 survivors of acute myocardial infarction and 1,122 controls aged 30-49 years without coronary heart disease completed questionnaire and gave blood sample
    - Nonsignificant trend in 510 aged and sex matched pairs of siblings (mean age 59 years) in whom 1 had survived myocardial infarction and 1 had no coronary heart disease

Source: Danesh J, et al. BMJ 1999;319(7218):1157-62.

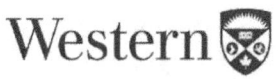

HELICOBACTER PYLORI Infection and Its Associated Diseases

- Association between atrial fibrillation and *H. pylori* infection reported in a cardiology practice

Source: Montenero AS, et al. Heart 2005;91(7):960-1.

- **Negative**
    - Inflammatory bowel disease
        - *H. pylori* infection associated with lower risk of inflammatory bowel disease (IBD)
            - Based on systematic review
            - Systematic review of 23 studies evaluating rate of *H. pylori* infection in 5,903 patients with IBD
            - *H. pylori* in 27.1% with IBD vs. 40.9% in patients without IBD
            - Relative risk 0.64, 95% CI 0.54-0.75
            - Results limited by significant heterogeneity

Source: Luther J, et al. Inflamm Bowel Dis 2010;16(6):1077-84.

- Gastroesophageal reflux disease
    - Prevalence of *H. pylori* infection LOWER in patients with gastroesophageal reflux disease (GERD) than in patients without GERD
        - Based on systematic review of 20 studies

Source: Raghunath A, et al. BMJ 2003 5;326(7392):737.

    - Barrett esophagus
        - No clear association between Helicobacter pylori infection and Barrett esophagus
            - Based on systematic review of case-control studies
            - Systematic review of 12 case-control studies evaluating prevalence of *H. pylori* infection comparing 550 patients with Barrett esophagus vs. 2,979 controls

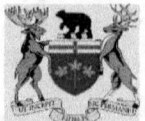

HELICOBACTER PYLORI Infection and Its Associated Diseases

- 9 studies included controls with normal endoscopy; 3 studies used healthy blood donors as control
- H. pylori infection rates comparing cases vs. controls
  - 42.9% vs. 43.9% in overall analysis (not significant)
  - 23.1% vs. 42.7% in subgroup analysis of 9 studies with endoscopically normal patients as controls (p = 0.03)
  - 71.2% vs. 48.1% in subgroup analysis of 3 studies with healthy blood donors as controls (p = 0.03)
  - In BE patients, the prevalence of H. pylori infection was significantly lower in the esophagus than in the stomach (3.3% vs. 24.7%, OR=0.14, 0.03-0.67) in three studies

Source: Wang C, et al. Am J Gastroenterol 2009;104(2):492-500.

➢ Clinical

- Take a directed history for H. pylori disease
  o Present illness
    - Majority are asymptomatic (clinically silent)
    - May be associated with dyspepsia or symptoms of peptic ulcer disease (epigastric abdominal pain, upper gastrointestinal bleeding)
    - Acute *Helicobacter pylori* infection may be associated with diarrhea
      - Based on prospective study
      - 345 children aged 6 months to 12 years followed for 2 years with *H. pylori* serology every 4 months

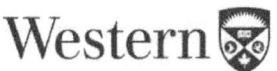

HELICOBACTER PYLORI Infection and Its Associated Diseases

- 12% annual incidence of *H. pylori* infection based on seroconversion
- Seroconversion associated with 2 times more diarrhea days in the subsequent year, strongest effect in first 2 months

Source: Pediatrics 2001 Nov;108(5):e87 full-text.

➢ Diagnosis

- Give who to test for H. pylori infection.
  - Past history
    - Ask about history of peptic ulcer disease (documented ulcer)
    - Ask about any prior testing or treatment for *Helicobacter pylori*
  - Social history: Smoking
    - *H. pylori* infection and smoking were major risk factors for peptic ulcer disease in cohort of 2,416 Danish adults.

Source: Rosenstock S, et al. Gut 2003;52(2):186-193.

  - Smoking associated with higher rate of failure of *Helicobacter pylori* eradication
    - Systematic review and meta-analysis of 22 studies with 5,538 patients
    - Smokers had nearly double the risk of eradication failure (summary odds ratio 1.95, 95% CI 1.55-2.45)
    - Absolute difference in eradication rates 8.4% (95% CI 3.3-13.5%) or NNH 12 (95% CI 7-30)

Source: Suzuki T, et al. Am J Med 2006;119(3):217-224, commentary can be found in Lau T. BMJ 2006;332(7556):1513.

  - Family history
    - Peptic ulcer disease

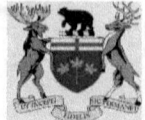

HELICOBACTER PYLORI Infection and Its Associated Diseases

- Gastric lymphoma
- H.pylori infection

About 50% of the world's population have an H. pylori infection, but only about 15% develop peptic (gastric or duodenal) when disease, and ~1% develop gastric cancer or MALT lymphoma. So, there a disconnect between H. pylori infection in the stomach, and H. pylori-associated diseases

- o Only test persons in whom you would be prepared to treat a positive test result for *H. pylori* infection
- ➤ Generally accepted indications for testing[1]
  - o Active peptic ulcer disease (regardless of whether patient is taking nonsteroidal anti-inflammatory drugs [NSAIDs] or aspirin)
  - o Past history of documented peptic ulcer (not previously treated for *Helicobacter pylori*)
  - o Gastric mucosa-associated lymphoid tissue (MALT) lymphoma
  - o Endoscopic resection of early gastric cancer
  - o Uninvestigated dyspepsia (in region with high *H. pylori* prevalence)
- ➤ Controversial indications
  - o Nonulcer dyspepsia (NUD)
  - o Gastroesophageal reflux disease (GERD)
  - o Persons using NSAIDs
  - o Unexplained iron deficiency anemia
  - o Populations at higher risk for gastric cancer
  - o Rule out:

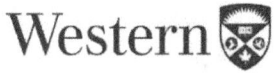

HELICOBACTER PYLORI Infection and Its Associated Diseases

- False positive serology (serology does not define active disease)
- Tests which may have false negatives with recent use of proton pump inhibitor, antibiotics, or bismuth
  - Urea breath test
  - Rapid urease test (Campylobacter-like organism test)
  - Histology
  - Culture

Source: Pattison CP et al. AJR Am J Roentgenol 1997;168(6):1415-20.

- No test considered gold standard for diagnosis[1]
  - Endoscopic

- Noninvasive tests include
  - Urea breath tests
  - Fecal antigen test
  - Antibody testing (serology)
  - Antibody testing (urine)

➤ Non-endoscopic testing

Test	Advantages	Disadvantages
Antibody testing	– Inexpensive – Widely available – Relatively high negative predictive value	• Positive predictive value depends on *Helicobacter pylori* prevalence • Not recommended after therapy
Fecal antigen test	– Identifies active infection – High positive and negative predictive value	• Polyclonal test less well-validated than urea breath test in posttreatment setting

HELICOBACTER PYLORI Infection and Its Associated Diseases

- Useful before and after therapy
- Unpleasant to collect stool

o Urea breath test (13C and 14C)
- Identifies active infection
- High positive and negative predictive value
- Useful before and after therapy
- Reimbursement and availability inconsistent

o Endoscopic tests
  - Culture
  - Histology
  - Polymerase chain reaction
  - Rapid urease test

o C-13 urea breath test may be most accurate test, including in patients with upper gastrointestinal bleeding and in children

➢ Endoscopic testing

Test	Advantages	Disadvantages
o Culture	- Not routinely recommended - High specificity - Permits determination	▪ Expensive ▪ Difficult to perform ▪ Not widely available ▪ Marginal sensitivity

			of antibiotic sensitivities
o	Histology	– High sensitivity and specificity	• Expensive • Needs infrastructure and trained personnel
o	PCR	– Not routinely recommended – High sensitivity and specificity – Permits determination of antibiotic sensitivities	• Methodology not standardized across labs • Not widely available
o	Rapid Urease testing (RUT)	– Inexpensive – Rapid results – High specificity and relatively high sensitivity in appropriately selected patients	• Sensitivity significantly reduced if used after treatment

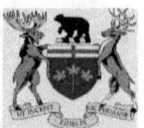

HELICOBACTER PYLORI Infection and Its Associated Diseases

> **Clinical Tips**
> A MCQ scenario speaks to the need for it to be proven that a previous H. pylori infection has been eradicated. Given the need to be certain the test is not falsely negative, watch out for
> - UBT – falsely negative if patient has been on PPIs, H2RA or antibiotics in the week before the test
> - Biopsy (EGD necessary) – based techniques if the test will be falsely negative and the H. pylori may have migrated to the gastric body; biopsy need to be taken from mucosa of both gastric antrum and body before you may be confident that the pathology report of "no H. pylori seen" signifies that the infection has truly been cured, and that the H. pylori are not simply hiding in the mucus adjacent to the mucosa of the gastric body.

- Treatment
    - Combine anti-H. pylori therapy with PPI to
        - ↑ anti-H. pylori effect of antibiotics
        - Accelerate improvement of ulcer healing and symptom relief
    - Optimal pH for outcomes for different conditions (18 hours per day)

≥ 3	GU, DU
4	GERD
5	H. pylori eradication
6	Non-variceal upper GI bleeding

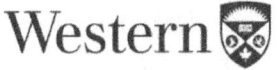

HELICOBACTER PYLORI Infection and Its Associated Diseases

- First-Line

Treatment Regimen	Duration	Eradication Rates
PPI BID, plus Clarithromycin 500 mg BID, plus Amoxicillin 1000 mg BID	10-14 days	70-85%
PPI BID, plus Clarithromycin 500 mg BID, plus Flagyl 500 mg BID	10-14 days	70-85%
PPI BID, plus Amoxicillin 1000 mg BID Followed by Clarithromycin 500 mg BID, plus Tindazole 500 mg BID	5 days followed by 5 days	90%
Bismuth 525 mg QID, plus Flagyl 500 mg QID, plus Tetracycline 500 mg QID, plus PPI or H_2RA BID	10-14 days	75-90%

    - Antibiotic resistance
        - Reported antibiotic resistance rates in United States for *Helicobacter pylori* treatment regimens from 1993 to 2002
            - 25%-37% for metronidazole
            - 10%-13% clarithromycin
            - 3.9%-5% for ≥ 2 antibiotics
            - 0.9%-1.4% for amoxicillin
        - Prior treatment with either macrolide or metronidazole for any reason significantly increases likelihood of *H. pylori* resistance to these drugs
    - Once daily regimens

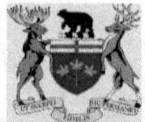

HELICOBACTER PYLORI Infection and Its Associated Diseases

- Once-daily treatment regimens may be inadequate (level 3 [lacking direct] evidence)
- Based on randomized trial without clinical outcomes
- 160 patients with *Helicobacter pylori* infection all given omeprazole 80 mg orally once daily for 10 days and metronidazole 750 mg orally once daily for 10 days and randomized to
  - No additional treatment
  - Amoxicillin 1.5 g orally once daily for 10 days
  - Clarithromycin 1 g orally once daily for 10 days
  - Azithromycin 500 mg orally once daily for 7 days
- Eradication rates
  - 8% with no additional treatment
  - 35% with amoxicillin
  - 78% with clarithromycin
  - 65% with azithromycin
- Clarithromycin group had highest rates of noncompliance and dropouts, primarily due to gastrointestinal disturbances

Source: Laine L, et al. Am J Gastroenterol 1999;94(4):962-6.

o Rescue treatment

Treatment Regimen	Duration	Eradication Rates
o Bismuth 525 mg QID, plus Flagyl 500 mg QID, plus Tetracycline 500 mg QID, plus PPI or H_2RA BID	14 days	70%

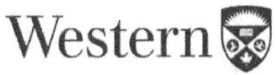

HELICOBACTER PYLORI Infection and Its Associated Diseases

- o PPI BID, plus Amoxicillin 1000 mg BID, plus Levofloxacin 250 mg BID — 10-14 days — 57-91%

- o PPI BID, plus Amoxicillin 1000 mg BID, plus Rifabutin 150 mg BID — 14 days — 60-80%

- o Common adverse effects (AEs)

Treatment	AEs
o PPI	- Headache - Diarrhea
o Clarithromycin	- GI upset - Diarrhea - Altered Taste
o Amoxicillin	- GI upset - Diarrhea - Headache
o Flagyl	- Metallic taste - Dyspepsia - Disulfiram-like reaction with alcohol
o Tetracycline	- GI Upset - Photosensitivity - Tooth Discoloration in children
o Bismuth	- Darkening of tongue and stool - Nausea - GI Upset

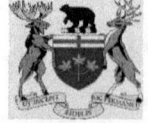

HELICOBACTER PYLORI Infection and Its Associated Diseases

- Adjuvant therapies
  - Probiotics
    - Systematic review of 4 trials
    - May reduce side effects (Diarrhea), but no effect on efficacy of *H. pylori* eradication

Source: Ann Pharmacother 2011 Jul;45(7-8):960.

  - Vitamins
    - Addition of vitamin C 500 mg plus vitamin E 200 units twice daily for 30 days to triple therapy regimen associated with increased *Helicobacter pylori* eradication rate (level 3 [lacking direct] evidence)
    - *H. pylori* eradication rate:
      - 82.5% with standard triple therapy plus vitamins C and E
      - 45% with standard triple therapy alone ($p < 0.005$, NNT 3)

Source: J Clin Pharm Ther 2012 Jun;37(3):282.

  - Bovine lactoferrin
    - Adding bovine lactoferrin to *Helicobacter pylori* eradication therapy associated with:
      - Increased eradication rates (level 3 [lacking direct] evidence)
      - Doesn't affect adverse effects (level 2 [mid-level] evidence)
  - Based on systematic review of 5 low-to-moderate quality trials (682 patients)
  - Bovine lactoferrin 200 mg twice daily for 1 week in addition to triple therapy
  - Comparing bovine lactoferrin supplementation vs. control

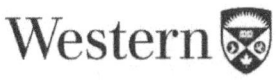

HELICOBACTER PYLORI Infection and Its Associated Diseases

- *H. pylori* eradication in 80% vs. 70.8% (OR 2.22, 95% CI 1.44-3.44, NNT 11)
  - Adverse events in 9.2% vs. 12.8% (not significant)

Source: Aliment Pharmacol Ther 2009 Apr 1;29(7):720.

- Mastic (chewing) gum
  - Mastic gum may have limited bactericidal activity against *Helicobacter pylori* (level 3 [lacking direct] evidence)
  - Based on randomized trial without clinical outcomes
  - 52 patients with *H. pylori* infection randomized to 1 of 4 treatments
    - Pure mastic gum 350 mg 3 times daily for 14 days
    - Pure mastic gum 1.05 g 3 times daily for 14 days
    - Pantoprazole 20 mg twice daily plus pure mastic gum 350 mg 3 times daily for 14 days
    - Pantoprazole 20 mg twice daily plus amoxicillin 1 g twice daily plus clarithromycin 500 mg twice daily for 10 days
  - Eradication rates based on urea breath test 5 weeks after completion of eradication regimen
    - 31% with pure mastic gum 350 mg
    - 38% with pure mastic gum 1.05 g
    - 0% with pantoprazole plus pure mastic gum
    - 77% with pantoprazole plus antibiotics

Source: Phytomedicine 2010 Mar;17(3-4):296.

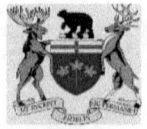

HELICOBACTER PYLORI Infection and Its Associated Diseases

- ➢ Selected Summary Background

Useful background: H. pylori
- o Meta-analysis does not show a statistical difference in H. pylori eradication rates using either triple or quadruple therapy (RR = 1.002; 95% CI 0.936-1.073) (Luther J Schoenfeld P, et al. *Am J Gastroenterol* 2008:S397.)
- o None of the H. pylori treatment guidelines endorse sequential therapy (Chey 09). Another meta-analysis showed 93% eradication rate with sequential therapy versus 74% for clarithromycin-based triple therapy (Jafri N, et al. *Ann Intern Med* 2008:2220-2223), particularly in persons with clarithromycin-resistant strains of H. pylori.
- o Meta-analysis has shown superiority of a 10-day course of levofloxacin-based triple therapy vs a 7 day course of bismuth-based quadruple therapy (rr = 0.51; 95% CI: 0.34-0.75) for persistent H. pylori infection (Saad R Schoenfeld P, et al. *Am J Gastroenterol* 2006:488-96.)
- o Rifampin has been used as an alternative to clarithromycin, with eradication rates of 38-91% (Chey WD, Wong BC. *Am J Gastroenterol* 2007:1808-1825). There may be rare but serious adverse effects (myelotoxicity and ocular toxicity)
- o Furazolide used in place of clarithromycin, metronidazole or amoxicillin gives eradication rates of 52-90% (Chey WD, Wong BC. *Am J Gastroenterol* 2007:1808-1825)
- o In persons with H. pylori (Hp) associated non-ulcer dyspepsia, eradication of Hp results in long term symptomatic relief in about 8% of patients

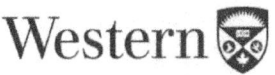

HELICOBACTER PYLORI Infection and Its Associated Diseases

- PCM (PPI – clarithromycin – metronidazole) and PCA (PPI – clarithromycin – amoxicillin) regimens are equivalent.
- It is useful for the physician to have available date on the local rates of Hp resistance to clarithromycin.
- "PPI – clarithromycin – containing therapy without prior susceptibility testing should be abandoned when the clarithromycin resistance rate in the region is more than 15-20%" (Malfertheiner et al., Gut 2012; 61: 646-664).
- Smoking reduces Hp – eradication rates by about 8%
- Extending the duration of triple therapy with PCM or PCA from 7 to 10-14 days increases the Hp – eradication rate by only ~ 5%
- Bismuth - containing quadruple therapy is also an alternate first-line empirical therapy since compliance with quadruple therapy is high and is particularly useful in areas of high clarithromycin resistance
- If Hp – eradication fails with PCM or PCA, use either
  - bismuth – containing quadruple therapy, or
  - levofloxacin – containing triple therapy (PLA, PPI, levofloxacin plus amoxicillin or PCL for 10 days)
- If Hp – eradication fails after first and then second line treatment, subsequent treatment. "…should be guided by antimicrobial susceptibility testing, whenever possible".
- For persons who cannot take amoxicillin (penicillin allergy), use PCM or bismuth – containing quadruple therapy

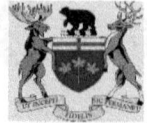

HELICOBACTER PYLORI Infection and Its Associated Diseases

- o Concomitant therapy (CT) is comprised of PPI, clarithromycin, metronidazole, amoxicillin more effective than standard triple therapy (pooled or, 2.86), and is less complex than ST
- o Sequential therapy is comprised of
  - PPI bid plus amoxicillin 1 gm bid for 5 days
  - followed by PPI bid plus clarithromycin 500 mg bid plus metronidazole or tinidazole bid - for the next 5 days
  - The place for ST remains to be established.
- o Hp tests have a sensitivity of ~95%, so before stating that a patient has a Hp negative duodenal ulcer, perform biopsy- and non-biopsy-based tests for Hp, and for biopsy-based ulcers, ensure that at least 6 gastric biopsies were taken (antrum, 2; angularis, 2; and body 2) within more than 2 weeks of stopping acid inhibitory therapy.

Please see: Thomson ABR. Chapter 61. In: Therapeutic Choices. Grey J, Ed. 6th Edition, Canadian Pharmacists Association: Ottawa, ON, 2011, Table 1: Drugs used for Dyspepsia and Peptic ulcer disease, page 821.

Please see: Thomson ABR. Chapter 61. In: Therapeutic Choices. Grey J, Ed. 6th Edition, Canadian Pharmacists Association: Ottawa, ON, 2011, Table 2: Helicobacter pylori Eradication Regimen, page 824-825.

Please see: Thomson ABR. Chapter 62. In: Therapeutic Choices. Grey J, Ed. 6th Edition, Canadian Pharmacists Association: Ottawa, ON, 2011, Table 1: Parenteral Drugs used in Management of Upper Gastrointestinal Bleeding, page 833.

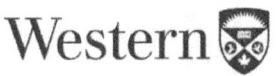

HELICOBACTER PYLORI Infection and Its Associated Diseases

- ➢ Confirming Eradication
- • Process
  - o May be most accurate when performed > 4 weeks after completion of antibiotic therapy
  - o Means of testing
    - Urea breath test
    - Endoscopic tests (only if endoscopy clinically indicated for other reasons)
      - Histology
      - Histology and rapid urease test
  - o AVOID antibody tests (serology), because only negative result is reliable (i.e., positive serology does not necessarily mean persistent active infection)

- • Prediction of Therapeutic Response
  - o First course of eradication therapy has greatest chance for eradicating *Helicobacter pylori*;
    - Subsequent courses less likely to be successful, especially if
      - Same antibiotics are used, or
      - If patient previously exposed to any antibiotics included in regimen
  - o Predictors of treatment failure following *H. pylori* eradication therapy:
    - Poor compliance with therapy
    - Antibiotic resistance
    - Smoking
    - Alcohol consumption
    - Diet

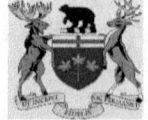

HELICOBACTER PYLORI Infection and Its Associated Diseases

- o Smoking associated with higher rate of failure of *H. pylori* eradication
    - Systematic review and meta-analysis of 22 studies with 5,538 patients
    - Smokers had nearly double the risk of eradication failure (summary odds ratio 1.95, 95% CI 1.55-2.45)
    - Absolute difference in eradication rates 8.4% (95% CI 3.3%-13.5%) or NNH 12 (95% CI 7-30)

Source: Suzuki T, et al. Am J Med 2006;119(3):217-24.

- o PPI rapid metabolizers (CYP2C19 genotype *1*1) may have lower eradication rates
    - Based on 67 patients aged 20-69 years treated with lansoprazole 30 mg, amoxicillin 750 mg, and clarithromycin 200 mg twice daily for 7 days
    - Eradication rates based on 13C urea breath test 1 month after treatment
        - 70% for rapid metabolizers (CYP2C19 genotype *1*1)
        - 94% for intermediate metabolizers (genotype *1*2 or *1*3)
        - 86% for poor metabolizers (genotype *2*2, *2*3, or *3*3)

Source: Ishida Y, et al. Int J Med Sci 2006;3(4):135-40.

- ➢ Clinical Impact of Eradication
    - o *Helicobacter pylori* eradication associated with healing of peptic ulcers
    - o Eradication of *H. pylori* may avoid long-term recurrences of gastric or duodenal ulcers
        - Prospective study of 247 ulcer patients treated with *H. pylori* regimens

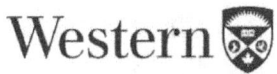

HELICOBACTER PYLORI Infection and Its Associated Diseases

- Of 75% patients with successful *H. pylori* eradication, no recurrences over mean 2.6 year follow-up

Source: Van der Hulst RW, et al. Gastroenterology 1997;113(4):1082-6.

- o *H. pylori* eradication may provide durable remission in patients with low-grade mucosa associated lymphoid tissue (MALT) lymphoma
  - Tumor regression rates of 60%-90% for localized gastric MALT lymphoma
  - 5-year recurrence rates of 3%-13%
- o *H. pylori* eradication may reduce risk for gastric cancer (level 2 [mid-level] evidence)
- o *H. pylori* eradication has unclear clinical effect in many situations
  - *H. pylori* eradication has modest benefit in patients with *H. pylori*-positive nonulcer dyspepsia (level 1 [likely reliable] evidence)
  - No clear evidence that eradication worsens or improves gastroesophageal reflux disease (GERD) symptoms
  - *H. pylori* infection has association with iron deficiency anemia but cause and effect relationship not established

➤ Reinfection Rates after Eradication

- o Reappearance rate of *H. pylori* infection 1.2% per patient year after eradication in 1 study
  - Based on prospective study

Source: van der Hulst RW, et al. J Infect Dis 1997;176(1):196-200.

- o 1.08% annual reinfection rate after eradication in highly endemic area in China

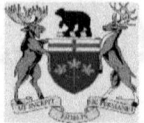

HELICOBACTER PYLORI Infection and Its Associated Diseases

- 184 patients with *H. pylori*-associated duodenal peptic ulcer had *H. pylori* eradication and followed 2 years
- 6 ulcers recurred, of which 4 were related to *H. pylori*
- 3 reinfections occurred within 6 months

Source: Mitchell HM, et al. Gastroenterology 1998;114(2):256-61.

> Special circumstances
  o H. pylori may be
  - Associated with, or causative of GU and DU
  - Worsen chance of developing ASA / NSAID-associated GU / DU
  - Worsen effect of smoking on slow healing, and higher risk of relapse of ulcer

  (Note: once associated H. Pylori infection has been cured, smoking loses these adverse on ulcer healing and relapse.
  - ↑ risk of ulcer relapse (80% for H. pylori +, 10% for H. pylori-)

- Give 3 recommended indications for *H. pylori* eradication therapy (ET) in the patient taking NSAIDs or ASA.
  o Reduce PUD formation
  o Reduce recurrent PUD
  o Reduce recurrent PUD bleeding (in ASA or NSAID high risk users) (ET does not prevent further PUD bleeding in high risk ASA/NSAID users on PPI)

Abbreviation: ET, eradication therapy

Adapted from: Lai LH, and Sung JJY. *Best Pract Res Clin Gastroenterol* 2007; 21(2): pg. 270.

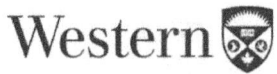

HELICOBACTER PYLORI Infection and Its Associated Diseases

Helicobactor pylori – positive Peptic Ulcer Disease (PUD)

- Therapeutic options
  - Uncomplicated peptic ulcer
    - PPI of your po bid for 2 weeks with 2 antibiotics followed by PPI od for 2 weeks
    - If patient experiences frequent recurrent recurrences
      - Perform UBT with patient off PPI for 1 week
      - If UBT positive, retreat H. pylori
      - If UBT negative, consider PI po od continuously as maintenance therapy

  - Complicated peptic ulcer
    - Complications of hemorrhage, obstruction, perforation
    - Treat PUD plus H. pylori infection as above for uncomplicated ulcer
    - Either repeat UBT off PPI therapy, and retreat and prove eradication of H. pylori, with no PPI maintenance therapy (PPI po od), or
    - PPI maintenance therapy (PPI od), because of
      - Risk (low) of reinfection with H. pylori
      - Risk (low) of reulceration even without reinfection with H. pylori
      - Possibility that the original ulcer may have been caused by ASA / NSAIDs plus H. pylori infection

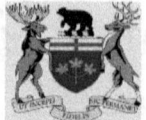

HELICOBACTER PYLORI Infection and Its Associated Diseases

> Caution alert
>
> - Every patient being considered for long-term use of ASA / NSAIDs / Coxibs should be tested (by UBT) and treated for H. pylori of positive
>
> - Depending upon patient (host) and medication considerations, some persons on long-term on PPI po od, even after eradication of any associated H. pylori infection.

- Give 4 clinical situations/syndromes which can be associated with fundic gland polyps.

    - Hypergastrinemia
    - H. Pylori infection
    - PPI use
    - Familial adenomatous polyposis (FAP; Attenuated FAP, 0.5-1.0% lifetime risk of gastric cancer)
    - Cowden syndrome
    - Idiopathic

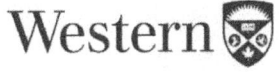

References and Suggested Reading

Bektas M, et al. The effect of Helicobacter pylori eradication on dyspeptic symptoms, acid reflux and quality of life in patients with functional dyspepsia. *Eur J Intern Med* 2009;20(4):419-423.

Chey WD, et al, Practice Parameters Committee of the American College of Gastroenterology. American College of *Gastroenterology* guideline on the management of Helicobacter pylori infection. *Am J Gastroenterol* 2007;102:1808-1825.

DeLyria, ES, et al. Vaccine-induced immunity against *Helicobacter pylori* in the absence of IL-17A. *Helicobacter.* 2011; 16(3): 169–178.

El-Nakeeb A, et al. Effect of Helicobacter pylori eradication on ulcer recurrence after simple closure of perforated duodenal ulcer. *Intern J Surg* 2009;7:126-129.

Every AL, et al. Evaluation of superoxide dismutase from *Helicobacter pylori* as a protective vaccine antigen. *Vaccine.* 2011; 29(7): 1514-1518.

Feenstra B, et al. Common variants near MBNL1 and NKX2-5 are associated with infantile hypertrophic pyloric stenosis. *Nat Genet.* 2012;44(3):334-337.

Fischbach L. Meta-analysis: effect of antibiotic resistance status on the efficacy of triple and quadruple first-line therapies for Helicobacter pylori. *Aliment Phamacol Ther* 2007;26(3):343-357.

Flach, et al. C-F. Proinflammatory cytokine gene expression in the stomach correlates with vaccine-induced protection against *Helicobacter pylori* infection in mice: an important role for interleukin-17 during the effector phase. *Infection and Immunity.* 2011; 79(2): 879-886.

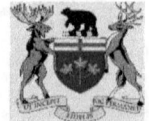

Fletcher EH, et al. Systematic review: Helicobacter pylori and the risk of upper gastrointestinal bleeding risk in patients taking aspirin. *Alim Pharmacol Ther* 2010;32(7):831-839.

Ford A, et al. Eradication therapy for peptic ulcer disease in Helicobacter pylori positive patients. *Cochrane Database Syst Rev* 2004; CD003840.

Gisbert JP, et al. Long-term follow-up of 1,000 patients cured of Helicobacter pylori infection following an episode of peptic ulcer bleeding. *Am J Gastroenterol.* 2012;107(8):1197-1204.

Graham DY, et a. Helicobacter pylori treatment in the era of increasing antibiotic resistance. *Gut.* 2010;59(8):1143-1153.

Greenberg ER, et al. 14-day triple, 5-day concomitant, and 10-day sequential therapies for Helicobacter pylori infection in seven Latin American sites: a randomised trial. *Lancet* 2011;378(9790):507-514.

Grubman A, et al. The innate immune molecule, NOD1, regulates direct killing of Helicobacter pylori by antimicrobial peptides. *Cellular Microbiol* 2010; 12(5): 626–639.

Guarner J, et al. Helicobacter pylori diagnostic tests in children: review of the literature from 1999 to 2009. *Eur J Ped* 2010;169(1):15-25.

Guideline for the Treatment of Helicobacter Pylori infection in adults. Edmonton (AB): Toward Optimized Practice (TOP) Program; 2009. Available from: www.topalbertadoctors.org/informed_practice/clinical_practice_guidelines/complete%20set/Helicobactor%20Pylori/h_pylori_guideline.pdf.

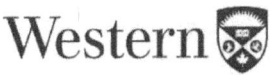

Hunt R, et al. World Gastroenterology Organisation Practice Guidelines: Helicobacter pylori in Developing Countries. *WGO*. 2010, 1-14.

Jafri N, et al. Meta-analysis: Sequential therapy appears superior to standard therapy for Helicobacter pylori infection in patients naïve to treatment. *Annals of Internal Medicine* 2008;103:2220-2223.

Jones N, et al. Helicobacter pylori in First Nations and recent immigrant populations in Canada. *Can J Gastroenterol* 2012;26(2):97-103.

Lai LH, et al. Helicobacter pylori and benign upper digestive disease. *Best Pract Res Clin Gastroenterol* 2007;21(2):261-279.

Luther JSP, et al. Triple versus quadruple therapy as primary treatment for Helicobacter pylori infection: A meta-analysis of efficacy and tolerability. *The Am J Gastroenterol* 2008; 103:S397.

Malfertheiner P, et al. Current concepts in the management of Helicobacter pylori infection: the Maastricht III Consensus Report. *Gut* 2007; 56:772-781.

Malfertheiner P. The intriguing relationship of Helicobacter pylori infection and acid secretion in peptic ulcer disease and gastric cancer. *Dig Dis* 2011;29(5):459-464.

Mazzoleni LE, et al. Helicobacter pylori eradication in functional dyspepsia: HEROES trial. *Arch Intern Med*. 2011;171(21):1929-1936.

McColl KE. Clinical practice. Helicobacter pylori infection. *N Engl J Med*. 2010;362(17):1597-1604.

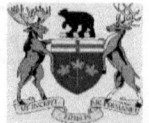

Peeters B, et al. Infantile hypertrophic pyloric stenosis--genetics and syndromes. *Nat Rev Gastroenterol Hepatol.* 2012;9(11):646-660.

Peura DA. Association between Helicobacter pylori infection and duodenal ulcer. *UpToDate.* www.uptodate.com 2014

Raju D, et al. Vacuolating cytotoxin and variants in Atg16L1 that disrupt autophagy promote Helicobacter pylori infection in humans. *Gastroenterology.* 2012;142(5):1160-1171.

Saad RJ. Persistent Helicobacter pylori infection after a course of antimicrobial therapy—what's next? *Clin Gastroenterol Hepatol* 2008;6:1086-1090.

Shanks AM, et al. Helicobacter pylori infection, host genetics and gastric cancer. *J Digest Dis* 2009;10(3):157-164.

Sheu BS, et al. Helicobacter pylori colonization of the human gastric epithelium: a bug's first step is a novel target for us. *J Gastroenterol Hepatol* 2010;25(1):26-32.

Suzuki H, et al. Helicobacter pylori eradication therapy. *Future Microbiol.* 2010;5(4):639-648.

Toller IM, et al. Carcinogenic bacterial pathogen Helicobacter pylori triggers DNA double-strand breaks and a DNA damage response in its host cells. *Proc Natl Acad Sci U S A.* 2011;108(36):14944-14949.

Tomtitchong P, et al. Systematic review and meta-analysis: Helicobacter pylori eradication therapy after simple closure of perforated duodenal ulcer. *Helicobacter.* 2012;17(2):148-152.

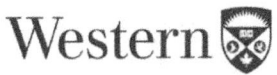

Varadarajulu S. Helicobacter pylori negative peptic ulcer disease. *UpToDate*. www.uptodate.com

Wee JLK, et al. Protease-activated receptor-1 down-regulates the murine inflammatory and humoral response to Helicobacter pylori. *Gastroenterology*. 2010; 138(2): 573-582.

Wilson KT. Immunology of Helicobacter pylori insights into the failure of the immune response and perspectives on vaccine studies. *Gastroenterology* 2007;133(1):288-308.

Wong GL, et al. High incidence of mortality and recurrent bleeding in patients with Helicobacter pylori-negative idiopathic bleeding ulcers. *Gastroenterology* 2009; 137:525-531.

Wu CY, et al. Early helicobacter pylori eradication decreases risk of gastric cancer in patients with peptic ulcer disease. *Gastroenterology* 2009;137:1641-1648.

Wündisch T, et al. Second cancers and residual disease in patients treated for gastric mucosa-associated lymphoid tissue lymphoma by Helicobacter pylori eradication and followed for 10 years. *Gastroenterology*. 2012;143(4):936-942.

Zelickson MS, et al. Helicobacter pylori is not the predominant etiology for peptic ulcers requiring operation. *Am Surg* 2011; 77:1054-1060.

Zulio A. The sequential therapy regimen for Helicobacter pylori eradication: a pooled-data analysis. *Gut* 2007;56:1353-1357.

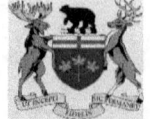

MINI UPDATE

Paraneoplastic Syndromes in Gastric Adenocarcinoma

Aze Wilson

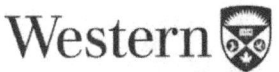

GASTRIC ADENOCARCINOMA

An interesting history

- Gastric adenocarcinoma (gastric CA) has been described as early as 1600 B.C.
- In hieroglyphic inscriptions and papyri manuscripts from ancient Egypt
- Hippocrates a 4th century B.C. a Greek physician, father of western medicine, believed cancerous pathology attacked the human body from the outside, penetrating the skin and infiltrating the soft tissues and internal organs
    - Physical experience with external organs only autopsies were prohibited in Greece, Egypt, Rome and were forbidden by the Cahtholic church for several centuries. Avicenna's medical encyclopedia
- Hippocrates theory persists through to the end of the 1st century A.D.
    - The belief that all diseases were from the absorption of black from the bowel into the blood persisted thru the middle ages to the end of the 1st century AD. Supported by lack of evidence b/c autopsies
    - Avicenna's Medical Encyclopedia describes gastric cancer but theory of how its pathophysiology does not differ from hippocrates. Avicenna is the most prominent exponent of arabic medicine at the time.
- 18th century: radical change in cancer origin theories
- Early 19th century:
    - Napolean Bonaparte suffers prolonged fever, abdominal pain, coffeeground emesis, diarrhea
    - At autopsy: "..on opening the organ along its long curvature, its capacity appeared..filled with a liquid resembling the sediment of coffee. The internal surface...was occupied by a cancerous ulcer...with scirhous thickening of the wall."

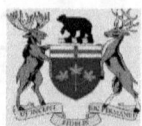

GASTRIC ADENOCARCINOMA

- Dr. Francesco Anonmarchi - 1821

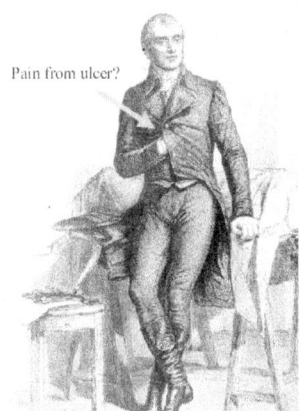

Pain from ulcer?

  - Late 19th century:
    - 1st gastric resection performed by Jules Emile Peau
    - 1st successful gastroduodenal anastomosis in 1881 by Theodor Billroth in Vienna
    - 1st total gastrectomy in 1897

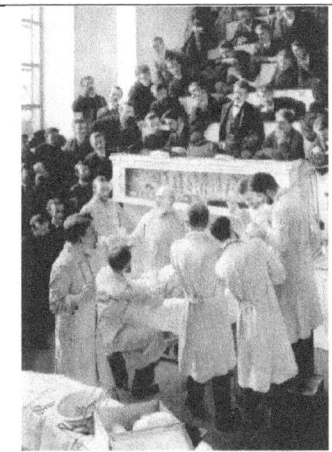

  - 20th century:
    - Millions of patients diagnosed with gastric adenocarcinoma

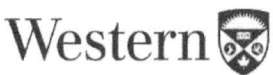

GASTRIC ADENOCARCINOMA

The Facts: Gastric Adenocarcinoma

- Demography
  - One of the most common cancers world-wide
    - 989,600 new cases/year
    - 738,000 deaths/year
    - 8% of new cancers/year
  - Was leading cause of cancer deaths world wide until 1980s, when it was overtaken by lung cancer
  - World wide incidence has been decreasing since World War II
    - Recognition of certain RFs
    - Popularization of refrigerators
      - Reducing salt-based preservation of food
      - Preventing bacterial and fungal contamination
      - Allowed for fresh food and vegetables to be more readily available, which may be a valuable source of antioxidants important for cancer prevention.
    - Availability of fresh produce
    - This decline began before the identification of H. pylori
  - Despite this decline, upward trend in young patients recently

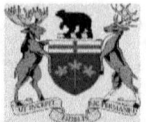

GASTRIC ADENOCARCINOMA

- ➢ Risk factors
    - o Helicobacter pylori (class 1 carcinogen, WHO)
    - o Diet high in
        - Salt
        - Nitrates —bacteria→ nitrites
    - o Smoking (RR~2)
    - o Low socioeconomic status
    - o Inherited predisposition
        - First degree relative ↑ RR 2-3x
        - Failial clustering in 10%

- ➢ Pathology
    - o Gastric cancer can be subdivided into two distinct pathologic entities:
    - o Intestinal form
        - Formation of gland-like tubular structures (mimicking intestinal glands)
        - Form of GCa that is declining worldwide
    - o Diffuse form
        - Linking to dietary and environment risk factors
        - More poorly differentiated poorer prognosis than intestinal form
        - Lacks glandular structures
        - Found at the same frequency worldwide
        - Occurs at a lower age than interstinal form

- ➢ Clinical features
    - o 80% asymptomatic unless gastric muscularis propria is penetrated
    - o In advanced disease:
        - Weight loss (62%)
        - Abdominal pain (52%)

GASTRIC ADENOCARCINOMA

- Nausea / vomiting
- GI bleeding
- Paraneoplastic syndromes
  - The poor prognosis is related to the disease usually being advanced by the time symptoms develop.

Paraneoplastic Syndromes

➤ Definition
  - Disorders that accompany benign or malignant tumours not directly related to mass effect or tissue invasion
  - Neoplastic cells can produce a variety of peptides that exert biologic actions at local and distant sites and can elicit responses that cause a variety of hormonal, hematologic, dermatologic, and neurologic clinical features.
  - Caution
    - Signs and symptoms of paraneoplastic syndromes may be easily overlooked in the context of the underlyingmalignancy

➤ In gastric adenocarcinoma
  - Deep vein thrombosis (DVT) and pulmonary embolus (PE)
    - Stomach
    - Pancreas
    - Lung
    - Prostate
  - Trousseau syndrome– peripheral vein thrombosis (PVT) with visceral carcinoma
  - Pathogenesis of ↑ risk of thrombosis in cancer (adenocarcinoma 20x > squamous cell cancer)
    - Mucins produced by adenocarcinomas may trigger PVT by reacting with leukocyte and

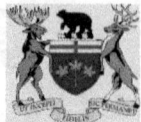

GASTRIC ADENOCARCINOMA

  platelet selectins → production of platelet-rich microthrombi.
- o DVT and pe are the most common thrombotic condtions in patients with malignancy.
- o About 15% of patients who develop DVT or PE will have cancer.

- Skin
  - o Lesar-Trelat syndrome
    - The sudden and explosive appearance or worsening of previously present diffuse seborrheic keratoses with inflammatory bases.
    - An ominous sign heralding the appearance of an internal malignancy.
    - Not specific to gastric cancer: also seen in
      - Adenocarcinoma
        - Liver
        - Pancreas
        - Colon / rectum
        - Breast
      - Lymphoma
    - Thought to be related to various cytokines and other growth factors produced by the neoplasm
    - May be associated with Acanthosis nigrans
  - o Acanthosis nigricans
    - Velvety hyperpigmented plaques in intertriginous areas
    - unusual locations
    - Florid
    - Associated with cancer of
      - Stomach
      - Lung
      - Liver
      - Kidney
      - Breast
      - Ovary
    - Benign causes

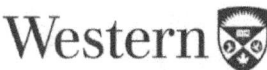

GASTRIC ADENOCARCINOMA

- Diabetes
- Obesity

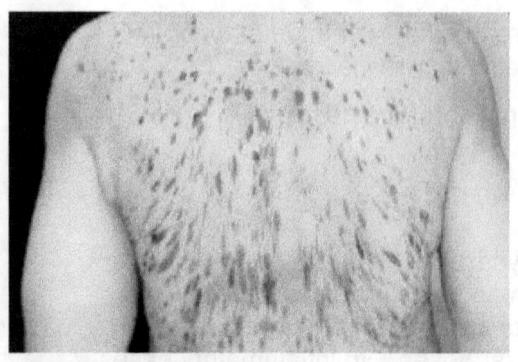

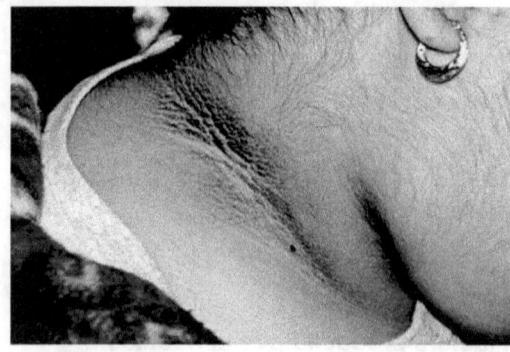

- ➢ Kidney
  - o Membranous nephropathy (MN)
    - 5-20% of adults with MN have a malignancy (solid> hematologic)
    - Malignancy risk 2-12 average population
    - Tumor antigens in glomeruli promote antibody deposition, complement activation, injury and proteinuria
    - Pathophysiology
      - Microangiopathic hemolytic anemia (MAHA)
      - Very rare
      - Forced through abnormal small blood vessels → fragmentation of RBCs

GASTRIC ADENOCARCINOMA

- Clinical signs:
    - Abrupt onset of severe MAHA
    - Associated with thrombocytopenia in 1/3 of cases
    - Direct contact with tumor microemboli
    - Contact with tumor produced tissue thromboplastin

- Differential
    - TTP / HUS
        - ADAMTS13 deficiency → unchecked accumulation of vonWillibrand factor / platelets in microvascular thrombi → consumption, hemolysis and end organ ischemia.
        - Plasma exchange removes the autoantibodies to ADAMSTS13 → replensihing the missing protease.
        - Autonatibody to ADAMTS13 → ADAMTS13 deficiency
    - DIC
        - Seen more commonly in pancreatic, lung and prostate cancer (MAHA is seen more frequently with gastric cancer
        - Normal coagulation profile
        - Improvement with heparin

Abbreviations: DIC, disseminated intravascular coagulopathy; TTP / HUS, thrombotic thrombocytopenic purpural hemolytic uremic syndrome;

Elliott MA et al. Eur J Hematol 2010:85: 43-50

- Treatment
    - Treat underlying cancer (chemoradiotherapy)
    - Supportive care
    - High mortality, especially if diagnosis is delayed, or mistaken for TTP / HUS or DIC

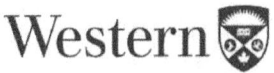

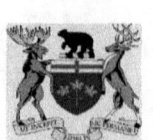

SMALL BOWEL

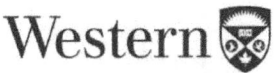

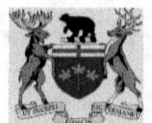

Bile Secretion and the Enterohepatic Circulation

Michael Sey

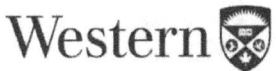

BILE SECRETION AND THE ENTEROHEPATIC CIRCULATION

Composition of Bile

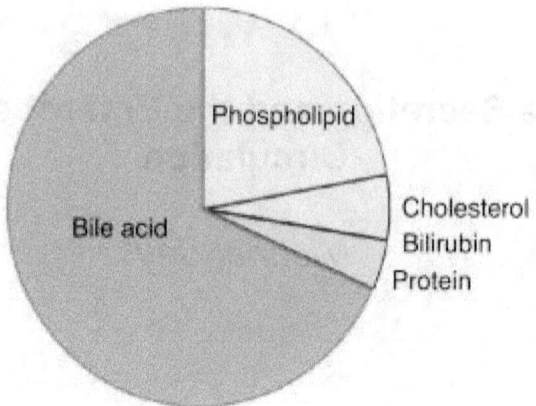

Functions of Bile

- Liver
  - ↑ hepatic secretion of cholesterol and phospholipids
  - Cholesterol homeostasis
  - ↑ excretion of xenobiotics
  - ↑ bile water flow (choleretic effect)

- Intestine
  - ↑ solubilization of cholesterol, triglycerides, phospholipids, fat-soluble vitamins
  - Interact with pancreatic colipase
  - ↑ activity of lipase
  - Mucosal defense
    - Jejunum
      - Bacteriostatic
    - Ileum
      - ↑ expression of antimicrobial genes

BILE SECRETION AND THE ENTEROHEPATIC CIRCULATION

- Stones
  - Gallbladder — ↓ formation of calcium stones
  - Kidney — ↓ formation of oxalate stones

- Metabolic function
  - Regulate their own EHC
  - Signal nuclear and G-protein-coupled receptors → helps to maintain homeostasis of fat, glucose and energy

Bile Acid Synthesis in Hepatocyte

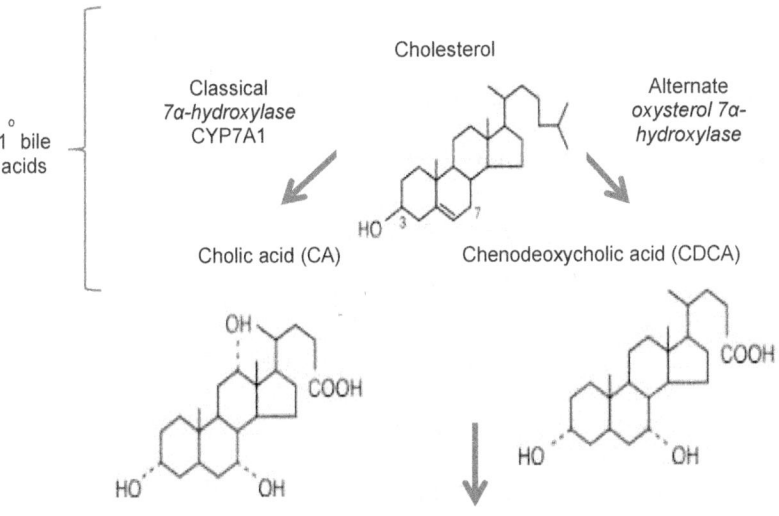

Bile Acid Secretion

- Give the name of 3 canalicular bile acid transporters, and indicates which diseases arise from their defects.

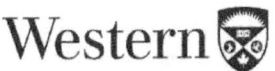

BILE SECRETION AND THE ENTEROHEPATIC CIRCULATION

- MDRS intrahepatic cholestasis of pregnancy (PFIC3)
- MDR2 – DJS (Dubin Johnson Syndrome)
- BSP (PFIC2)

Disease	Protein (gene)	GGT	Bile acid	Histology
➤ PFIC 1	FIC1 (ATP8B1)	N	↑	
➤ PFIC 2	BSEP (ABCB11)	N	↑	Giant cell formation, portal fibrosis
➤ PFIC 3	MDR3 (ABCB4)	↑	↑	Extensive bile duct proliferation, periportal fibrosis

Abbreviation: GGT, gamma glutamyl transferase

Intestinal Luminal Circulation

- Fasting state:
    - Bile acid synthesized, secreted, and stored in gall bladder in concentrated state
- Fed state:
    - Luminal CCK stimulates gall bladder contraction and sphincter of Oddi relaxation
    - This leads to secretion of concentrated bile into duodenum
    - Role of bile acids in the intestinal lumen

BILE SECRETION AND THE ENTEROHEPATIC CIRCULATION
Ileal Reabsorption & and Fecal Elimination

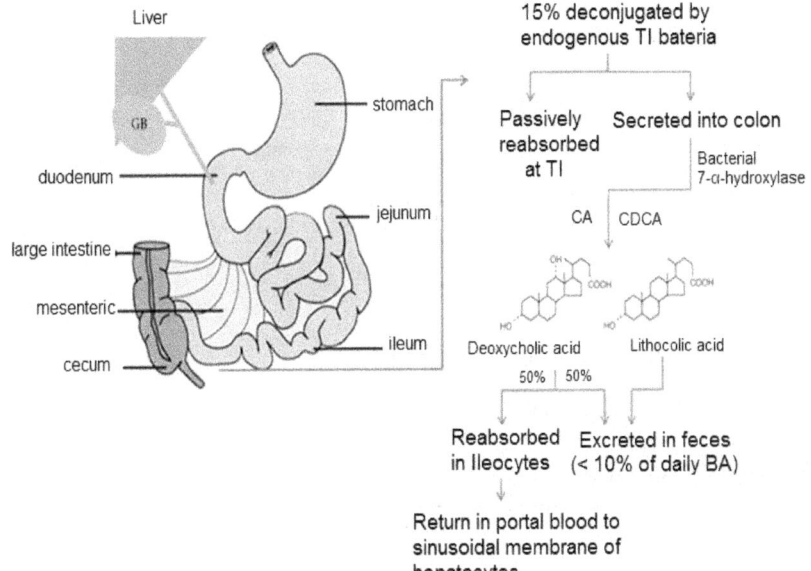

- > 90% of bile acids are recycled
- Total body bile acid recirculated 2-3x per meal
- Bile supply is a function of bile synthesis and recirculation

Disorders of Bile Secretion and Circulation

➤ Bile production
- Rare genetic disorders
  - 7 α-hydroxylase deficiency

➤ Bile secretion
- PFIC 1, 2, 3
- Benign recurrent intrahepatic cholestasis (BSEP)

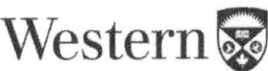

BILE SECRETION AND THE ENTEROHEPATIC CIRCULATION

- o Intrahepatic cholestasis of pregnancy (MDR3)
- o Dubin Johnson syndrome (MDR2)
- o Biliary tract obstruction
    - Stones
    - Strictures
    - Tumors

> Luminal transit
- o SIBO

> Bile absorption
- o Post cholecystectomy diarrhea
- o TI disease/resection

Abbreviations: SIBO, small intestinal bacterial overgrowth; TI, terminal ileum

Biliary Tract Obstruction

- o With partial obstruction, bile acids are regurgitated back into hepatocytes
    - Backflow into systemic circulation
    - Accumulation of bile acids→pruritis
- o Secreted bile acids are still efficiently absorbed at TI
    - Increased systemic bile acids→pruritis
    - Cholestyramine breaks cycle by increasing luminal losses of bile acid

Small Intestinal Bacterial Overgrowth (SIBO)

- o Normally bacteria limited to distal SI (deconjugate 15% of bile acids)
- o SBBO results in bacteria in proximal SI
    - ↑ deconjugation of bile acids

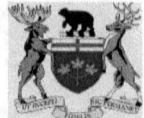

BILE SECRETION AND THE ENTEROHEPATIC CIRCULATION

- ↑ passive absorption of bile acids
- ↓ luminal [bile acid]
- Diarrhea/steatorrhea

Post-Cholecystectomy Diarrhea

- o Usually of no consequence
  - Duodenal storage
- o Post-cholecystectomy diarrhea (~10%)
  - TI transporters
  - Cholerheic enteropathy
    - Bile acid stimulate chloride secretion via Ca dependent mechanisms and secondary water loss
    - Primarily due to CDCA, DCA

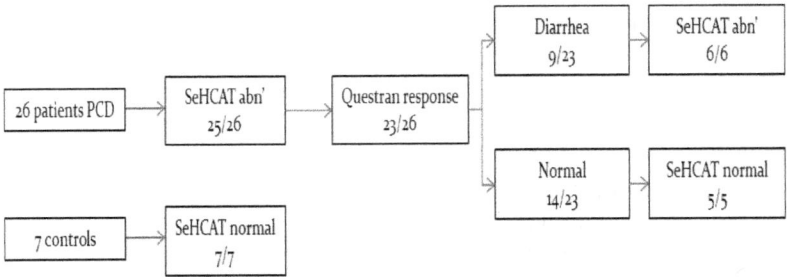

Source: Sciarretta et al. Am J Gastroenterol 1992;87:1852-4.

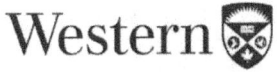

BILE SECRETION AND THE ENTEROHEPATIC CIRCULATION

Ileal Resection

- Resection < 100 cm
    - ↓ TI absorptive capacity → ↑ bile acid delivery to colon → cholerheic enteropathy
    - ↓ negative feedback → ↑ bile acid synthesis
    - Tx: cholestyramine
- Resection > 100 cm
    - Loss of TI bile acid absorptive capacity
    - Loss of entero-hepatic circulation
    - Depletion of bile acid stores
    - Total body bile acid a function of synthesis rather than circulation
    - Tx: low fat diet, medium chain triglycerides

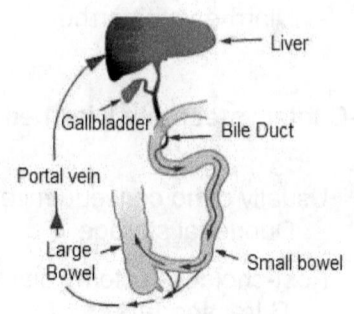

BILE SECRETION AND THE ENTEROHEPATIC CIRCULATION

- Give the reason why a resection of < 100 cm of ileum result in choleretic diarrhea, whereas a > 100 cm resection results in steatorrhea?

    - The neutral and the acidic pathways for the production of bile acids from cholesterol are capable of increasing their usual secretion rates by ~ 25%
    - When there is a small reduction in the EHC (enterohepatic circulation [of bile acids [BA]), such as might occur from an ileal resection of < 100 cm, the hepatic conversion of BA increases, and sufficient BA may be secreted across the CM and into the bile ducts and lumen of the duodenum to maintain a normal CMC (critical micellar concentration [of bile acids]).
    - Bile acid micelles and vesicles form, and lipids are absorbed.
    - Because of the loss of some of the ileum. Some BA escape reabsorption and spill in increased amounts into the colon.
    - In the colon the increased [BA] stimulated cGMP and secretion of Cl⁻, leading to a watery bile-acid induced (choleretic) diarrhea

- Give the change in pathophysiology which occurs with a loss of > 100 cm of ileum, leading to steatorrhea.

    - When there is a major loss of ileum (> 100 cm), the mount of malabsorbed BA is so great that liver cannot compensate for the large loss of BA by increasing the hepatic conversion of cholesterol to bile acids.

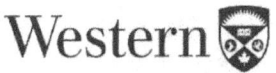

BILE SECRETION AND THE ENTEROHEPATIC CIRCULATION

- o Thus, the CMC is not achieved, and fat malabsorption (steatorrhea) occurs.

Response to treatment with cholestyramine in 171 patients with bile acid malabsorption.

Type of bile acid malabsorption*	7-day retention of SeHCAT <5%	7-day retention of SeHCAT 5% – <10%	7-day retention of SeHCAT 10% – <15%	
Type I	40 of 58	5 of 7	6 of 7	
Type II	29 of 39	12 of 14	2 of 4	
Type III	20 of 32	5 of 7	0 of 4	
Total	89 of 129	22 of 28	8 of 14	
	(69% CI**: 60%–77%)	(79% CI: 63%–94%)	(57% CI: 31%–83%)	
Excluding 21 patients with adverse effects of cholestyramine:				
Type I	35 of 49	4 of 6	6 of 7	72% responders
Type II	26 of 33	11 of 13	2 of 3	
Type III	19 of 29	5 of 6	0 of 4	
Total	80 of 111	20 of 25	8 of 14	
	(72% CI: 64%–80%)	(80% CI: 59%–93%)	(57% CI: 29%–82%)	

Printed with permission: Borghede et al. Eur J Intern Med 2011;22:137-40.

Useful background

The rate-limiting stop for the classical pathway of bile acid synthesis and secretion is the enzyme CYP7A1. As the throughput of the bile acids (BA) increases in the cytosol of the ileocyte or hepatocyte, CYP7A, falls and bile acid synthesis and secretion fall.

- Describe the FGF-dependent, SHP-dependent and mitochondrial cholesterol dependent negative feedback regulation of bile acid synthesis and secretion.

  - ➢ Classical ileocyte and hepatocyte CYP7A1 pathway

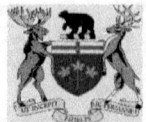

BILE SECRETION AND THE ENTEROHEPATIC CIRCULATION

- Overall
  - ↑ BA
  - ↓ BA synthesis
- FGF12: ↑ BA in cytosol of ileocyte → activate FXR → ↑ FGF_{12} → ↓ hepatic CYP7A1
  - ↓ hepatic synthesis of BA
- SHP/HNF4 α and LRH-1; ↑ BA in cytosol of hepatocyte → activate FXR → SHP
→ ↑ HNF4α ⎫→ hepatic CYP 7A1 → ↓ hepatic synthesis of BA ⎭
→ ↓ LRH-1
  - Activation of c-Jun (JNK) pathway

➢ Alternate pathway

↑ cholesterol in mitochondria

Abbreviations: HNF4α, hepatocyte nuclear factor 4α; JNF, c-Jun NH_2-terminal kinase; LRH, liver receptor homology; FGF19, fibroblast growth factor-19; FXR, farnesoid X receptor; SHP, small heterodimer partner a nuclear receptor

- When bile acids (BA) are conjugated in the liver to the amino acids glycine and taurine, the conjugated BA become more hydrophilic and less hydrophobic, so then passive absorption in the proximal intestine is less.
- Less passive absorption of conjugated BA in the proximal intestine maintains an adequate concentration of BA in the intestinal lumen to provide for continued solubilisation, digestion and absorption of lipids.

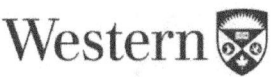

BILE SECRETION AND THE ENTEROHEPATIC CIRCULATION

- As the BA pass along the length of the small intestine, there becomes less and less exogenous or endogenous lipids to be absorbed, and the BA needs to be reabsorbed.

- The reabsorption of bile acids, their return to the liver, resecretion by the hepatocyte, and return to the lumen of the small intestine represents the EHC (enterohepatic absorption of bile acids).

- The endogenous microbacteria in the lumen of the terminal ileum deconjugates the primary and secondary bile acids.

- Enteric bacteria dehydroxylate Ba (primary (1°) → secondary (2°) BA), and deconjugate 1°/2° BA; enteric bacteria also epimerize the 7α-hydroxy group of CDCA (chenic acid), forming UDCA (ursodeoxycholic acid, 3α, 7β – dihydroxy BA).

- About 95% of BA in the lumen of the intestine are reabsorbed and recycled to the liver, representing the high efficiency of the EHC.

- The ~5% of the luminal bile acids that are not reabsorbed and recycled spill into the colon bacterial 7α-dehydroxylate in the colon produce 2° from 1° bile acids:

    CA → DCA (50% absorbed by colon)

    CDCA → LCA

    → UDCA

Abbreviations: BA, bile acid; CA, cholic acid; CDCA, chenodeoxycholic acid (aka chenic acid); DCA, deoxycholic acid; LCA, lithocholic acid; UDCA, ursodeoxycholic acid

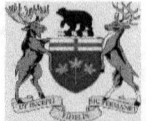

BILE SECRETION AND THE ENTEROHEPATIC CIRCULATION

- Give the physiological basis for the choleretic effect of UDCA.

Unconjugated dihydroxy bile acids such as UDCA are partially reabsorbed from the duct lumen across the luminal membrane of the cholangiocytes.

- ○ ASBT on the Cholangiocyte luminal membrane also quickly shunts conjugated BA back to the hepatocyte for resynthesis.
- ○ The UDCA quickly returns to the hepatocytes through the periductular capillary plexus.
- ○ The uptake of the protonated (H^+) unconjugated UDCA generates HCO_3.
- ○ The UDCA is quickly resecreted into the bile by the hepatocyte canalicular membrane.
- ○ The HCO3- produced from the uptake of the protonated UDCA through the cholehepatic shunt causes a bicarbonate-rich (i.e. reuptake of BA by active [ASBT] and by passive process of the luminal membrane of the cholangiocytes) choleresis.
- ○ Because this bicarbonate-rich choleresis depends on the uptake of the protonated unconjugated BA, this rapid reabsorption and resecretion of the BA because of uptake by the Cholangiocyte is, of course, causing BA-dependent bile flow.

- In the context of the EHC (enterohepatic circulation) of BA (bile acids), give the difference in the function of hepatocytes in zone I versus zone 3.

	BA absorption	BA secretion
Zone I, periportal	During fasting	Recycle BA
Zone III, pericentral (aka perivenous)	During feeding	Newly synthesized BA

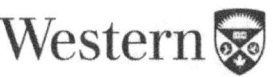

BILE SECRETION AND THE ENTEROHEPATIC CIRCULATION

- Give the physiology of bile acid-dependent and independent canaliculated secretion of water (bile flow / secretion).
    - Bile acid (BA)-dependent flow
        - Transport of BA across hepatocyte canalicular membrane by
            - BSEP
            - MRP_2
            - See "cholehepatic shunt, below
    - BA-independent flow
        - MRP_2 (multidrug resistance-associated protein 2) transport of GSH (reduced glutathione)
        - GGTP (gamma glutamyl transpeptidase, which catabolizes GSH in lumen)
        - AE_2 (chloride [Cl^-] bicarbonate [HCO_3^-] anion exchanger isoform2, which secretes HCO_3^- from cholangiocyte into the lumen of duct

Abbreviations: BSEP, bile salt export protein; MRP_2, multidrug resistance-associated protein-2

Useful background: BA metabolism

o	Size of BA pool	– 2 g to 4 g (50 to 60 mmol per Kg body weight)
o	Cycles of BA pool	– Per meal 2 to 3
		– Per day 6 to 10
o	Absorption of Ba per day	– 10 to 30 g (pool size x number of cycles)
o	Colonic loss of BA per day	– 200 to 600 mg
o	Hepatic synthesis of BAA per day to	– >> 95%

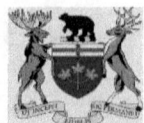

BILE SECRETION AND THE ENTEROHEPATIC CIRCULATION

match daily fecal losses

- ○ Efficiency of EHC — (loss / pool size x number of cycles → 500 mg / 4g x 10 cycles per day → 0.5 g / 40 g x 100%)

➢ Transport proteins for bile acids in the EHC

	BBM	BLM	Cytosol
➢ Ileocyte	○ ASBT (apical sodium bile acid transporter)	— OST αβ (organic solute transporter)	➢ FXR (farnesoid X receptor) — FXF19 (fibroblast growth factor 19)
	SM	CM	
➢ Hepatocyte	○ NTCP (Na$^+$-taurocholate cotransporting polypeptide)	— BSEP (bile salt export pump)	
➢ Cholangiocyte	○ ASBT	— OST α/β	
➢ Renal proximal tubular cell	○ ASBT	— OST α/β	

Abbreviations: AM, apical membrane of hepatocyte (aka canalicular membrane); BBM, brush border membrane of ileocyte; BLM, basolateral membrane of ileocyte;

A word of note:

There is bile acid-dependent and BA-independent bile flow, as well as Na$^+$-dependent bile acid clearance.

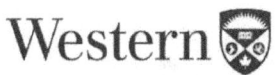

BILE SECRETION AND THE ENTEROHEPATIC CIRCULATION

- Give 3 inborn errors of bile acid or phospholipid transport, and for each name the defective transporter.

    - PFIC type 1
        - Progressive familial intrahepatic cholestasis
    - PFIC type 2
        - BSEP (ABCB11) deficiency
    - PFIC type 3
        - MDR3 (ABCB4) deficiency
    - BRIC syndrome
        - Benign recurrent intrahepatic cholestasis syndrome
    - Bile acids in the ileocytes bind to and activate FXR (a number of the family of sterol nuclear receptors)
    - FXR alters the activity of
        - Enzymes in the ileocyte cytosol: 7α – hydroxylase
        - Transporters in hepatocyte
            - BBM – sodium-dependent bile salt transporter
            - SM NTCP (sodium-dependent)
            - CM BSEP (bile salt export protein)

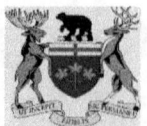

MINI UPDATE

IBD and Pregnancy

Mahmoud Mosli

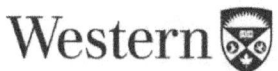

- Give the special considerations for the treatment of the IBD patient who is pregnant.

FDA pregnancy Category for Medications used in the Treatment

Medications	FDA pregnancy Category
Mesalamine	B
Corticosteroids	C
Azathioprine/ Mercaptopurine	D
Methotrexate	**X**
Metronidazole	
Ciprofloxacin	
Olsalazine	C
Sulfasalazine	B
Cyclosporine	C
Infliximab	B
Adalimumab	B
Tacrolimus	C
Thalidomide	**X**

Beware: No methotrexate or thalidomide in pregnancy: take double measures to prevent pregnancy if patient is on either methotrexate or thalidomide

Gisbert et al, Inflamm Bowel Dis 2010;16:881–895; Beaulieu et al. "Inflammatory bowel disease in pregnancy". World J Gastroentrol 2011 June 14; 17(22): 2696-2701.

Background

- 70% of females with IBD are in the child bearing age group
- Fertility has become a major concern for patients with IBD

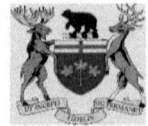

MINI UPDATE

- When conception occurs when the IBD is in remission, 75% will remain in remission
  - Active, the frequency of adverse outcomes is measured, such as *preterm birth small or premature baby*
  - *Miscarriage*
- It is generally recommended to women with IBD to conceive at a time when their IBD is in remission
  - This increased adverse effect is related to the active disease and its treatment
- In the CESAME study of 215 pregnancies in 204 IBD women, no significant differences were found between those women.

Outcome	Thiopurines	Other drugs	No drugs
- Live births	64%	67%	60%
- Prematurity	22%	16%	15%
- Low birth weight (<2500 g)	16%	14%	7%
- Congenital abnormalities	4%	7%	0%

Coelho et al "Pregnancy outcome in patients with inflammatory bowel disease treated with thiopurines: cohort from the CESAME Study". Gut 2011;60:198-203.

- Individual Medications
  - 5- ASA agents
    - All aminosalicylates (sulfasalazine, mesalamine, balsalazide) are FDA pregnancy category, B except for olsalazine which is pregnancy category C; these drugs are considered to be safe in pregnancy.

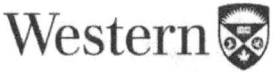

- Steroids[2]
  - FDA pregnancy category C
  - The very small risk of cleft lip and palate is outweighed by the benefit of controlling the mother's IBD, and therefore can be used to treat flare ups

- Azathioprine / 6-MP
  - FDA pregnancy category D drugs
  - Azathioprine crosses the placenta, but the immature fetal liver lacks the enzyme "inosinate pyrophosphorylase" needed to convert azathioprine to its active metabolite; mercaptopurine
  - This lack of inosinate pyrophosphorylase likely protects the fetus from toxic drug exposure during the crucial period of organogenesis
  - These drugs are likely safe during breast-feeding

- Methotrexate
  - FDA pregnancy category **X**
  - It teratogenic, and therefore should not be used in women considering conception
  - First trimester
    - Methotrexate is a folic acid antagonist
    - Use during the critical period of organogenesis (6 to 8 weeks post conception) is associated with multiple congenital anomalies.
    - This is called "methotrexate embryopathy" or "the fetal aminopterin-methotrexate syndrome"
  - Second/ third trimester
    - May be associated with fetal toxicity and mortality

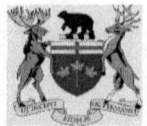

MINI UPDATE

- **Metronidazole**
  - FDA pregnancy category B
  - Not recommended during lactation

- Infliximab / Adalimumab/ Certolizumab
  - FDA pregnancy category B
  - IgG1 immunoglobulin's pass the placental barrier in the second and third trimester of pregnancy
  - Infusion of IFX during the third trimester just before delivery results in clinically significant levels of the antibody in the infant, and the half-life of these antibodies in newborns is prolonged
  - Pregnant patients should avoid therapeutic antibody treatments after 30 weeks' gestation
  - If necessary the expectant mother can be bridged with steroids to control the disease activity until delivery
  - Certolizumab differs from infliximab and adalimumab in that it is a Fab fragment of an antitumor necrosis factor alpha monoclonal antibody, and therefore it may not be necessary to stop certolizumab in the third trimester
  - Anti-TNF-agents can be safely restarted after delivery
  - Infants can receive routine vaccinations but live virus vaccines (e.g. rotavirus) should be avoided for the first 6 months (unless infliximab levels have been documented to be absent)

- Ciprofloxacin
  - FDA pregnancy category C
  - Ciprofloxacin crosses the placenta and is not recommended during lactation

- Cyclosporine
  - FDA pregnancy category C
  - Treatment with cyclosporine for steroid-refractory UC during pregnancy can be considered safe and effective

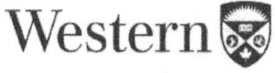

- Therefore, use of cyclosporine should be considered in cases of severe UC as a means of avoiding urgent surgery and reaching a gestational age when the fetus can be safely delivered
- However, breast-feeding is contraindicated for patients receiving cyclosporine

References and Suggested Reading

Mahadevan U, Kane S. "American Gastroenterological Association Institute technical review on the use of gastrointestinal medications in pregnancy". Gastroenterology. 2006;131:283–311.

Schnitzler et al. "Outcome of Pregnancy in Women with Inflammatory Bowel Disease Treated with Antitumor Necrosis Factor Therapy". Inflamm Bowel Dis 2011;17:1846–1854

Gisbert et al. "Safety of Immunomodulators and Biologics for the Treatment of Inflammatory Bowel Disease During Pregnancy and Breast-feeding". Inflamm Bowel Dis 2010;16:881–895)

Cornish et al "A meta-analysis on the influence of inflammatory bowel disease on pregnancy". Gut 2007;56:830–837.

"Certolizumab pegol: new drug. As a last resort in Crohn's disease: continue to use other TNF alpha inhibitors". Prescrire Int. 2009;18(101):108-10.

Magro F et al "Management of inflammatory bowel disease with infliximab and other anti-tumor necrosis factor alpha therapies". BioDrugs. 2010;24 Suppl 1:3-14.

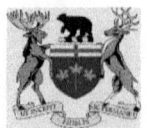

MINI UPDATE

European evidence-based consensus on the prevention, diagnosis and management of opportunistic infections in IBD

Aze Wilson

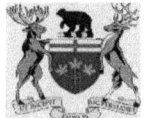

- Definition of an immunocompromised individual:
  - Defective in phagocytic, cellular or humoral immunity which increases risk for opportunistic infection
  - Being Immunocompromised (IC)
  - Non-HIV immunocompromised persons
    - Congenital causes
    - Cancer
    - Anti-metabolites or corticosteroids
  - Persons with HIV infection
  - Persons with conditions that cause limited immune deficits eg.
    - Chronic renal failure
    - Diabetes mellitus
    - Hyposplenism

Abbreviations: CDC, Centre for Disease Control

- IC in GI conditions

- Inflammatory bowel diseases (IBD)
  - Risk factors for being IC in IBD
    - Use of drugs
      - Corticosteroids
      - Immunosuppressants
      - Biologicals
    - Malnutrition
    - ↑ Age
    - Co-morbid illness
    - Foreign travel

- Hepatitis C virus (HCV) Infection
  - No consensus on screening for HCV in IBD
    - Same incidence of HCV in general population

(Loras et al AJG 2009; Chevaux IBD 2010)

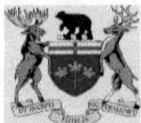

MINI UPDATE

- o Immunosuppressants (IM) for IBD are not necessarily contraindicated in active HCV
- o HCV should be treated according to standard practice without stopping IM
    - ?anti-TNF improves virologic response to INF/rib
    - IFN for HCV may worsen CD not UC

- Hepatitis B virus (HBV) Infection
  - o Prevention
    - HBV vaccination is recommended in all HBV – IBD patients
    - Efficacy of the HBV vaccination is affected by the amount of IM given
      - Higher doses may be needed to achieve immunity
      - Serological response should be measured after vaccination
  - o Treatment
    - Before and during IM tx, HBsAg+ carriers (past infection) should receive therapy with antiviral agents regardless of degree of viremia
    - All IBD patients should be tested for HBV to rule out HBV infection
      - In acute infection
        - Treat HBV
        - Delay IM until after treatment of HBV
      - In chronic active HBV
        - preferentially treat with nucleoside/tide analogs, not with IFN (interferon, which may ↑ activity of IBD)

Abbreviation: IM, immunosuppressing medications

- HIV
  - o Testing for HIV prior to starting IM, especially in high risk patients

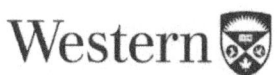

- Treat HIV for usual indications and with usual treatment (referral recommended to appropriate infectious disease / HIV- AIDs specialist)
- IM are not necessarily contra-indicated in HIV+ IBD patients

Herpesviruses (HSV, VZV, EBV, CMV) & HPV & JCV & Flu

- Cytomegalovirus (CMV) infection
  - Screening for latent CMV is not necessary in all IBD patients
  - Latent CMV
    - Not a contraindication for IM in IBD
  - Treatment with IM has been associated with reactivation of latent CMV, but causes
    - No colitis
    - No systemic infection
  - CMV colitis
    - Excludein refractory IBD
  - If CMV colitis is found in IBD
    - Stop IM
    - Start appropriate anti-viral

- Herpes simplex virus (HSV)
  - Screening +/- chemoprophylaxis for HSV infection is not necessary
  - Past or latent HSV infection
    - Not a contraindication for IM in IBD
  - Self-limited oral-labial or genital infection
    - Continue IM for IBD
    - Start anti-viral therapy for HSV
  - Severe systemic infection while on IM for IBD

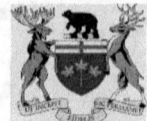

- Stop IM
- Start antiviral therapy for HSV

- VZV
  - Vaccination
    - If no previous vaccination for chicken pox, shingles and VZV
      - Immunize (live viruses)
      - Immunisation with VZV vaccine should be performed **>3 weeks prior** to initiating IM
  - Treatment
    - During active VZV
      - Do not start IM
      - If IM already started
        - Start anti-viral
        - Stop IM
        - Restart IM after the resolution of vesicles and fever

- EBV (Epstein Barr Virus)
  - Screening is not necessary prior to initiating IM
  - Severe EBV infection while or IM for IBD
  - EBV-related lymphoma developing while on IM
    - Stop IM

- Human Papilloma virus (HBV) Infection
  - Current or past HPV infection is not a contraindication for IM in IBD
  - Regular gynecological screening for cervical cancer is recommended in IBD women, on IM for IBD

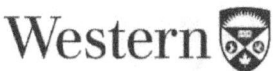

- In patients with extensive cutaneous warts or condylomata
  - Stop IMs
- Routine HPV vaccination (non-live) is recommended for women according to national guidelines
  - Females 11-12, before onset of sexual activity
  - Females 13-18 if vaccination was missed
  - No benefit in women >26

- JC virus (JCV)
  - No recommendations can be made re screening
  - Progressive multifocal leukoencephalopathy (PML) is caused by JC virus
    - Latently found in 60-80% of adult Europeans
  - No recommendations can be made re: screening
  - Patients with profound immunosuppression with new onset neurological symptoms should undergo contrast-enhanced cranial MRI and lumbar puncture (LP)

- Influenza
  - Patients on IMs are at increased for developing influenza infection
  - IBD patients on IMs should receive **annual** vaccination with inactivated influenza vaccine
  - Seroconversion is not affected by IMs American Centre for Disease Control & Prevention

- Parasitic and Fungal Infections
  - Corticosteroids and anti-TNFs
    - Are potent inhibitors of T cell function
    - ↑ infection with
      - Aspergillus sp
      - Candida sp

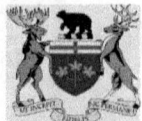

MINI UPDATE

- Crypotococcus
- P jiroveci
- Strongyloides
- T gondii
    - The risk is unknown of parasitic and fungal infection in IBD
    - Systemic infections are rare, but mortality high
    - No vaccines for fungal or parasitic infections
    - Prevention is key: when visiting endemic areas – avoid farms, pigeon lofts, extended stay
    - If severe infection develops, stop IM and treat as per national standards

- Pneumocystis jiroveci (PCJ)
    - No vaccines for prevention of P jiroveci pneumonia
    - For patients on triple IMs, with one being anti-TNF
        - Standard prophylaxis with septra (I SS tab daily or 1DS tab 3/week)
    - No consensus on double IMs
        - Infectious disease experts voted for prophylaxis on 1 IM / 2 IMs, where as gastroenterologists voted against, using their expert opinion from extrapolation of HIV / transplant data

- Tuberculosis
    - IMs increases ↑ risk for TB in IBD patients, especially anti-TNF agents
    - Anti-TNF patients may develop atypical TB
        - >50% extrapulmonary
        - >25% disseminated)
    - TB mortality ~13%
    - Perform careful evaluation for latent TB before anti-TNF started

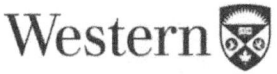

- Should also be considered before corticosteroid or other IMs in high risk patients
    - RFs, cxr, TBst
- Patients with latent TB should be treated with a complete regimen for latent TB
- For latent TB and active IBD
    - No increased risk for isoniazid associated hepatotoxicity
- For persistent fever or non-specific clinical deterioration during IM
    - Exclude TB
    - Stop anti-TNF for atleast 2 mon
    - Rule out multi-drug resistant TB
    - 5-ASA, Imuran, Azathioprine, Methotrexate or steroids do **NOT** need to be stopped, as long as, multi-drug resistant TB has been ruled out.

- Pneumococcal infection
    - Patients with IBD on IM are at ↑ risk for pneumococcal infections.
    - IBD patients on IM tx with pneumonia should be tested for L pneumophila
    - IBD patients on IM tx should receive a single revaccination with pneumovax q3-5 years if still immune compromised
        - Steroids and anti-TNF
            - NO affect on vaccine-induced seroconversion after immunization
            - Methotrexate vaccine-induced seroconversion
    - IBD patients on IM
        - ↑ risk for severe infections with Salmonella and Listeria
            - Prevention is key: food hygiene (avoid raw eggs, unpasteurized milk, under cooked or raw meats)

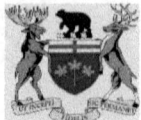

MINI UPDATE

- o IBD patients on IM
  - Stop IM until resolution of the active infection

- **C. difficile**
  - o IBD is an independent risk factor for C difficile
  - o Screening for C difficile is recommended at **every** flare in patients with colonic disease
  - o Unknown whether IM should be stopped

Special Circumstances

- o IBD patients travelling on IM frequently or to less developed countries
  - Pre-travel consultation with ID specialist/gastroenterologist
  - Avoid regions where live attenuated vaccine are required (e.g. yellow fever, varicella, PO polio, BCG)
  - Live vaccines acceptable if on steroid ' 20 mg é d or higher doses ' 14 days
  - Avoid liver attenuated vaccines for 3 months after stopping IM, or
  - 1 mon after stopping prednisone
  - Hold IM for 3 weeks prior to live vaccination
  - Non-live vaccines are safe, but may be less effective on IM (DPT, IV polio, flu, pneumovax, hep A/B,
- o IM tx patients travelling frequently or to less developed countries
  - IC IBD patients should pay greater attention to precautions regarding food and water during travel
  - Have a lower threshold for starting quinolone for Traveller's diarrhea
  - IC IBD patients travelling for >1mo to an endemic area should have a TB skin test (TST) before departure and if TST-negative initially, repeat 8-10 weeks after return.

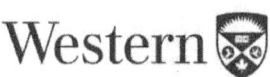

Considerations re Vaccination before introducing immunosuppression (IM)

- o Consider risk factors
  - Past history
    - Bacterial infections
    - Fungal infections
    - Varicella infection
  - Risk of latent or active TB
  - Immunisation status for HBV
  - History of travel
  - Future plans to travel

- o Investigations
  - Chest x-ray
  - TB skin test
  - VZV serology
    - In patients without a reliable history of immunisation or illness
    - VZV vaccine if serology for VZV is negative
  - HBV serology
    - HBV vaccine if seronegative
  - HIV serology
  - HPV vaccine in appropriate age/gender
  - Vaccination
    - Vaccine annually
  - Pneumococcal vaccine q 3-5 years
  - Routine vaccines
    - DPT

Reference

Rahier JF et al. Second European evidence-based consensus on the prevention, diagnosis and management of opportunistic infections in inflammatory bowel disease. Journal of Crohn's and Colitis (2014) 8, 443–468

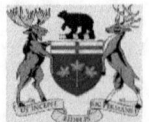

MINI UPDATE

COLON

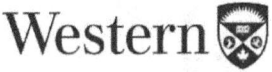

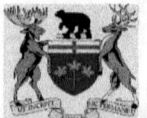

MINI UPDATE

Clostridium Difficile Infection

Mohammed Aljawad

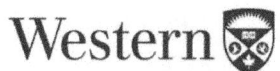

C. DIFFICILE INFECTION

Background

Antibiotic-Associated Diarrhea (AAD), Pseudomembranous Enterocolitis (PMEC) and Clostridium difficile-Associated Diarrhea and Colitis (CDADC).

Useful background
- There is overlap between AAD, PMEC and CDADC
- PMC (pseudomembraneous colitis) or PME (pseudomembraneous enteritis): the pseudomembrane is comprised of inflammatory and cellular debris, may be seen only on biopsy and not on colonoscopy, and may be associated with underlying ulceration.
- PMEC (PMC and PME) is caused by non-invasive C. difficile, S. aureus, and non-infectious conditions such as the seriously ill ICU patient.
- Predisposition to C. difficile indicates antineoplastic chemotherapy, HIV and IBD (even in the absence of use of antibiotics).
- Diagnostic tests include
  - Tissue culture cytotoxicity assay
  - EIA (enzyme-linked Immunoassays) for toxin A and B
  - Culture followed by testing for toxin A and B
  - PCR 9polymerase chain reaction) to detect the genes for the toxins
  - Colonoscopy: AAD plus PMC = C. diffcile colitis (sigmoidoscopy is not adequate, since 20% of PMC involves only the right side of the colon)
- ~20% of C. diffcile diarrhea patients recur after initially successful treatment with metronidaazole or vancomycin. Because post-infectious IBS (irritable

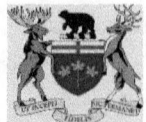

C. DIFFICILE INFECTION

bowel syndrome) may present with similar symptoms, reculture is appropriate.

- Risk factors

  - C.diffcile is a "big deal" organism these days, because of
  - Its widening disease scope, as well as its morbidity and mortality.
  - The usual
    - Recent use of antibiotics
    - Dirty hospitals
    - Dirty hands
  - Hand washing with the alcohol-containing dispensers which are now found throughout most hospitals!! (only soap and water destroys C.difficile)
  - Newly recognized
    - Anybody-that means even healthy persons in the community
    - Recent use of PPIs
    - Post-partum women
    - Patients with UC and CD

Abbreviations: UC, ulcerative colitis; CD, Chronic disease; PPIs, proton pump inhibitors

- Organism
  - A gram-positive, cytotoxin-producing, anaerobic, spore-forming bacterium
  - NAP1/ B1/ 027 strain, a new, hypervirulent strain, responsible for multiple C difficile outbreaks since the early 2000s.
    - Characteristics
      - Production of binary toxin
      - Larger quantities of toxins A and B than other strains
      - Resistant to fluoroquinolones

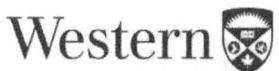

C. DIFFICILE INFECTION

- Diagnosis based on symptoms and confirmatory test

- Symptoms
  - ≥ 3 unformed stool in 24 hrs

- Laboratory confirmation
  - Toxigenic C. Diff
  - Toxins
  - ± pseudomembranous colitis (PMC), on endoscopy and biopsy

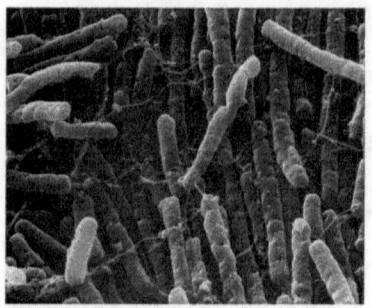

Clostridium Difficile

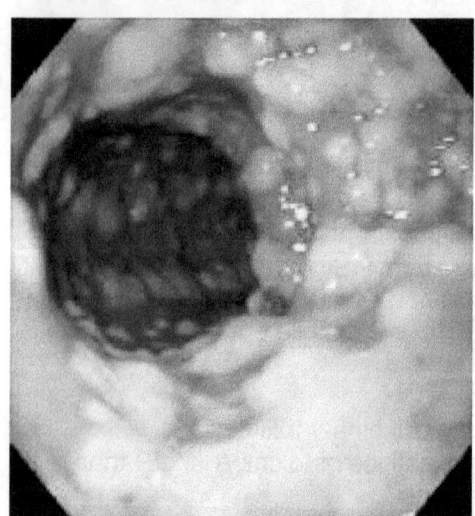

Pseudomembranous colitis (PMC)

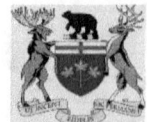

C. DIFFICILE INFECTION

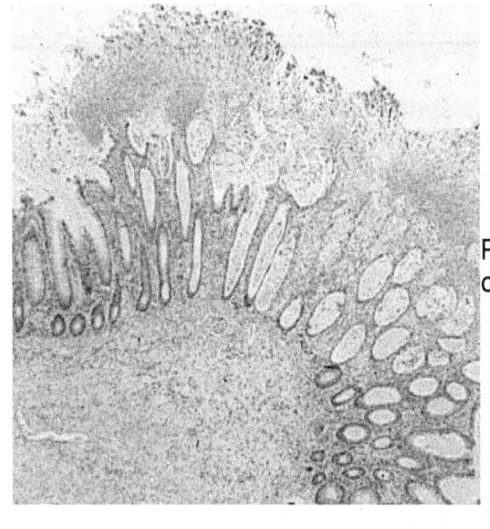

Pseudomembranous colitis (PMC)

- Epidemiology
    - Present in 90% of infants < 1 year old
    - The carrier rate among healthy adults is about 3%
    - Colonization occurs in 20 to 50% of adults in hospitals and long term care facilities
    - Accounts for 20-30% of antibiotics associated diarrhea

- Transmission
    - 21% of patients who initially had negative test results acquired the organism during admission
    - C. difficile cultured from environmental surfaces in 49% of hospital rooms of symptomatic patients
    - Present in 59% of the health care workers, hands caring for these patients

McFarland LV, Mulligan ME, Kwok RY, Stamm WE. Nosocomial acquisition of Clostridium difficile infection. *N Engl J Med*. 1989 Jan 26;320(4):204-10.

C. DIFFICILE INFECTION

> Clinical variants

- Give the 4 clinical and endoscopic variants of C. difficile infection.

Type of infection	Diarrhea	Other symptoms	Physical examination	Sigmoidoscopic examination
> Asymptomatic carriage	Absent	Absent	Normal	Normal
> C. difficile associated diarrhea (CAAD) with colitis	o Multiple loose bowel movements per day o Fecal leukocytes present o Occult bleeding may be seen o Heamatochezia rare	Nausea, anorexia, fever, malaise, dehydration, leukocytosis with left shift	Abdominal distention, tenderness	Diffuse or patchy nonspecific colitis

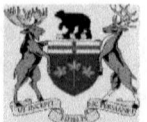

C. DIFFICILE INFECTION

	Diarrhea	Other symptoms	Physical examination	Sigmoidoscopic examination
➢ Pseudo-membranous colitis (PMC)	o Diarrhea more profuse than in colitis without pseudo-membranes o Fecal leukocytes present o Occult bleeding may be seen o Hematochezia rare	Nausea, anorexia, fever, malaise, dehydration, leukocytosis with left shift; symptoms may be mire severe than in colitis without pseudo-membranes	Marked abdominal tenderness, distension	Characteristic raised, adherent, yellow plaques, diameter up to 2 cm; rectosigmoid spared in 10% of case; pseudomembranes may not be noted unless colonoscopy performed

Type of infection	Diarrhea	Other symptoms	Physical examination	Sigmoido-scopic examination
➢ Fulminant colitis	o Diarrhea may be severe OR diminished (due to paralytic ileus and colonic dilatation) o Surgical consult required; colectomy can be life-saving	Lethargy, fever, tachycardia, abdominal pain; dilated colon/ paralytic ileus may be demonstrated on plain abdominal film	May present as acute abdomen; peritoneal signs suggest perforation	Sigmoidoscopy and colonoscopy contraindicated; flexible proctoscopy with minimal air insufflation may be diagnostic

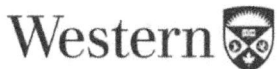

C. DIFFICILE INFECTION

- Pathogenesis

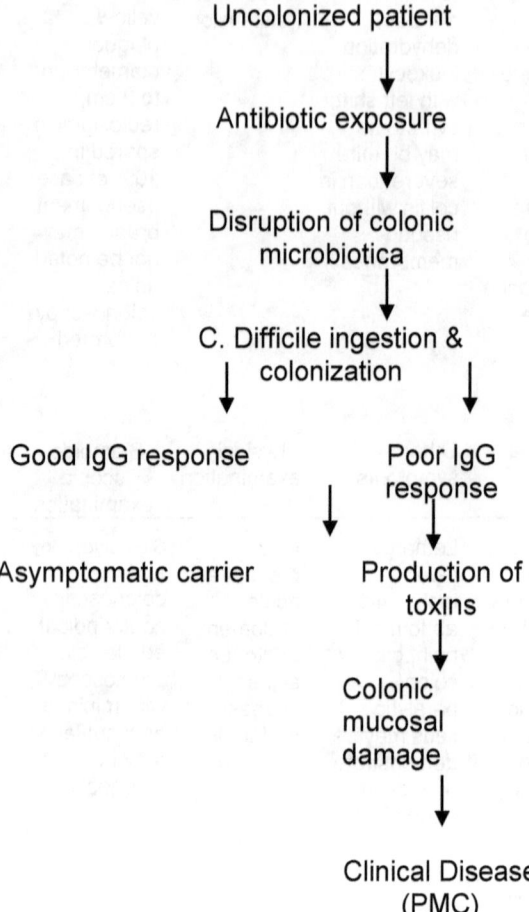

C. DIFFICILE INFECTION

- Give the way in which a Clostridium difficile infection (CDI) causes pseudomembranous colitis in a patient with a history recent of antibiotic use.
    - Antibiotics deplete regular gut microbiotica, which normally outnumber the C.*difficile* which is present.
    - C.*difficile* can resist antibiotics as a spore and then will outgrow normal microbiotica when antibiotics are discontinued.
    - Toxins A and B are produced by the greater numbers of C.*difficile* ,causing diarrhea.

> Risk factors
> - Antibiotic usage
> - Poor hand washing
> - Hospital or nursing home care
> - Advanced age
> - Severe illness (associated IBD (crohn, ulcerative colitis)
> - Gastrointestinal manipulation
>   - Surgery
>   - Tube-feeding
>   - Enemas
>   - Proton-pump inhibitors (PPIs)
> - Anti-neoplastic agents

> Prevention
> - Hand washing
> - Antibiotic restriction
> - Gloves and gowns use
> - Single-use rectal thermometers
> - Environmental cleaning and disinfection

> More on the importance of hand washing
> - Conventional hand washing with soap and water is optimal
> - Alcohol-based hand rubs are

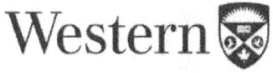

C. DIFFICILE INFECTION

- Associated with an increase in C. difficile infection
- Inferior to soap and water; in fact, alcohol rubs may be ineffective

Oughton MT, Loo VG, Dendukuri N, et al. *Infect Control Hosp Epidemiol.* 2009;30(10):939-44; Rupp ME, Fitzgerald T, Puumala S, et al. *Infect Control Hosp Epidemiol.* 2008;29(1):8-15.

➢ More on antibiotic use
  o The most widely recognized and modifiable risk factor
  o Increases with duration and number of antibiotics

Antibiotics associated with Clostridium difficile infection*

Frequent	Infrequent	Rare
o Ampicillin plus clavulanic acid, amoxicillin	- Ampicillin	▪ Vancomycin
o Second- or third – generation cephalosporins	- Sulfonamides with or without trimethoprim	▪ Penicillin or antistaphlo-coccal penicillin
o Clindamycin	- Erythromycin	▪ First-generation cephalosporin
o Fluoroquinolones	- Aminoglycosides	
o Antipseudomonal penicillin	- Metronidazole	
	- Tetracycline	

*Owens RC Jr, Donskey CJ, Gaynes RP, et al. Antimicrobial – associated risk factors for clostridium difficile infection. *Clin Infect Dis.* 2008;46 Suppl 1:S19-31.

➢ Treatment

• Give the treatment of C. difficile infection (CDI).

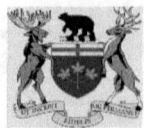

C. DIFFICILE INFECTION

- General management
  - Stop offending antibiotics
  - Contact precaution, especially hand hygiene
  - Supportive therapy
  - Treatment is not indicated for asymptomatic / carrier patient

(A) Mild CDI
  - Stop offending antibiotics if possible
    - 15% of CDI respond to cessation of antibiotics alone (Olson MM, Shanholtzer CJ, Lee JT Jr, Gerding DN. Ten years of prospective Clostridium difficile-associated disease surveillance and treatment at the Minneapolis VA Medical Center, 1982-1991.*Infect Control Hosp Epidemiol.* 1994;15:371-81
  - Antibiotics (bacteriostatic)
    - Metronidazole 500 mg po tid, or 250 mg po qid, for 10 to 14 days
    - If metronidazole ineffective and symptoms persist, vancomycin 125 mg po qid, for 10 to 14 days
    - If patient requires antibiotics for non- C. Difficile indication, continue metronidazole or vancomycin ("concomitant antibiotics") for 1 week after other antibiotics for non- C. difficile infection is stopped.
    - Note; Risk of VRE (vancomycin-resistant enterococci) is similar with both metronidazole and vancomycin.
  - Repeat stool cultures

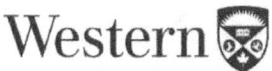

C. DIFFICILE INFECTION

- Not indicated if symptoms subsided (50% will have C. difficile spores for up to 6 weeks in persons who have become asymptomatic)
- Not indicated to treat C. difficile spore; even if person is toxin-positive, they may be an asymptomatic carrier.

Clinical Caution

- Vancomycin given PO or PR (by enema) is absorbed through the inflamed colonic mucosa in CDI, so you must **monitor** serum creatinine for renal toxicity.

Clinical Caution

- Recurrence of symptoms after treatment for initial CDI does not automatically mean disease related to CDI, even if stool cultures are positive by stool toxin assay.
- This is because the patient may be an asymptomatic C. difficile carrier.

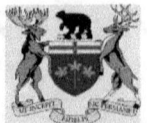

C. DIFFICILE INFECTION

SO YOU WANT TO BE A GASTROENTEROLOGIST!

Because CDI is a common and serious complication of hospitalization and poor hand hygiene, including poor contact precaution by staff, alcohol-based hand sanitizers are being increasing placed in / outside patient rooms.

- Give a reason why this practice may be challenged.
    - C. difficile spores are destroyed by soap and wate
    - Washing with alcohol allows spores to survive, germinate and potentially cause more CDI

Relapse or reinfection of difficile leading to recurrent symptoms occurs in about 25% of persons.

- Give 3 risk factors for recurrent CDI.
    - Age > 65 years
    - Need for concomitant antibiotics (antidote for medical condition, plus antibiotic for CDI)
    - Co-morbidities
    - ↓ host immune response (low anti-toxin antibody levels)
    - Exposure to asymptomatic carriers

Note: Answering development of antibiotic resistance is not correct recurrence of CDI after initial treatment with metronidazole does not signify metronidazole resistance.

(B) Severe CDI
- No consensus definition

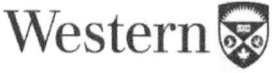

C. DIFFICILE INFECTION

- 2010 IDSA guidelines definition for CDI
    - WBC > 15,000 cells / μL, or
    - Serum creatinine ≥ 1.5 x pre-infection level
- 2013 ACG guidlines definition for severe CDI
    - Serum albumin <3g/dl plus ONE of the following:
        - WBC ≥15,000 cells/mm^3
        - Abdominal tenderness
- Severe complicated (2013 ACG guidelines)
    - Any of the following attributable to CDI:
        - Admission to intensive care unit for CDI
        - Hypotension with or without required use of vasopressors
        - Fever ≥38.5 °C
        - Ileus or significant abdominal distention
        - Mental status changes
        - WBC ≥35,000 cells/mm^3 or <2,000 cells/mm^3
        - Serum lactate levels >2.2 mmol/l
        - End organ failure (mechanical ventilation, renal failure, etc.
    - Scoring system (maximum 8 points)
        - One point each for
            - Age. > 60 years > 38.3 °C
            - WBC > 15,000 WBC/μL within 48 hours of enrollment
            - Serum albumin < 2.5 mg/dL
        - Two points each for
            - PMC (pseudomembranous colitis) on endoscopy
            - Admission to ICU
    - Severe disease ≥ 2 points

Source : Clin Infect Dis 2007;45:302-7

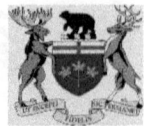

C. DIFFICILE INFECTION

- Complications
  - Patient
    - Shock
    - Death (within 30 days)
  - Colon
    - Megacolon
    - Perforation
    - Need for colectomy
  - Risk of complications for the hypervirlent stain of C. difficile, NAP (north American Pulsed Field type I), 11%
- Treatment
- 1- Severe CDI:
  - Vancomycin 125 mg po qid for 10-14 days
  - For severe disease, vancomycin (VAN) is superior to metronidazole (Met)

	VAN	MET
Cure rate for severe CDI	97%	76%

Zar FA, et al. A comparison of vancomycin and metronidazole for the treatment of Clostridium difficile-associated diarrhea, stratified by disease severity. *Clin Infect Dis.* 2007;45(3):302-7. Epub 2007 Jun 19

2- Severe complicated

- NO megacolon, abdominal distension, ileus or shock
  - Vancomycin 500 mg PO qid AND Metronidazole 500 mg IV

- Severe and complicated WITH signigicant abdominal distension, megacolon, ileus or shock

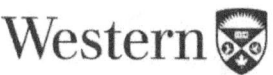

C. DIFFICILE INFECTION

- Vancomycin po 500 mg qid + IV metronidazole 500 mg q 8 h
- Vancomycin enema 500 mg in 100 mL of normal saline q 6 h
- Colectomy – indication
  - Failure of medical therapy for complicated cases after 5 days of antibiotics
  - Toxic megacolon
  - Perforation
  - Sepsis with organ dysfunction
  - shock/hypotension requiring vasopressor
  - Lactate > 5
  - peritoneal signs
  - WBC > 50,000

Procedure : subtotal colectomy with end-ileostomy

Source : 2013 ACG guidlines
2010 IDSA guidlines

(C) Recurrent CDI

➢ Definitions
  - Treatment failure: patient still has diarrhea after at least 6 days of antibiotic therapy
  - Relapse ("recurrence"): the patient responded to a course of antibiotic therapy, but subsequently has symptom recurrence when off antibiotics
  - Relapse usually occurs 1 to 3 wks after termination of Rx
  - Occurs in approximately 25% of cases
  - Patient with one episode of recurrent C. difficile 40-65% chance of additional episodes

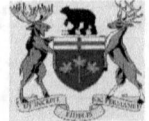

C. DIFFICILE INFECTION

Antibiotic	Treatment failure	Relapse/ recurrence
- Metronidazole	18%	29%
- Vancomycin	3%	20%

- First relapse: repeat initial regimen, unless severe presentation
- Associations with metronidazole failures
  - Transfer from another hospital
  - CDI on hospital admission
  - Recent use of cephalosporin
- Second relapse:
  - Vancomycin for any level of severity, to avoid neurotoxicity due to repeated courses of metronidazole
  - Tapered Vancomycin regimen: After initial 14 days course of vancomycin in a regimen appropriate to the degree of illness, follow with
    - A tapering course of vancomycin:
      - 125 mg po bid for 7 d, then
      - 125 mg po od daily for 7 d, then
      - 125 mg po every 2-3 d for 2-8 wk
    - Pulsed vancomycin follow with a pulse-dose course of vancomycin: 125, 250, or 500 mg every 3 d for 4-6 wk

Kelly CP, LaMont JT. Clostridium difficile--more difficult than ever. N Engl J Med. 2008;359(18):1932-40.

- Rifaximin
  - Rifaximin 400 mg bid for 14 days when patient is asymptomatic, and immediately after completion, of a course of vancomycin
  - No further recurrence in 7 out of 8 patients who had more than 4 relapses

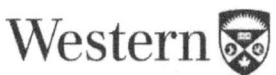

C. DIFFICILE INFECTION

Johnson S, Schriever C, Galang M, et al. *Clin Infect Dis*. 2007;44(6):846-8.

- o Fidaxomicin
  - Fidaxomicin (F) may prove to be superior to vancomycin (V), especially for recurrent disease (for example, per protocol, 13% vs 24%, p=0.004)

Source : Cornely OA et al. Clin Infect Dis 2012; 55(Suppl 2): S154–S161.

- o Anion-binding resins
  - Cholestyramine and colestipol, as adjunctive therapy for relapsing infection
  - Cholestyramine 4 g qid, taken 3 hr after vancomycin, for 14 days
  - Not effective as primary therapy for C. difficile colitis

Tedesco FJ. Treatment of recurrent antibiotic-associated pseudomembranous colitis. *Am J Gastroenterol*. 1982;77(4):220-1.

- o Probiotics
  - Saccharomyces Boulardii used combined with antibiotic only to treat recurrence
  - Bactermeia and fungemia may occur, especially with
    - Severe comorbidities
    - Immunosuppressive medication
    - Recent surgical intervention

Rask KJ, Williams MV, Parker RM, McNagny SE. Obstacles predicting lack of a regular provider and delays

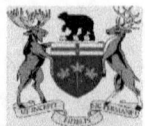

C. DIFFICILE INFECTION

in seeking care for patients at an urban public hospital. *JAMA*. 1994;271(24):1931-3.
McFarland LV. Meta-analysis of probiotics for the prevention of antibiotic associated diarrhea and the treatment of Clostridium difficile disease. *Am J Gastroenterol*. 2006;101(4):812-22.

- **Immunotherapy**
  - Monoclonal antibodies (MAb) to toxin A and B
    - Adjuvant to antibiotics (Ab), to reduce rate of recurrence
  - IVIG (intravenous immunoglobulin) – no proven therapy

- **Fecal transplantation**
  - Can be considered in the third recurrence after a pulsed regimen
  - Recipient:
    - Vancomycin 500 mg pot id for 7 days, followed by single oral lavage with 4 liters of PEG
    - 300 g of stool suspended in 300 mL of sterile normal saline, given for 5 days by enema, colonoscopy or NG tube
  - Cure rate of approximately 95%

Borody TJ, Warren EF, Leis SM, et al. Bacteriotherapy using fecal flora: toying with human motions. *J Clin Gastroenterol*. 2004;38(6):475-83. Bakken JS et al. Clin Gastroenterol Hepatol 2011;9:1044–1049.

Clinical alert

- In patient with Crohn disease or ulcerative colitis who experiences symptoms suggestive of a recurrence of their IBD, always test for C. difficile infection.

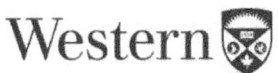

C. DIFFICILE INFECTION

➢ Summary of CDAD/ PMC
  o Increasing in incidence and severity
  o Hospitals and health care workers are major source of spreading the infection
  o No longer seen just in those who have been on antibiotics
  o No longer seen just in hospitals and other institutions
  o Primary failure and recurrence rate is high
  o Eradication is difficult

References and Suggested Reading

2013 ACG Guidlines. Surawicz CM et al. Guidelines for Diagnosis, Treatment, and Prevention of Clostridium difficile Infections Am J Gastroenterol 2013; 108:478–498

Cohen SH, et al. Clinical practice guidelines for Clostridium difficile infection in adults: 2010 update by the society for healthcare epidemiology of America (SHEA) and the infectious diseases society of America (IDSA). *Infect Control Hosp Epidemiol.* 2010;31(5):431-55.

Johnson S, et al. Interruption of recurrent Clostridium difficile-associated diarrhea episodes by serial therapy with vancomycin and rifaximin. *Clin Infect Dis.* 2007;44(6):846-8.

Kuehne SA, et al. The role of toxin A and toxin B in Clostridium difficile infection. *Nature* 2010;4677:11-713.

Louie TJ, et al. Fidaxomicin versus vancomycin for Clostridium difficile infection. *N Engl J Med.* 2011;364(5):422-31.

Oughton MT, et al. Hand hygiene with soap and water is superior to alcohol rub and antiseptic wipes for removal of Clostridium difficile. *Infect Control Hosp Epidemiol.* 2009;30(10):939-44.

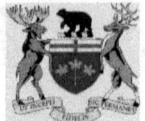

MINI UPDATE

Hereditary Colon Cancer: FAP and HNPCC

Brian Yan

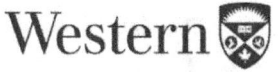

Outline

- Overview of colon cancer genetics
- FAP
- HNPCC
- MUTYH Associated Polyposis

Colon Cancer Genetics

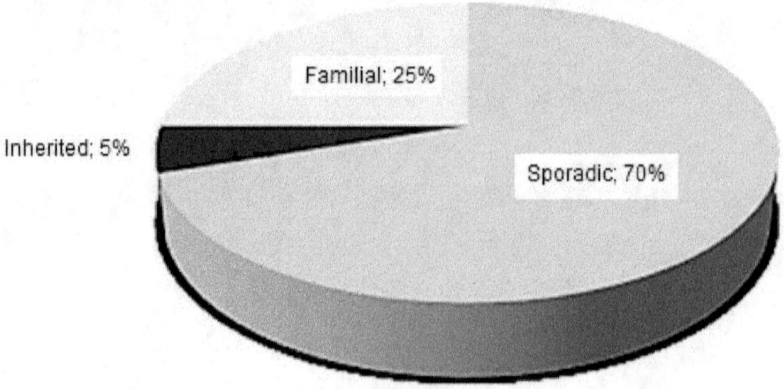

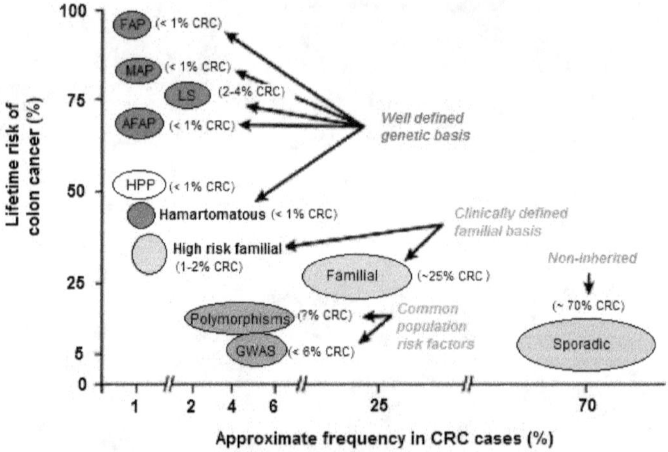

Printed with permission: Jasperson KW, et al. Gastroenterology. 2010;138(6):2044-58.

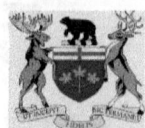

MINI UPDATE

- ➤ Types of Mutations:
  - o Germline mutations
    - – Mutations in sperm, ova, zygote
      - ▪ Inherited from previous generation
      - ▪ Spontaneous
  - o Somatic mutations
    - – Mutation during growth/development of tissue
      - ▪ Spontaneous
- ➤ Mechanism of mutations
  - o Point mutations
  - o Altered DNA methylation
  - o Gene rearrangements
  - o Amplifications
  - o Deletions

Colon Cancer Genetics – Terminology

- o Oncogenes: makes cells grow
  - – mutated oncogene → constitutive activation → uncontrolled proliferation
    - ▪ e.g. ras (K-ras), c-myc
- o Suppressor genes: inhibits growth, promote apoptosis
  - – function lost when both alleles are lost - 2-hit hypothesis
    - ▪ e.g. APC, p53
- o Mismatch Repair (MMR)
  - – correct DNA replication errors
    - ▪ e.g. hMSH2, hMLH1 in HNPCC
- o Modifier genes
  - – influence cell function
    - ▪ e.g. COX-2, PPAR

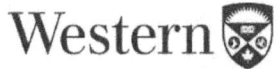

Adenoma → Carcinoma Sequence

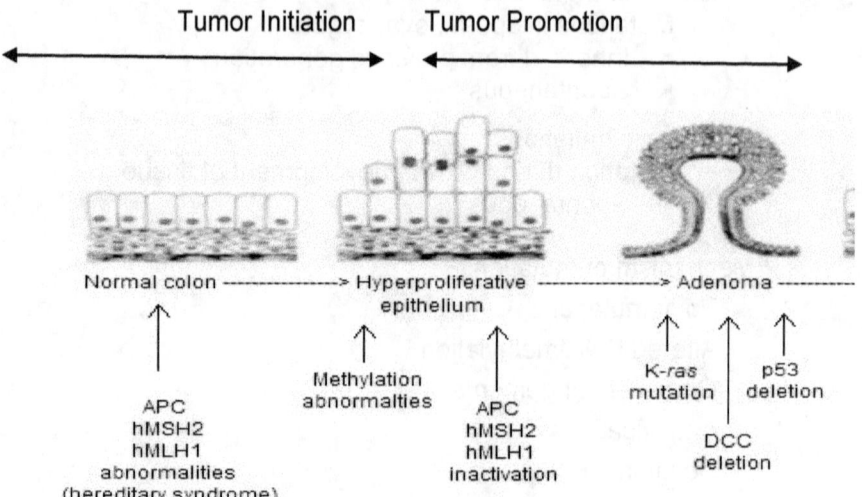

Multistep Carcinogenesis in the Colon

First put forth by Fearon ER and Vogelstein B. Cell 1990;61(5):759-67.

Chromosomal instability

Microsatellite instability

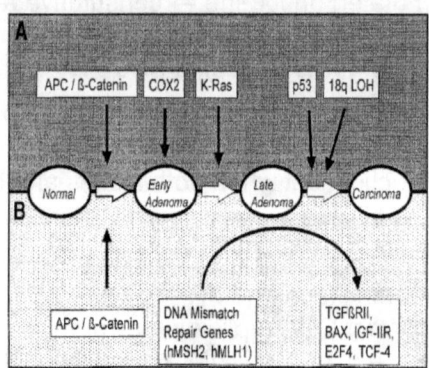

Printed with permission: Chung DC. Gastroenterology 2000;119(3):854-65.

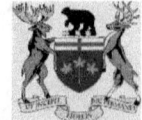

MINI UPDATE

Polyposis Syndromes
- Characterized by:
  - distinct clinical manifestations
    - multiple polypoid lesions of the GI tract
  - most are inherited
  - varying degrees of increased colon cancer risk

Polyposis Syndromes (GENES)

➢ Non-Hereditary GI Polyposes
  - Hyperplastic
  - Lymphoid
    - Reactive lymphoid hyperplasia
    - Lymphoma
  - Lipomatosis
  - Angiomatosis
  - Leiomyomatosis
  - Pneumatosis cystoides intestinalis
  - Cronkhite-Canada syndrome

➢ Hereditary GI Polyposes
  - Adenomatous polyposes syndromes
    - Familial adenomatous polyposis (APC)
    - Gardner, Turcot, Attenuated (APC)
    - MUTYH Associated Polyposis
  - Hamartomatous polyposes syndromes
    - Peutz Jeghers syndrome (STK11)
    - Familial juvenile polyposis (SMAD4 or BMPR1A)
    - Cowden's disease (PTEN)
    - Intestinal ganglioneuromatosis (varying syndrome genes)
    - Ruvalcaba-Myrhe-Smith syndrome (PTEN)
    - Tuberous sclerosis (TSC1)

➢ Hereditary Non Polyposis Syndrome: HNPCC

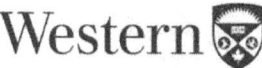

C. DIFFICILE INFECTION

Familial Adenomatous Polyposis (FAP)
- Most common polyposis syndrome
- AD inheritance
  - 80-100% penetrance
  - 1:8300 - 1:14,025 live births
- Germline mutations of APC gene
  - 80% will dmonstrate mutation
  - 2-hit hypothesis:
    - One mutated APC allele inherited → subsequent loss/mutation of normal allele = polyposis
  - 15-25% of patients do not have family history suggesting spontaneous germline mutation

APC Gene

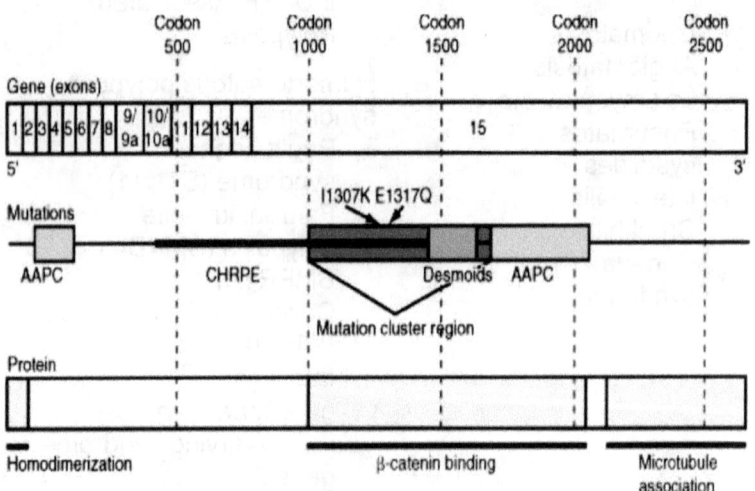

- 15-exon gene
- large protein - 2843 amino acids; 310 kilodaltons
- cell adhesion, signal transduction, transcriptional activation

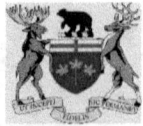

MINI UPDATE

- o 300 different mutations identified
  - Insertions, deletions, nosense mutations → premature stop codons truncated APC gene product

APC Structure and Function

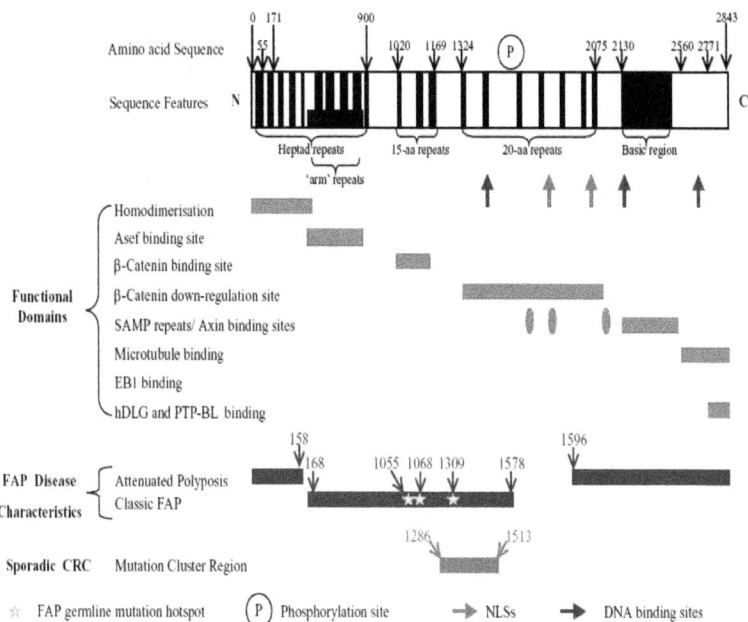

"Use your skills and abilities to contribute to a greater good and find a purpose beyond position, and beyond money."

Sylvia Chrominska

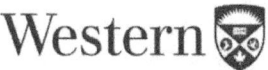

APC/β-Catenin Pathway

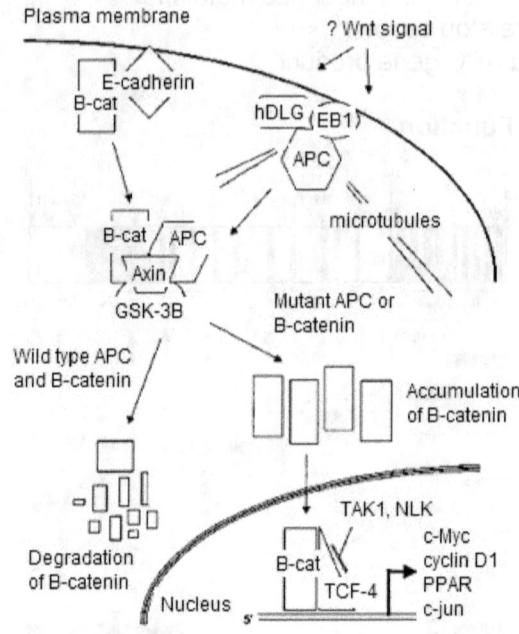

- Wingless/Wnt signaling pathway
- signal transduction pathway necessary for embryonic development
- mutated APC → increased β-catenin
- β-catenin binds to transcription factor
- T-cell factor-4 (TCF-4)
  - stimulates proliferation
  - induces resistance to proliferation
  - upregulates oncogenes (c-myc)

Printed with permission: Chung DC. Gastroenterology 2000;119(3):854-65.

MINI UPDATE

Genetic testing is part of the standard management of families with FAP.

- Give the methods used for genetic testing in FAP to confirm the diagnosis of FAP in suspected cases, and to determine if a person from a family with FAP is a gene carrier.

    o *In vitro* protein truncation in FAP
    - Detects the presence of truncating mutations in vitro
    - Detects a mutation in 80% to 90% of affected families known to have FAP
    - Near 100% effective in family members once the presence of a mutation has been found in an affected person

    o Gene sequencing
    - Often preceded by single-strand conformational polymorphism (SSCP) or denaturing gradient gel electrophoresis (DGGE) to narrow the area of the gene where sequencing is to be performed
    - Up to 95% effective in finding a disease-causing mutation if it is present
    - Near 100% effective in family members once the presence of a mutation has been found in an affected person

    o Linkage testing
    - Used if other methods unsuccessful
    - Two or more affected persons from two generations must be living for DNA to be obtained

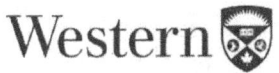

- Effective in >95% of families, with >98% accuracy with present linkage markers
- Genotype-phenotype correlations:
  - These have not yet been found to be of precise use in the clinical setting
  - The following correlations have been made:
  - CHRPE (congenital hypertrophy of the retinal pigment epithelium): present in families with mutations distal to exon 9 of the APC gene
  - Dense polyposis: present with mutations in the mid portion of exon 15
  - AFAP/AAPC: found with mutation in the extreme proximal or distal end of the gene
  - Osteomas and desmoids (Gardner's syndrome): more commonly found with mutations in the distal portion of exon 15

Abbreviations: CHRPE, congenital hypertrophy of the retinal pigment epithelium; DGGE, denaturing gradient gel electrophoresis; SSCP, single-strand conformational polymorphism

Adapted from: Doxey BW, Kuwada SK, Burt RW. *Clin Gastroenterol Hepatol*. 2005;3(7):633-41; and Burt R, Neklason DW. *Gastroenterology* 2005;128(6):1696-716.

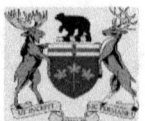

MINI UPDATE

SO YOU WANT TO BE A GASTROENTEROLOGIST

- Give the role of APC gene function, nuclear β-catenin, the Wnt signal pathway, the LEF (lymphoid enhancer factor) / T-cell factor family in the development of CRC.
    - Normal
        - APC (tumor suppressor) gene
        - Association with E-cadherin → cell-cell adhesion
        - Binds β-catenin → ↑ phosphorylation
        - ↓ β-catenin - ↓ stimulation of Wnt-Tcf signal pathway
            - ↓ proliferation
            - ↑ apoptosis
    - APC gene mutation
        - ↓ cell-cell adhesion
        - ↓ β-catenin phosphorylation
            - ↑ unphosphorylated β catenin complex with LEF / TCF
            - ↑ Wnt-Tcf
        - Target genes
            - ↑ proliferation
            - ↓ apoptosis

Clinical Features of FAP

- ≥ 100 adenomas throughout the colon
- 50% have adenomas by age 15
- 95% have adenomas by age 35
- Colon cancer risk - 100%
- Mean age colon cancer 39 yrs
    - Giardiello et al., Gastroenterology, 2001

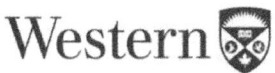

C. DIFFICILE INFECTION

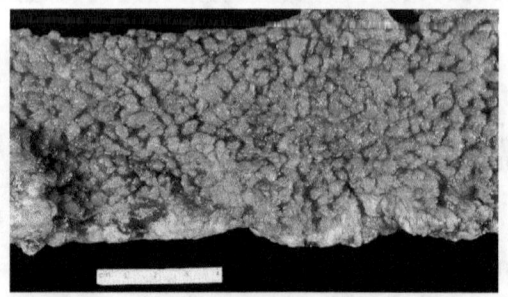

FAP: Familial Adenomatous Polyposis

Extracolonic Manifestations of FAP

Other	Cancer

o Eye
    − CHRPE (Congenital hypertrophy of the retinal pigment epithelium)
	o Brain
	    − Medulloblastoma (FAP)
	    − Glioblastoma (HNPCC)

o ENT − Nasopharyngeal angiofibromas	o Thyroid

o Mouth, jaw
    − Radiopaque jaw lesions
    − Supernumerary teeth
	o Duodenum
	o Periampullary region
	o Pancreas
	o Hepatoblastoma
	o Biliary tree

o Desmoid tumors o Osteomas	

MINI UPDATE

Cancer Risk in FAP

Cancer	Lifetime Risk
o Colon	~100%
o Duodenal/periampullary	5-12%
o Gastic	~0.5%
o Pancreatic	~2%
o Thyroid	~2%
o CNS	<1%
o Hepatoblastoma (age < 5)	1.6%

Genetics

- o Mutation of the tumour suppressor gene on the long arm of chromosome 5 q21 – q22 region
- o MUTYH is a base-excision-repair gene on chromosome 1
- o 70% of the germline defects in APC are inherited, while 15-25% occur spontaneously
- o Mutations or deletions in the APC gene are present in 90% of FAP and 30% of AFAP

Variants of FAP

- o Gardner's = FAP + extracolonic manifestations
- o Turcot's = familial polyposis + primary CNS tumors
    - medulloblastomas (APC mutations) - FAP/Turcot's
    - glioblastomas (HNPCC mutations) - HNPCC/Turcot's
- o Attenuated adnomatous polyposis coli (AAPC)
    - fewer adenomas (<100)

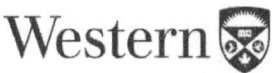

- Polyps by median age 35-45
- Cancer by median age 55
  - often R-sided (like HNPCC)
  - flat adenomas
  - germline APC mutations
    - proximal and distal ends of gene
  - Lifetime risk of CRC 69%

FAP Screening Guidelines

- Mutation screening of at risk individuals age 10-12
  - at risk = 1st degree relatives of FAP patients
- If no mutation → annual flex sig age 12-50
- Upper endoscopy q1-3 years starting at time of colectomy or age 20
  - upper GI polyps rare prior to onset of colonic disease
  - side viewing duodenoscope should be used
- Annual thyroid exam starting at age 10-12
- ? periodic abdo US after age 20 (pancreatic cancer)
- Periodic CT head in families with CNS neoplasms

Source: Sleisenger & Fordtran's - 7th ed; Giardiello FM, et al. *Gastroenterology*, 2001 ;121(1):198-213; Bronner MP, et al. *Mod Pathol*, 2003 ;16(4):359-65; Canadian Association of Gastroenterology (CAG); American College of Gastroenterology (ACG); American Society for Gastrointestinal Endoscopy (ASGE)

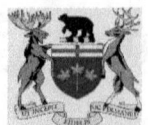

MINI UPDATE

MUTYH Associated Polyposis

- ➢ M(UT)YH Gene Mutations
  - o Germline mutations in MYH base excision repair gene discovered
    - – Al-Tassan et al. *Nat Genet*, 2002
  - o Role of MUTYH:
    - – base excision repair glycosylase involved in the repair of oxidative damage to guanine
    - – Prevents G/C to T/A transversions
      - ▪ Frequently occurs in APC coding regions
      - ▪ Transversions seen for k-RAS in 70% of individuals with MAP (mitogen-activated protein)
  - o 25-30% of AFAP patients with >10-15 adenomas have MUTYH biallelic mutations
    - – Sieber OM, et al., *N Engl J Med*, 2003 ;348(9):791-9.
    - – Sampson et al., *Lancet*, 2003 ;362(9377):39-41.

- ➢ MUTYH Polyposis Genetics
  - o Bi-allelic mutation in MUTYH
    - – Mutations in two hotspots, Y165C or G382D, account for 70% of all Caucasian mutations
    - – Full gene sequencing if these are negative
    - – Significant polyposis similar to AFAP/FAP with (-) mutations in APC should be tested for MUYTH mutations
  - o Autosomal RECESSIVE
    - – Siblings of affected patients have 25% of having MUTYH mutation
    - – Unlike FAP, parents and children are rarely affected

- ➢ MUTYH Phenotype
  - o Phenotype mimics attenuated FAP

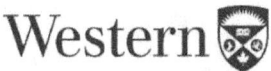

- CRC penetrance: 19% at 50, 43% at 60, 80% lifetime
  o Polyposis typically by 40's
    - Adenomatous, Hyperplastic, SSA
  o UGI polyps in 11-17%
    - Duodenal Cancer in 4%
  o Possible increase in: ovarian, bladder, skin, sebaceous glands, and breast
  o Clinical diagnostic criteria NOT established
  o Genetic testing warranted in individuals with 10 adenomatous polyps without identifiable mutations in APC

➤ MUYTH Management
  o Colonoscopy q2-3y: start mid 20's in at risk individuals
  o Subtotal colectomy if cancer, lots of polyps, large polyps, or HGD
  o UGI tract screening as per FAP
    - EGD q1-3y starting age 25

- Give 20 **extracolonic manifestations** of FAP.

  o Gastrointestinal other than colon
    - Stomach
      ▪ Fundic gland polyps
    - Duodenum
      ▪ Ampullary cancer
      ▪ Duodenal cancer

  o Extraintestinal associations of the **Gardner syndrome** variant of FAP

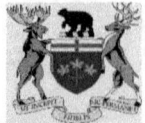

MINI UPDATE

- Osteomas
    - Jaw (in 90% of ES)
    - Cysts
    - Impacted teeth
    - Extra teeth
    - Skull
    - Long bones

- Exostoses

- Soft tissue tumors (benign)
    - Desmoid
    - Fibromas
    - Lipomas
    - Diffuse mesenteric fibromatosis
    - $300/10^5$ person-years
    - Treat with NSAIDs and tamoxifin chemotherapy, colectomy small bowel transplantation
    - May be a lethal association

- Cysts
    - Epidermoid (aka inclusion cysts)
    - Sebaceous

- Endocrine tumors
    - Thyroid papillary tumor
    - Adrenal

- Eye
    - CHRPE (congenital hypertrophy of the retinal pigmented epithelium)
    - Multiple in 63%
    - Bilateral in 87%

- Teeth
    - Supernumerary teeth
- Skin

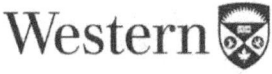

C. DIFFICILE INFECTION

- Desmoid tumors
- Epidermoid cysts
- Fibromas
- Lipoma
- Sebaceous cysts
  - Mesentery
    - Mesenteric fibromatosis
  - Bone
    - Osteomas
      - Skull
      - Jaw
  - Turcot syndrome (associated with FAP)
    - Medulloblastoma

  - And still more: "familial tooth agenesis" is caused by mutation in APC pathway (AXIN2)
    - Both adenomatous and hyperplastic colonic polyps

MCQ Trick

- Remember: FAP in its classical form may be associated with dental abnormalities and osteomas of the jaw, without being considered to be a Gardner variant.
- Also remember, osteomas and CHRPH may occur in MUTYH

Abbreviations: CHRPE, congenital hypertrophy of retinal pigmented epithelium (pigmented spots on the fundus of the eye)

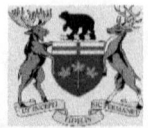

MINI UPDATE

SO YOU WANT TO BE A GASTROENTEROLOGIST!

- About 60% to 90% of FAP patients have periampullary adenomatous polyps, and about 10% will develop duodenal cancer.
- Clearly, FAP patients require surveillance with SV-EGD (side-viewing EGD, esophagogastroduodenoscopy).
- Risk stratification for the development of duodenal cancer is based on the Spigelman classification
- This Spigelman classification provides guidance for EGD surveillance of these duodenal adenomas. Until EUS has refined our appreciation for any change in the currently recommended EGD surveillance guidelines, this remains the standard of care.
- Screening with SV-EGD should begin at 2 years of age, and then be followed by regular SV-EGD surveillance.

Give the recommended interval of duodenoscopic screening (visualization and biopsy) of duodenal polyps in FAP, using the **Spigelman staging criteria**.

Score	1	2	3
Polyp count	1-4	5-20	>20
Polyp size (mm)	1-4	5-10	>10
Histologic type	Tubular	Tubulovillous	Villous
Grade of intraepithelial neoplasia	Low-grade	Intermediate*	High-grade

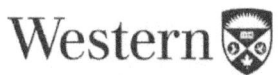

C. DIFFICILE INFECTION

Grade	Surveillance interval (years)
O	5
I, II	3
III	1
IV	3-6 months – pylorus preserving, pancreas sparing duoden

Stage 0: 0 points, Stage I: 1-4 points, Stage II: 5-6 points, Stage III: 7-8 points, and stage IV: 9-12 points

*Intermediate grade is not existent in actualized classifications of intraepithelial neoplasia

Printed with permission: Schulmann K, et al. *Best Pract Res Clin Gastroenterol* 2007; 21(3): pg 413.

Turcot Syndrome
- o Definition: ".... a syndrome of familial colonic polyposis with primary tumors of the central nervous system" (Feldman M., et al. Sleisenger and Fordtran's Gastrointestinal and Liver Disease. 9th Edition. Saunders/Elsevier, Philadelphia, 2010, page 2184).

MINI UPDATE

SO YOU WANT TO BE A GASTROENTEROLOGIST!

- o The **Turcot syndrome** is considered to be variant of FAP, and as such has a mutation in the APC gene.

- Give the reason why the Turcot syndrome may be misclassified, and should be considered either as a variant of HNPCC, or an overlap of both FAP and HNPCC.

    - o In Turcot syndrome, the gene mutations are in FAP, or in DNA MMR, the same germline mutation seen in HNPCC.

- Give the difference in the CNS presentation of Turcot syndrome, depending upon which germline mutation is present.
    - o Gene mutation in
        - APC
            - Medulloblastomas
        - DNA MMR
            - Glioblastoma multiforme tumors (familial tooth agenesis)
    - o It may be surprising to learn, but there are actually at least two attenuated adenomatous polyposis syndrome.

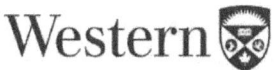

C. DIFFICILE INFECTION

> **Exam Alert**
> - In the clinical examiner tells you that the patient has colonic polyps and hands you a fundoscope.
> - She/he is expecting you to look for pigmented lesions in the ocular fundus, suggesting CHRPE in the Gardner variant of FAP.

> **Useful Quote**
>
> "The presence of multiple [CHRPE] lesions appears to be a reliable marker for gene carriage in FAP" (Feldman M., et al. Sleisenger and Fordtran's Gastrointestinal and Liver Disease. 9th Edition. Saunders/Elsevier, Philadelphia, 2010, page 2180).

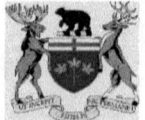

MINI UPDATE

SO YOU WANT TO BE A GASTROENTEROLOGIST – NERD

- o The second most lethal complication of the Gardner variant of FAP is desmoid tumor (diffuse mesenteric fibromatosis).
- o A strong family history of FAP increases the risk of having desmoid tumors.
- o Treatment may include an NSAID, tamoxifen, sulindac plus tamoxifen, progesterone; chemotherapy; resection, and even small bowel transplantation.

- Give the **Church staging system** for desmoid tumors in the Gardner variant of FAP.

    Staging system for desmoid tumors in Gardner variant of FAP.

Findings	I	II	III	IV
Symptoms	No	Mild	Moderate*	Severe
Size, cm	< 10	< 10	10-20	> 20
Growth	No	No	Slow	Rapid

*May be associated with symptoms of obstruction of the bowel or ureter

Adapted from: Feldman M., et al. Sleisenger and Fordtran's Gastrointestinal and Liver Disease. 9th Edition. Saunders/Elsevier, Philadelphia, 2010, Table 122.16, page 2182.

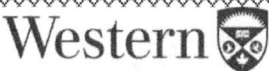

C. DIFFICILE INFECTION

➢ Management

- Give the clinical management of FAP (familial adenomatous polyposis)
  - Genetic testing
    - Consider genetic testing between ages 10 to 12 years, as it will first be clinically useful.
    - May need to begin in first decade of life to determine who should be screened for hepatoblastoma

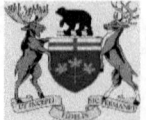

MINI UPDATE

SO YOU WANT TO BE A GASTROENTEROLOGIST!

- Genetic testing in FAP is important because there may be skipped generations, and 20% of FAP patients may have gene mutation.
- It is important in the screening of the family to know the genetic mutation in the index patient (performed on DNA from peripheral blood WBCs), and to better focus on which mutation to look for in the next-of-kin, and to provide better genetic counseling.

- While all the family needs to be tested, if resources are a limiting factor, give the family groups that should be tested in FAP and MUTYH.
    - FAP autosomal dominant (1 in 2)
        - Parents and children
    - MUTYH autosomal recessive (1 in 4)
        - Siblings and spouses

- Give the postulated mechanism for the benefit of NSAIDs / ASA / Coxibs in the regressive of adenomatous polyps.
    - With adenomatous polyps → ↑ COX-2 expression
    - ↑ COX-2 → ↓ apoptosis
    - NSAIDs / ASA / Coxibs → ↓ COX-2
        - ↑ apoptosis
            - ↑ conversion of sphingomyelin to ceramide
        - ↑ arachidonic acid →
            - ↓ PPAR and gene
            - ↑ arachidonic acid

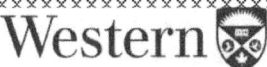

C. DIFFICILE INFECTION

- GI tract screening
  - Colon cancer risk > 90%
  - Sigmoidoscopy in gene carriers every 1 to 2 years, beginning at age 10 years, or in all at-risk persons if genetic testing is not done or not informative.
  - Colonoscopy every 2 years beginning at age 20 in families with AFAP/AAPC, or sometimes earlier, depending on the age of polyp emergence in other family members
  - Upper GI endoscopy
    - Upper GI tract (5-10% cancer risk for duodenal or peri-ampillary, 0.5% for gastric)
    - Begin when colon polyps emerge or by age 25 years
    - Repeat every 1 to 3 years, depending on the number of polyps, their size and histology
    - Side viewing should be performed as part of the examination to carefully identify and examine the duodenal papilla.
  - Small bowel
    - Diagnostic imaging should be done before colectomy.
    - Should be done if numerous or large adenomas are present in the duodenum
    - Frequency determined by number and size of lesions found
  - Pancreas (2% cancer risk) -periodic US (abdominal ultrasound) after age 20
  - Hepatoblastoma (1.6 % of children <5 yrs) EUS (endoscopic ultrasound), AFP (alpha-fetoprotein) during first decade of life
  - Non GI tract screening

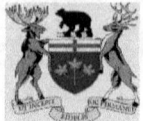

MINI UPDATE

- Thyroid (2%) – annual thyroid exam starting age 20
- Cerebellar meduloblastoma (<1%) – possible periodic head CT

Adapted from: Half EE, and Bresalier RS. *Curr Opin Gastroenterol* 2004;20(1):32-42.

- Give the recommended method, age to begin, interval of screening, and management of the person with FAP.

Screening method	Age to begin	Interval	Management
o Colonoscopy or flexible sigmoidoscopy	– 10-12 years, or late teens if attenuated FAP	▪ If polyps are detected, screen annually until colectomy	Colectomy is recommended when polyps become too numerous to monitor safely, or if polyps are ≥ 1 cm or exhibit advanced histology. Removal of the rectum should be based on polyp burden and family history.
o Flexible sigmoidoscopy	– Within two years after colectomy	▪ Every 6 months to 3 years depending on polyp size and number	Chemoprevention with NSAIDs may be considered
o EGD with end and side viewing instrument	– 20-25 years or at the onset of colonic polyps	▪ 3 yrs if stage[1] 0, II ▪ 2 yrs if stage[1] III	Chemoprevention with NSAIDs is less effective for

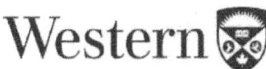

C. DIFFICILE INFECTION

Screening method	Age to begin	Interval
	• 6-12 months if stage IV	upper GI adenomas
o Physical examination	– 10 to 12 years	• Annually
o Physical exam, hepatic ultrasound, and alphafetoprotein	– 6 months	• Every 6 months during first decade of life
o Determined by location of suspected desmoids, often abdominal CT	– When palpable mass or relevant symptoms present	

[1]Spigelman staging criteria

Printed with permission: Burt RW. *2007 AGA Institute Postgraduate Course.* pg. 236.

HNPCC

- ➢ Epidemiology
    - o 2-4% of CRC
    - o Polyposis is rare
    - o CRC in 50-80%
        - – younger age
        - – Proximal tumors

- ➢ Genetics
    - o Germline mutation in DNA mismatch repair genes
    - o Maintain genomic stability
        - – Repair single base pair mismatches
        - – Repair insertion or deletion loops

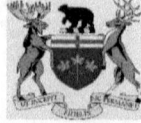

MINI UPDATE

- Differences in Cancer Risk with Mutations

Mutation	Frequency	CRC Risk	Other cancer risk
hMSH2	90%	50-80%	40-60% endometrial
hMLH1			
hMSH6	10%	Lower than hMSH2/hMLH1	Higher than hMSH2/hMLH1
hPMS2	Rare	15-20%	15% endometrial 25-30% any Lynch Ca
EpCAM	6%		

- Diagnosis
  - Clinical Diagnosis
    - Amsterdam 1 and 2
      - 50% of families with HNPCC fail to meet Amsterdam 1 criteria
    - Bethesda
      - Identify pts at risk who require further testing
      - Genetic testing for individuals at risk: can miss 28% of HNPCC cases
    - 4 MMR genes and EpCAM
  - Test Tumor for MMR mutations (MSI analysis or IHC)
    - 90% of HNPCC tumors will be +
    - 15% of sporadic CRC will be + from somatic hypermethylation of hMLH1

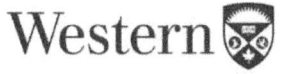

C. DIFFICILE INFECTION

> **Terminology Caution**
> o While Lynch syndrome is one of the hereditary colon cancer syndromes, it is not a cause of multiple polyposis, so is **not** one of the polyposis syndrome.

➢ Guidelines

- Give the clinical guidelines for the diagnosis of Lynch Syndrome

- **Amsterdam I criteria**

At least three relatives with *colorectal cancer* including all of the following:
  o At least two successive generations be involved
  o One should be a first degree relative of the other two
  o At least one colorectal cancer case diagnosed before the age of 50 years
  o FAP should be excluded in any cases of colorectal cancer
  o Tumors should be verified by pathological examination

- **Amsterdam II criteria**

Thre relatives with *Lynch-associated cancer* (colorectal, endometrial, small bowel, ureter, or renal pelvis) including all of the following:
  o At least two successive generations should be involved
  o One should be first relative of the two

MINI UPDATE

- Cancer in one of the affected individuals should be diagnosed before the age of 50 years
- FAP should be excluded in any cases of colorectal cancer
- Tumors should be verified by pathological examination

Amsterdam Criteria (3-2-1)

- **≥ 3** first degree relatives with CRC / Lynch-associated tumor
- ≥2 generations affect with CRC / Lynch-associated tumor
- **≥ 1** < 50 yr old
- **≥ 1** first degree relative of the other family members
- **No** FAP

Useful background: In families not meeting the Amsterdam criteria, three approaches have been suggested:

➤ The frequent presence of micro-satellite errors in tumour tissue is called micro-satellite instability (MSI)
  - MSI is present in >90% of colon cancers in HNPCC. MSI is present in only about 15% of sporadic colon cancers, and occurs usually by a different mechanism.
  - MSI is easily detected in tumour tissue and is often used as a marker that leads to the suspicion of HNPCC. l
  - It has been suggested that MSI testing be done on tumours when one of the "Bethesda criteria" are met. They are as follows:
  - Individuals with cancer in families that meet the Amsterdam criteria

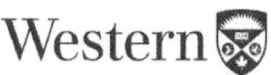

- Individuals with two HNPCC-related cancers, including synchronous and metachronous colorectal cancers or associated extracolonic cancers*

> Apply MSI testing to the colon cancer tissue in the following situations and when positive, perform mutation findings in DNA from peripheral blood:
- CRC diagnosis <50 yrs
- CRC plus one first-degree relative with colon or endometrial cancer
- CRC plus a previous colon or endometrial cancer
- With this method, 24% of colon cancer cases will undergo MSI testing of the tumour, and 4% of colon cancer cases will have mutation finding in the MMR gene

> Use a specific logistic model applied to an extended family that includes kindred structure and known cancer cases
- If the model predicts >20% chance of HNPCC, go directly to mutation finding.
- If the model predicts <20% chance of HNPCC, first do MSI and if positive, go to mutation finding

The Amsterdam criteria for HNPCC do not include the extracolonic cancers (Lynch tumors) which may occur in these families

- The Bethesda guidelines contain reference to both the colonic and extracolonic cancers, and serve as guidelines as to who with CRC should be tested for microsatellite instability (MSD).
- The Bethesda criteria were developed to identify persons whose tumours should be tested for microsatellite instability, the tumour fingerprint, the DNA MMR gene mutation.

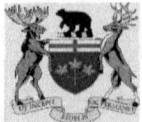

MINI UPDATE

- Go directly to MMR mutation finding if one of the first three Bethesda criteria for testing tumour tissue is positive, but use age <50 years, rather than 45 yrs. In one study this approach gave a sensitivity of 94%, and a specificity of 49%.

    o Over 95% of families in whom mutations have been found have mutations of either the MSH2 or MSH1 genes, which are responsible for replication error repair. These types of errors usually occur during DNA replication. They are most often one or several base pairs in length. Mutation of the MMR genes leads to rapid accumulation of relocation error, and frequently are found in DNA repeats, singlets, doublets, or triplets, called microsatellites

    o Individuals with CRC and a first-degree relative with CRC and/or diagnosed at age <45 yrs, and an adenoma diagnosed at age <45 yrs

    o Individuals with CRC or endometrial cancer diagnosed at age <45 yrs

    o Individuals with right-sided colorectal cancer with an undifferentiated pattern (solid/ cribriform) on histopathology diagnosed at age <45 yrs

    o Individuals with signet-ring-cell-type colorectal cancer diagnosed at age <45 yrs

    o Individuals with adenomas diagnosed at age <40yrs

    o Endometrial, ovarian, gastric, hepatobiliary, or small bowel cancer or transitional cell carcinoma of the renal pelvis or ureter

    o Genetic errors that accumulate when the MMR genes are mutated and dysfunctional are quite specific and include genes such as TGF-beta and BAX

    o Mutations in any one of the MMR genes leads to HNPCC

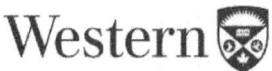

C. DIFFICILE INFECTION

Adapted from. Bresalier RS, and Schiller, L. *Sleisenger & Fordtran's gastrointestinal and liver disease: Pathophysiology/Diagnosis/Management* 2006: pg. 2774.; and Printed with permission: Burt R. *2007 AGA Institute Postgraduate course*: 237.

Bethesda Criteria (for testing tumour tissue)

- Persons who have had 2 Lynch tumours
- Persons with a Lynch tumour with a first degree relative under 50
- Persons with a Lynch tumour in at least 2 first- or second-degree relatives at any age
- CRC diagnosed before age 50
- CRC with MSI-related histological features diagnosed before age 60

➤ **Revised Bethesda guidelines**
- Colorectal cancer diagnosed in a patient who is less than 50 years of age
- Synchronous, metachronous colorectal cancer, ot other Lynch related cancer* regardless of age
- Colorectal cancer with MSI-H histology (presence of tumor infiltrating lymphocytes, Crohn's-like lymphocytic reaction, mucinous/signet-ring differentiation, or medullary growth pattern) diagnosed in a patient less than 60 years of age.
- Colorectal cancer diagnosed in one or more first-degree relatives with Lynch-related tumor*, with one of the cancer being diagnosed under age 50 years.
- Colorectal cancer diagnosed in two or more first- or second-degree relatives with Lynch-related tumors*, regardless of age

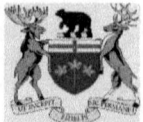

MINI UPDATE

*Includes endometrial, ovarian, gastric, small bowel, urinary tract, pancreas, brain, and sebaceous gland

[1] Lynch syndrome related cancers for these guidelines include colorectal, endometrial, stomach, ovarian, pancreas, ureter and renal pelvis, biliary tract, brain (usually glioblastoma), sebaceous gland adenomas, and keratoacanthomas.

[2] MSI associated histologic features include tumour infiltrating lymphocytes, Crohn-like lymphocytic reaction, mucinous/signet-ring differentiation, or medullary growth pattern.

Printed with permission: Burt RW. *2007 AGA Institute Postgraduate Course:* pg. 237.

Please also see Feldman M., et al. Sleisenger and Fordtran's Gastrointestinal and Liver Disease. 9th Edition. Saunders/Elsevier, Philadelphia, 2010, Table 123.5, page 2206.

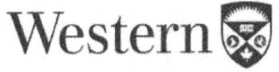

C. DIFFICILE INFECTION

➤ Management of HNPCC

Condition: Inheritance	Gene	Lifetime Cancer Risks		Non-Malignant Features
Lynch syndrome: Autosomal dominant	kMLH1	Colon	50-80%	Physical or non-malignant features, besides keratinocarcinomas and sebaceous adenomas / carcinomas, are rare
	kMLH2	Endometrium	40-60%	
	kMSH6	Stomach	11-19%	
	kPMS2	Ovary	9-12%	
	EpCAM	Hepatobiliary tract	4-5%	
		Upper urinary tract	4-5%	
		Pancreatic	3-4%	
		Small bowel	1-4%	
		CNS (glioblastoma)	1-3%	

➤ Why HNPCC polyps might be missed
- HNPCC polyps may occur sporatically
- The family may not have been carefully detailed (especially forgetting to use the Bethesda criteria and include high risk "Lynch" extraintestinal cancers).
- The clinical suspicion of HNPCC may not be properly recorded on the pathology requisition.

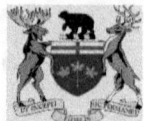

MINI UPDATE

- o Failure to diagnosis HNPCC has serious consequences for the patient and their family (not to mention the physician, who may be exposed to malpractice claims).
- o Sometimes the pathologist may consider that an adenomatous polyp is truly an HNPCC polyp from the histopathology.

(Please see Feldman M., et al. Sleisenger and Fordtran's Gastrointestinal and Liver Disease. 9th Edition. Saunders/Elsevier, Philadelphia, 2010, Table 123.6, page 2206).

> Pathology

- Give 5 characteristic pathologic features of tumours that are highly suggestive of microsatellite instability (MSI) (Lynch syndrome).
    - o Endoscopic
        - Multiple
        - Synchronous
        - Metachronous
        - Right-sided
    - o Microscopic
        - Lymphocytes infiltrating the CRC tumour
        - Mucinous histology ("signet ring")
        - Poor differentiation
        - Lack of "dirty" necrosis

Please see Feldman M., et al. Sleisenger and Fordtran's Gastrointestinal and Liver Disease. 9th Edition. Saunders/Elsevier, Philadelphia, 2010, Table 122.1, page 2172, Surveillance Recommendations After Colonoscopic Polypectomy".

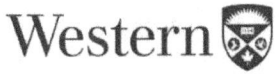

C. DIFFICILE INFECTION

- **Muir-Torre Syndrome**
  - Extracolonic cancer in HNPCC is known as the Muir-Torre variant
  - A rare subset of HNPCC associated genetically with
    - MSI
    - Loss of expression
      hMLH1
      hMSH2
  - Associated cancers
    - Skin
      - Keratoacanthomas
      - Sebaceous adenomas
    - Carcinomas
      - Basal call
      - Squamous
  - GI tract
    - Stomach
    - Small intestine
    - Biliary tree
  - GU
    - Ovary
    - Uterus
    - Ureter
  - CNS
    - Brain

MINI UPDATE

- Give 5 of the screening and management guidelines for Lynch syndrome.

Cancer	Screening	Age to start	Interval	Treatment
o Stomach	EGD	30-35 yrs	Every 1-2 yrs	
o Small bowel[2]	Small bowel enteroclysis	30-35 yrs	Every 1-2 yrs	
o Colon	Colonoscopy	20-25 yrs (or 10 yrs before the earliest diagnosis in the family)	Every 1-2 years	Consider colectomy if cancer or advanced adenoma is found.
o Endometrial/ Ovarian	Endometrial biopsy (for pre-menopausal women) and transvaginal ultrasound (preferably day 1-10 of cycle) for premenopausal women CA125	30-35 yrs (or 5-10 yrs before the earliest diagnosis in the family) 30-35 yrs	Annually Every 6-12 mon	Consider prophylactic TAH/BSO after childbearing Consider oral contraceptives for premeno-pausal women.

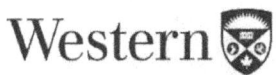

C. DIFFICILE INFECTION

Cancer	Screening	Age to start	Interval
o CNS	MRI	CNS symptoms	Every 1-2 yrs
o Urinary tract	Pelvic and abdominal US	30-35 yrs	Annually
	Urinalysis with cytology	30-35 yrs	
o Biliary tract, gallbladder	Liver function tests	30-35 yrs	Every 1-2 yrs

Abbreviations: TAN/BSO, total abdominal hysterectomy, bilateral salpingo-oophorectomy; CNS, central nervous system; EGD, esophagogastroduodenoscopy.

Printed with permission: Burt RW. *2007 AGA Institute Postgraduate Course.* pg. 240.

NCCN Guidelines for Extracolonic Cancer Surveillance in Lynch Syndrome

- o Gastric and duodenal cancer
    - Upper gastrointestinal endoscopy wwith side-veiwing examination at age 25-30 years with repeat examination in 1-3 years
- o Urothelial cancer
    - Annual urinalysis
- o CNS cancers
    - Annual physical examination. No recommendations have been made
- o Pancreatic cancer
    - Annual physical examination. No recommendations have been made

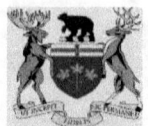

MINI UPDATE

- o Endometrial and ovarian cancer
  - Patient education and response to endometrial cancer symptoms
  - Referral to gynecologic oncologist for surveillance (annual endometrial sampling
  - Transvaginal ultrasound, and serial CA-125 measurements starting by age 30-35 years before the earliest age in the family)
  - Consider prophylactic total abdominal hysterectomy and salpingo-oophrectomy after completion of childbearing or during colectomy

Printed with permission: Venesio, T et al. *Gastroenterology* 2004; 126: 1681-5.

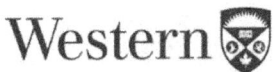

C. DIFFICILE INFECTION

References and Suggested Reading

Ahnen DJ, et al. Approach to the patient with colonic polyps. *UpToDate.* www.uptodate.com, 2014

Ahnen DJ. The American College of Gastroenterology Emily Couric Lecture--the adenoma-carcinoma sequence revisited: has the era of genetic tailoring finally arrived? *Am J Gastroenterol* 2011;106(2):190-198.

Almansa C., et al. Association between visual gaze patterns and adenoma detection rate during colonoscopy: a preliminary investigation. *Am J Gastroenterol* 2011;106:1070-1074.

Aminalai A., et al. Live image processing does not increase adenoma detection rate during colonoscopy: a randomized comparison between FICE and conventional imaging (Berlin Colonoscopy Project 5, BECOP-5). *Am J Gastroenterol* 2010;105:2383-2388.

Anke ML, et al. Effect of a retrograde-viewing device on adenoma detection rate during colonoscopy: the TERRACE study. *Gastrointestinal Endoscopy* 2011;73:480-489.

Armstrong D, et al. Point of care, peer comparator colonoscopy practice audit: The Canadian Association of Gastroenterology quality program- endoscopy. *Can J Gastroenterol* 2011;25:13-20.

ASGE Technology Committee, Mamula P, et al. Colonoscopy preparation. *Gastrointest Endos* 2009;69(7):1201-1209.

Augsten M, et al. A digest on the role of the tumour microenvironment in gastrointestinal cancers. *Cancer Microenviron* 2010;3:167-176.

Backman V, et al. Light-scattering technologies for field carcinogenesis detection: a modality for endoscopic prescreening. *Gastroenterology* 2011;140:35-41.

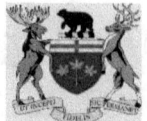

MINI UPDATE

Bannert C, et al. Sedation in screening colonoscopy: impact on quality indicators and complications. *Am J Gastroenterol* 2012;107(12):1837-1848.

Bellam N, et al. TGF-beta signaling alterations and colon cancer. *Cancer Treat Res* 2010;155:85-103.

Belsey J, et al. Meta-analysis: the relative efficacy of oral bowel preparations for colonoscopy 1985-2010. *Aliment Pharmacol Ther* 2012;35(2):222-237.

Benjamin L, et al. The impact of suboptimal bowel preparation on adenoma miss rates and the factors associated with early repeat colonoscopy *Gastrointest Endos* 2011;73(6):1207-14.

Benson M, et al. A Comparison of Optical Colonoscopy and CT Colonography Screening Strategies in the Detection and Recovery of Subcentimeter Adenomas. *Am J Gastroenterol* 2010;105:2578-2585.

Bonadona V, et al. Cancer risks associated with germline mutations in MLH1, MSH2, and MSH6 genes in Lynch syndrome. *Journal of the Am Med Assoc* 2011;305:2304-2310.

Bourke MJ and Rex DK. Tips for better colonoscopy from two experts. *Am J Gastroenterol* 2012;107(10):1467-1472.

Brown SR, et al. Chromoscopy versus conventional endoscopy for the detection of polyps in the colon and rectum. *Cochrane Database of Systematic Reviews*. 2010; 10: CD006439.

Buddingh KT, et al. Locaion in the right hemi-colon is an independent risk factor for delayed post-polypectomy hemorrhage: a multi-center case-control study. *Am J Gastroenterol* 2011;106:1119-1124.

Burke CA, et al. A comparison of high-definition versus conventional colonoscopies for polyp detection. *Dig Dis Sci* 2010;55:1716-1720.

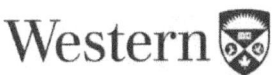

Butte JM, et al. Rate of residual disease after complete endoscopic resection of malignant colonic polyp. *Dis Colon Rectum* 2012;55(2):122-127.

Carlson CM, et al. Lack of follow-up after fecal occult blood testing in older adults: inappropriate screening or failure to follow up? *Arch Intern Med* 2011;171(3):249-256.

Corporaal S, et al. Low-volume PEG plus ascorbic acid versus high-volume PEG as bowel preparation for colonoscopy. *Scand J Gastroenterol* 2010;45:1380-1386.

Cristina A, et al. Association Between Visual Gaze Patterns and Adenoma Detection Rate During Colonoscopy: A Preliminary Investigation. *Am J Gastroenterol* 2011;106:1070–1074.

Dalerba P, et al. Single-cell dissection of transcriptional heterogeneity in human colon tumors. *Nat Biotechnol* 2011;29(12):1120-1127.

de Jonge V, et al. Systematic literature review and pooled analyses of risk factors for finding adenomas at surveillance colonoscopy. *Endoscopy* 2011;43(7):5605-72.

de Wijkerslooth TR, et al. Immunochemical fecal occult blood testing is equally sensitive for proximal and distal advanced neoplasia. *Am J Gastroenterol* 2012;107(10):1570-1578.

DeMarco D.C., et al. Impact of experience with a retrograde-viewing device on adenoma detection rates and withdrawal times during colonoscopy: The Third Eye Retroscope study group. *Gastrointestinal Endoscopy* 2010;71:542-550.

East JE, et al. Dynamic patient position changes during colonoscope withdrawal increase adenoma detection: a randomized, crossover trail. *Gastrointest Endos* 2011;73:456-463.

East JE, et al. Sporadic and syndromic hyperplastic polyps and serrated adenomas of the colon: classification,

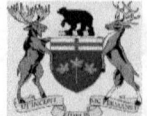

MINI UPDATE

molecular genetics, natural history, and clinical management. *Gastroenterol Clin North Am* 2008;37:25-46.

Efthymiou M, et al. Biopsy forceps is inadequate for the resection of diminutive polyps. *Endoscopy* 2011;43:312-316.

Enestvedt BK, et al. 4-Liter split-dose polyethylene glycol is superior to other bowel preparations, based on systematic review and meta-analysis. *Clin Gastroenterol Hepatol* 2012;10(11):1225-1231.

Ghosh S, et al. Practice audit in gastroenterology- the route to improving quality and safely. *Can J Gastroenterol* 2011;25:12

Giardiello FM, et al. Peutz-Jeghers syndrome and management recommendations. *Clin Gastroenterol Hepatol* 2006;4:408-415.

Glynne-Jones R, et al. Multimodal treatment of rectal cancer. *Best Pract Res Clin Gastroenterol* 2007;21(6):1049-1070.

Goodman A. Minorities benefit from more sophisticated colon cancer screening. *Oncol News Intl* 2010;19:7.

Gross CP, et al. Assessing the impact of screening colonoscopy on mortality in the medicare population. *J Gen Intern Med* 2011;26(12):1441-1449.

Gupta N, et al. Accuracy of in vivo optical diagnosis of colon polyp histology by narrow-band imaging in predicting colonoscopy surveillance intervals. *Gastrointest Endosc* 2012;75(3):494-502.

Gurudu SR, et al. Adenoma detection rate is not influenced by the timing of colonoscopy when performed in half-day blocks. *Am J Gastroenterol* 2011;106(8):1466-1471.

Gurudu SR, et al. Sessile serrated adenomas: demographic, endoscopic and pathological

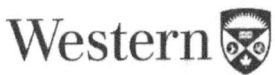

characteristics. *World J Gastroenterol* 2010;16:3402-3405.

Hassan C, et al. Performance improvements of imaging based screening tests. *Best Pract Res Clin Gastroenterol* 2010;24:493-507.

Hazewinkel Y, et al. Colonoscopy: basic principles and novel techniques. *Nat Rev gastroenterol Hepatol* 2011; 8: 554-564.

Heresbach D, et al. A national survey of endoscopic mucosal resection for superficial gastrointestinal neoplasia. *Endoscopy* 2010;42:806-813.

Hewett DG, et al. Colonoscopy and diminutive polyps: hot or cold biopsy or snare? Do I send to pathology? *Clin Gastroenterol Hepatol* 2011;9:102-105.

Hewett DG, et al. Miss rate of right-sided colon examination during colonoscopy defined by retroflexion: an observational study. *Gastrointest Endos* 2011;74:246-52.

Ignjatovic A, et al. What is the most reliable imaging modality for small colonic polyp characterization? Study of white-light. Autofluorescence, narrow-band imaging. *Endoscopy* 2011;43:94-99.

Inadomi J. Interval Cancers After Colonoscopy: The Importance of Training. *Am J Gastroenterol* 2010;105:2597-2598.

Ivan J, et al. The Submucosal Cushion Does Not Improve the Histologic Evalutaion of Adenomatous Colon Polyps Resected by Snare Polypectomy. *Clin Gastroenterol Hepatol* 2011;9:910-913.

Johnson CD, et al. Accuracy of CT colonography for detection of large adenomas and cancers. *N Engl J Med* 2008 Sep 18;359(12):1207-1217.

Jovanovic I, et al. The submucosal cushion does not improve the histologic evaluation of adenomatous colon

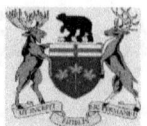

MINI UPDATE

polyps resected by snare polypectomy. *Clin Gastroenterol Hepatol* 2011;9:910-913.

Kahi CJ, et al. Prevalence and variable detection of proximal colon serrated polyps during screening colonoscopy. *Clin Gastroenterol Hepatol* 2011;9:42-46.

Kaminski M.F., et al. Quality indicators for colonoscopy and the risk of interval cancer. *N Engl J Med* 2010;362:1795-1803.

Kessler WR, et al. A quantitative assessment of the risks and cost savings of forgoing histologic examination of diminutive polyps. *Endoscopy* 2011;43(8):683-691.

Keswani RN. Single-ballon colonoscopy versus repeat standard colonoscopy for previous incomplete colonoscopy: a randomized, controlled trial. *Gastrointest Endos* 2011;73:507-512.

Kilgore TW, et al. Bowel preparation with split-dose polyethylene glycol before colonoscopy: a meta-analysis of randomized controlled trials. *Gastrointest Endos* 2011;73:1240-1245.

Ko CW, et al. Serious complications within 30 days of screeing and surveillance colonoscopy are uncommon. *Clin Gastroenterol Hepatol* 2010;8:166-173.

Kuiper T, et al. Endoscopic trimodal imaging detects colonic neoplasia as well as standard video enscopy. *Gastroenterology* 2011;140:1887-1894.

Laiyemo AO, et al. Likelihood of missed and recurrent adenomas in the proximal versus the distal colon. *Gastrointest Endos* 2011;74(2):253-261.

Lawrance IC, et al. Bowel cleansing for colonoscopy: prospective randomized assessment of efficacy and of induced mucosal abnormality with three preparation agents. *Endoscopy* 2011;43:412-418.

Lee A, et al. Queue position in the endoscopic schedule impacts effectiveness of colonoscopy. *Am J Gastroenterol* 2011;106(8):1457-1465.

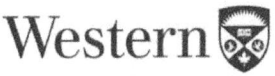

Lee JM, et al. Effects of hyosine N.-butyl bromide on the detection of polyps during colonoscopy. *Hepatogastroenterology* 2010;57:90-94.

Leedham SJ, et al. A basal gradient of Wnt and stem-cell number influences regional tumour distribution in human and mouse intestinal tracts. *Gut* 2012; 62(1):83-93

Leffler DA, et al. An alerting system improves adherence to follow-up recommendations from colonoscopy examinations. *Gastroenterology* 2011;140(4):1166-1173.

Leufkens AM, et al. Effect of a retrograde-viewing device on adenoma detection rate during colonoscopy: the TERRACE study. *Gastrointestinal Endoscopy* 2011;73:480-489.

Maas M, et al. Wait-and-see policy for clinical complete responders after chemoradiation for rectal cancer. *J Clin Oncol* 2011;29(35):4633-4640.

Mannath J, et al. Polyp recurrence after endoscopic mucosal resection of sessile and flat colonic adenomas. *Dig Dis Sci* 2011;56:2389-2395.

Mariani P, et al. Concordant analysis of KRAS status in primary colon carcinoma and matched metastasis. *Anticancer Research* 2010;30:4229-4233.

Marmo R, et al. Effective bowel cleansing before colonoscopy: a randomized study of split-dosage versus non-split dosage regimens of high-volume versus low-volume polyethylene glycol solutions. *Gastrointestinal Endoscopy* 2010;72:313-320.

Melton SD, et al. Biomarkers and molecular diagnosis of gastrointestinal and pancreatic neoplasms. *Nat Rev Gastroenterol Hepatol* 2010;7:620-628.

Moss A, et al. A randomized, double-blind trial of succinylated gelatin submucosal injection for endoscopic resection of large sessile polyp of the colon. *Am J Gastroenterol* 2010;105:2375-2382.

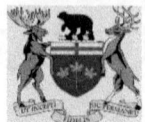

MINI UPDATE

Moss A, et al. Endoscopic mucosal resection outcomes and prediction of submucosal cancer from advanced colonic mucosal neoplasia. *Gastroenterology* 2011;140:1909-1918.

Müller SA, et al. Randomized clinical trial on the effect of coffee on postoperative ileus following elective colectomy. *Br J Surg* 2012;99(11):1530-1538.

Murthy S, et al. Novel colonoscopic imaging. *Clin Gastroenterol Hepatol* 2012;10(9):984-987.

Neerincx M, et al. Colonic work-up after incomplete colonoscopy: significant new findings during follow-up. *Endoscopy* 2010;42:730-735.

Nyberg C, et al. The safety of osmotically acting cathartics in colonic cleansing. *Nat Rev Gastroenterol Hepatol* 2010;7:557-564.

Nyberg C, et al. Adverse events associated with use of the three major types of osmotically acting cathartics. *Nat Rev gastroenterol Hepatol* 2010;7:558.

Nyberg C, et al. Risk factors for acute phosphate nephropathy. *Nat Rev gastroenterol Hepatol* 2010;7:559.

Pasha SF, et al. Comparison of the yield and miss rate of narrow band imaging and white light endoscopy in patients undergoing screening or surveillance colonoscopy: a meta-analysis. *Am J Gastroenterol* 2012;107(3):363-370.

Pohl J, et al. Pancolonic chromoendoscopy with indigo carmine versus standard colonoscopy for detection of neoplastic lesions: a randomized two-centre trial. *International Journal in Gastroenterology* 2011;60:485-490.

Radaelli F, et al. Warm water infusion versus air insufflation for unsedated colonoscopy: a randomized controlled trial. *Gastrointestinal Endoscopy* 2011;72:701-709.

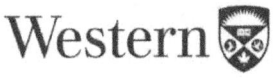

Ramsoekh D, et al. A back-to-back comparison of white light video endoscopy with autofluorescence endoscopy for adenoma detection in high-risk subjects. *International Journal in Gastroenterology* 2010;59:785-793.

Regula J, et al. Targeting risk groups for screening. *Best Pract Res Clin Gastroenterol* 2010;24:407-416.

Richard H Lash, et al. Sessile serrated adenomas: prevalence of dysplasia and carcinoma in 2139 patients. *Journal of Clinical Pathology* 2010;63:681-6.

Risio M. Reprint of : The natural history of adenomas. *Best Pract Res Clin Gastroenterol* 2010;24:397-406.

Roy HK, et al. Colonoscopy and optical biopsy: bridging technological advances to clinical practice. *Gastroenterology* 2011;140:1863-1867.

Sanduleanu S, et al. Interval cancers after colonoscopy-insights and recommendations. *Nat Rev Gastroenterol Hepatol* 2012;9(9):550-554.

Sato T, et al. Long-term expansion of epithelial organoids from human colon, adenoma, adenocarcinoma, and Barrett epithelium. *Gastroenterology* 2011;141(5):1762-1772.

Sauk J, et al. High-definition and filter-aided colonoscopy. *Gastroenterol Clin North Am* 2010; 39(4): 859-881.

Schreiner MA, et al. Proximal and Large Hyperplastic and Nondysplastic Serrated Polyps Detected by Colonoscopy Are Associated With Neoplasia. *Gastroenterology* 2010;139:1497-1502.

Sedlack RE. Training to competency in colonoscopy: assessing and defining competency standards. *Gastrointest Endosc* 2011;74(2):355-366.

Selinger CP, et al. Flexible sigmoidoscopy does not significantly increase polyp and cancer detection yield when used to supplement CT colonography. *Digestion* 2012;85(1):55-60.

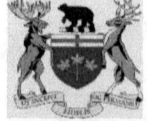

Spiegel BM, et al. Development and validation of a novel patient educational booklet to enhance colonoscopy preparation. *Am J Gastroenterol* 2011;106:875-883.

Suak J, et al. High-definition and filter-aided colonoscopy. *Gastroenterol Clin North Am* 2010;39:859-881.

Subramanian V, et al. High definition colonoscopy vs. standard video endoscopy for the detection of colonic polyps: a meta-analysis. *Endoscopy.* 2011; 43: 499-505.

Subramanian V, et al. Meta-analysisL the diagnostic yield of chromoendoscopy for detecting dysplasia in patients with colonic inflammatory bowel disease. *Aliment Pharmacol Ther* 2011;33:304-312.

Tee HP, et al. Prospective randomized controlled trial evaluating cap-assisted colonoscopy vs standard colonoscopy. *World J Gastroenterol* 2010;16:3905-3910.

Thackeray EW, et al. Colon neoplasms develop early in the course of inflammatory bowel disease and primary sclerosing cholangitis. *Clin Gastroenterol Hepatol* 2011;9:52-56.

Van B, et al. Faster recovery of gastrointestinal transit after laparoscopy and fast-track care in patients undergoing colonic surgery. *Gastroenterology* 2011;141(3):872-880.

Van Dam L, et al. Performance improvements of stool based screening tests. *Best Pract Res Clin Gastroenterol* 2010;24:479-492.

van Roon AH, et al. Diagnostic yield improves with collection of 2 samples in fecal immunochemical test screening without affecting attendance. *Clin Gastroenterol Hepatol* 2011;9(4):333-339.

Waye JD, et al. A retrograde-viewing device improves detection of adenomas in the colon: a prospective efficacy evaluation. *Gastrointestinal Endoscopy* 2010;71:551-556.

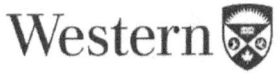

Waye JD. Wide view and retroview during colonoscopy. *Gastroenterol Clin North Am* 2010;39:883-900.

West NJ, et al. Eicosapentaenoic acid reduces rectal polyp number and size in familial adenomatous polyposis. *International Journal in Gastroenterology* 2010;59:918-925.

Willett CG. Adjuvant therapy for resected rectal cancer. *UpToDate.* www.uptodate.com

Win AK, et al. Cancer risks for relatives of patients with serrated polyposis. *Am J Gastroenterol* 2012;107(5):770-778.

Woodward TA, et al. Predictors of complete endoscopic mucosal resection of flat and depressed gastrointestinal neoplasia of the colon. *Am J Gastroenterol* 2012;107(5):650-654.

Zbuk Kevin M, et al. Hamartomatous polyposis syndromes. *Nat Clin Pract Gastroenterol Hepatol* 2007; 4(9):492-502.

Zhang X., et al. Aspirin use, body mass index, physical activity, plasma C-peptide, and colon cancer risk in US Health professionals. *Am J Epidemiol* 2011; 174(4):459-67.

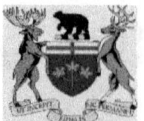

MINI UPDATE

LIVER, HEPATOBILIARY TREE AND GALLBLADDER

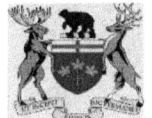

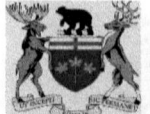

MINI UPDATE

Liver Diseases in Pregnancy

Michael Sey

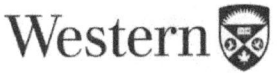

MINI UPDATE

General Approach

Liver disease occurring during pregnancy

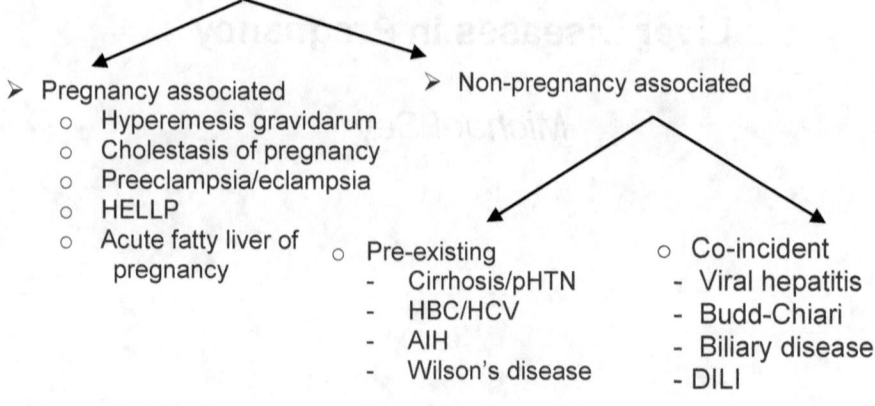

- ➤ Pregnancy associated
  - Hyperemesis gravidarum
  - Cholestasis of pregnancy
  - Preeclampsia/eclampsia
  - HELLP
  - Acute fatty liver of pregnancy

- ➤ Non-pregnancy associated
  - Pre-existing
    - Cirrhosis/pHTN
    - HBC/HCV
    - AIH
    - Wilson's disease
  - Co-incident
    - Viral hepatitis
    - Budd-Chiari
    - Biliary disease
    - DILI

Source: Joshi D, et al. *Lancet.* 2010;375:594-605.

➤ Changes in hepatic physiology during pregnancy

- ↓ SVR, ↑ SBP
- ↑ HR, ↑ CO

⟹ Mimic changes of rhosis

- ↑ BV (50%), peaking in 2nd trimester

⟹ Dilutional effect on biochemistry

Abbreviation: BV, blood volume; CO, cardiac output; HR, heart rate ; SBP, systemic blood pressure; SVR, systemic vascular resistance

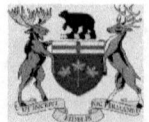

LIVER DISEASES IN PREGNANCY

- Changes in signs and laboratory values during pregnancy
    - Physical exam
        - Spider angiomata
        - Palmar erythema
        - ↑ abdominal girth
    - Laboratory
        - ↔ AST
        - ↔ ALT
        - ↑ ALP
        - ↔ GGT
        - ↔ Bilirubin
        - ↓ Albumin
        - ↔ INR
        - ↔ Platelets
    - Diagnostic imaging

    Fetal risks of ionizing radiation at different gestational ages (GA)

GA (days)	Risk
0-9	Death
13-50	Teratogenesis IUGR
51-280	IUGR CNS abnormalities ?Cancer risk

    Abbreviation: IUGR, intrauterine growth retardation

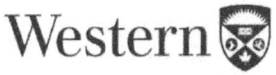

MINI UPDATE

Amount of radiation

Imaging	Dose (mRad)
- CXR	▪ 1
- AXR	▪ 200-300
- UGIS	▪ 50-400
- Barium enema	▪ 700-1600
- CT abdomen	▪ 250
- ERCP	▪ 50-500

- Annual radiation exposure 360 mRad/year in US
- Recommended pregnancy exposure < 500 mRad during pregnancy

Sleisenger & Fordtran's Gastrointestinal and Liver Disease 9th ed. 2010. UpToDate. Diagnostic imaging procedures during pregnancy. 2011.

- o General Advice
    - Good for mom = good for fetus
    - Consider using non-ionizing radiation if possible
        - Ultrasound
        - MRI
            - Avoid gadolinium because of its placental transfer (FDA Category C)
            - Theoretical risk of thermal injury before gestational week 12
    - Balance risk of imaging with risk of missed diagnosis or diagnostic delay in not imaging
    - Use appropriate shielding
- o Liver biopsy
    - Not indicated

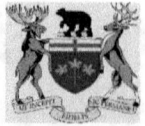

LIVER DISEASES IN PREGNANCY

- Shows mild steatosis and cholestasis

- EGD
  - Consider EGD if persistent symptoms beyond 18 weeks in order to rule out mechanical obstruction

Hyperemesis Gravidarum

- Definition:
  - Intractable Nausea/ vomiting
  - Dehydration
  - Ketosis
  - ≥5% weight loss

- Incidence and time course
  - 0.3 – 2% of all pregnancies
  - Onset within 1st trimester
  - Typically resolves by 18 weeks

- Risk factors:
  - High BMI
  - Multiple gestation
  - Molar pregnancy
  - Psychiatric illness
  - Diabetes mellitus

- Pathophysiology
  - Etiology unknown; speculations include
    - Hormonal (estrogen, progesterone, bHCG)
    - Delayed gastric emptying
    - Gastric H. pylori infection

- Treatment
  - Supportive care
  - Fluid and electrolyte replacement

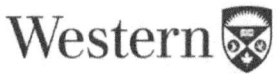

MINI UPDATE

- Thiamine for prevention of Wernicke's encephalopathy
- Anti-emetics

Medication used to treat hyperemesis Gravidarum

Medication	Mechanism	FDA Category
o Dilectin		?
o Gravol	Histamine antagonist	B
o Maxeran	Dopamine antagonist	B
o Ondansetron	5HT3 antagonist	B
o Stemetil	Dopamine antagonist	C

Pre-eclampsia/Eclampsia

➢ Definition:
- SBP >140/90, on two occasions 6 h apart
- Proteinuria >300 mg/24h
- Onset 2nd or 3rd trimester (after 20 week)
- Even if there are no signs of preeclampsia at the time of delivery, about 30% of cases of HELLP will develop after delivery

➢ Demography
- Incidence 5-10% of all pregnancies
    - 5% to 10% of women with pre-eclampsia develop HELLP
    - 85% of women with HELLP have pre-eclampsia
    - More common at Extremes of age (<16, >45)

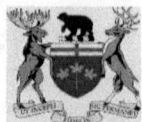

LIVER DISEASES IN PREGNANCY

- More common with molar pregnancy/multiple gestation

- Prevalence
  - Preeclampsia occurs in about 4% of pregnancies, and HELLP occurs with about 12% of women with severe eclampsia

- Risk factors
  - Personal or family history of pre-eclampsia
  - Primiparity
  - Systemic hypertension

- Pathophysiology
  - Unknown
  - Placental insufficiency theory
    - Abnormal placenta formation due to failure of trophoblastic invasion of uterus
    - Inability to increase placental perfusion as pregnancy progresses
    - Endothelial dysfunction with
      - ↑ soluble fms-like tyrosine kinase 1 (sFlt1)
      - Placental growth factor 9PIGF)
      - Soluble endoglin (sEng)
    - These factors lead to
      - Placental vasoconstriction
      - Inhibition of angiogenesis
  - Pathophysiology relates to the fetal and maternal sides of the placenta
  - On the fetal side
    - The high capacity low resistance placental vessels do not develop → fetal ischemia and intrauterine growth retardation

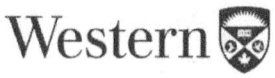

- On the maternal side
  - There is ↑ release of anti-angiogenic and ↓ release of pro-angiogenic factors → maternal vessel vasoconstriction
  - ↑ sensitivity to vasoconstrictors
  - Damage to the endothelium of the maternal blood vessels
  - Deposition of fibrin
  - Ischemic infarcts
  - Acute hepatic necrosis (in 10-20% of pre-eclamptic women)

➢ Clinical features

The HELLP (hemolysis, elevated liver enzymes, low platelet) syndrome is a pre-eclampsia liver disease. So, think of HELLP in this context, pre-eclamptic liver disease, with

- Required for diagnosis
  - Hypertension (sustained systolic blood pressure of ≥ 140/90 after week 20 of pregnancy, in a women whose blood pressure was previously normal)
  - Hypertension-associated end organ damage (eg, liver damage in HELLP syndrome)
  - Proteinuria (≥ 300 mg urinary protein per 24 hr, or 30 mg/dL urine [dipstick #1])

• Mother
  - CNS
    - Visual field changes
    - Focal neurological deficits
    - Seizure (eclampsia)

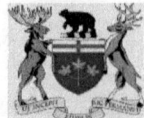

LIVER DISEASES IN PREGNANCY

- o GI/ liver
    - RUQ pain
    - N+V
    - If liver is involved, then eclampsia is defined as being "severe"

    - o Associations
        - Hyperreflexia
        - Peripheral edema
        - DIC (disseminated intravascular coagulation)
        - Abruption placentae
        - Budd-Chiari syndrome (hepatic vein thrombosis)

- Fetus
    - o Fetal hypoxia may develop quickly, with sudden intrauterine death, so early delivery of the fetus is recommended. Fetal mortality is 3-23%, and maternal mortality is up to 3.5%.

➢ Investigation

- o Blood tests
- o In HELLP, there are the usual laboratory findings of hemolysis (H).
- o The elevated liver tests (EL) include a wide range of changes in ALT/ AST, further increased in alkaline phosphatase, and jaundice in 5-40% depending on the extent of patchy ischemic necrosis and fibrin deposition, and hemolysis.
- o The thrombocytopenia (LP) may be associated with low fibrinogen, increased fibrin degradation products and renal dysfunction.
- o Ultrasound – filling defects from hepatic infarction
- o Liver Biopsy
    - Not usually indicated

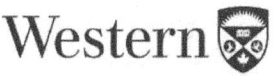

MINI UPDATE

- Periportal hemorrhage
- Thrombi
- Necrosis: pathy → confluent
- Hematoma → hepatic rupture

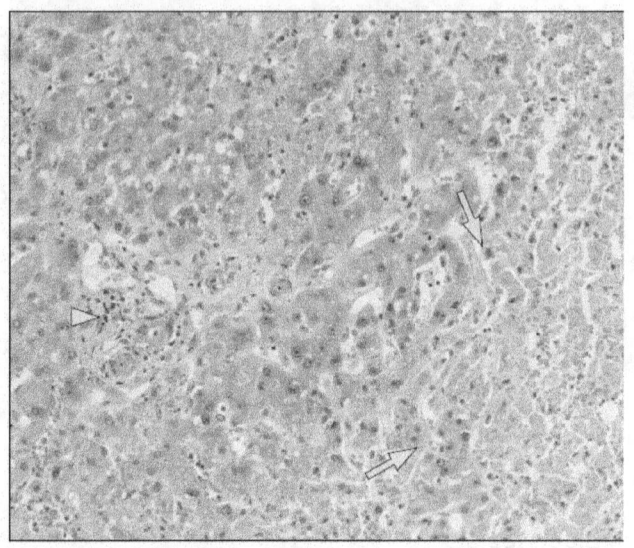

Joshi D, James A, Quaglia A, et al. Liver disease in pregnancy. *Lancet.* 2010;375:594-605.

- Treatment
  - Control blood pressure (typically, Magnesium is used)
  - Liver involvement = for severe preeclampsia (ie, liver involvement)
  - Delivery
  - Liver profile normalizes within 2 weeks of delivery

LIVER DISEASES IN PREGNANCY

HELLP (hemolytic anemia, elevated liver enzymes [low platelets thrombocytopenia])

- Definition:
    - 3rd trimester/post partum
    - Often associated with preeclampsia
- Demography
    - 0.6% pregnancies
    - Accounts for ~20% of material deaths
    - 5-10% of women with pre-eclampsia develop HELLP
    - 85% of women with HELLP has pre-eclampsia
    - Up to 30% occur post-partum
        - Pre-eclampsia and the HELLP syndrome usually occur in the 3rd trimester, but in 28% HELLP occurs in the early post-partum period.
    - ↑ maternal age
        - ↑ parity
        - Caucasian
        - Mortality rate, 50%
            - Mother, 20%
            - Fetus, 20%
        - Maternal and fetal mortality from a free rupture is 50-100%.
- Pathophysiology:
    - Unknown
    - Possibly on a spectrum with pre-eclampsia
    - Overlap with
        - TTP/ HUS
        - AFLP

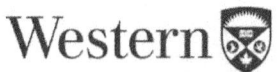

MINI UPDATE

Abbreviation: AFLP, acute fatty liver of pregnancy, TTP/HUS, thrombotic thrombocytopenic purpura

- Both HELLP and AFLP may be associated with maternal defects in the mitochondrial oxidation of fatty acids arising from deficiency of LCHAD (long-chain 3-hydroxyacyl- CoA dehydrogenase).
  - LCHAD in fetus: "AFLP may develop regardless of maternal genotype if the fetus is deficient in LCHAD and carries at least one allele for the G 1528C LCHAD mutation" (S/F, page 635)..." In cases of AFLP the mother, father and child should be tested for the G1528C LCHAD mutation" (S/F, page 636)
  - ↓ carnitine palmitoyltransferase

- ➢ Clinical   HELLP
  - Often associated with preeclampsia
    - ↑ SBP (systolic blood pressure)
    - Proteinuria
    - Peripheral edema
  - Hemolytic anemia
  - Fever
  - Liver dysfunction
  - Associations (conditions in which HELLP also occurs)
    - Pre-eclampsia
    - Adenoma
    - HCC
    - Hemangioma

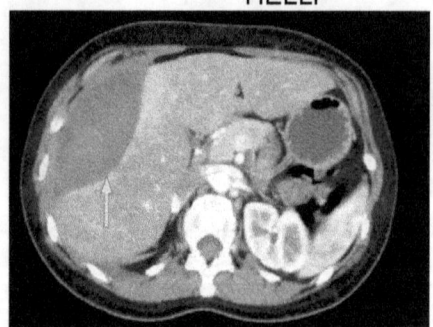

Joshi D, James A, Quaglia A, et al. Liver disease in pregnancy. Lancet. 2010;375:594-605.

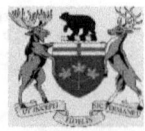

LIVER DISEASES IN PREGNANCY

- Complications
  - General
    - ARDS
    - Shock
    - Sepsis
    - Acute kidney injury (AKI)
  - Liver
    - Hepatic infarction
    - Hemorrhage
    - Hematoma
    - Rupture
    - Liver failure

➢ Laboratory
  - Hemolysis (from microangiopathic hemolytic anemia) → unconjugated hyperbilirubinemia
    - ↑ LDH
    - ↓ haptoglobulin
  - ↑ ALT, AST
  - ↓ platelets
  - ↑ WBC
  - In keeping with the hemolysis ("H") in HELLP, the peripheral blood smear may show schistocytes, and there may be increased serum LDH (lactate dehydrogenase), and although transaminases are often increased 6x (median, 249 U/L for serum aspartate aminotransferase), values > 1000 may occur.
  - The extent of laboratory abnormalities does not reflect the severity of HELLP

➢ Diagnostic imaging
  - Hepatic infarction
  - Hemorrhage

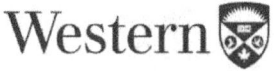

- o Hematoma
- o Rupture
- o While abdominal ultrasound may be reliable to detect intrahepatic complications of HELLP, imaging is not reliable to prove the absence of AFLP (the liver must contain > 30% before the abdominal ultrasound becomes reliably positive for steatosis).

➢ Treatment of HELLP:
- o Multidisciplinary approach
- o Supportive care
- o BP control
- o Close monitoring (ICU)
- o Steroids for fetal lung maturity
- o Delivery
  - Prompt resolution of illness
  - Rarely recurs in subsequent deliveries

➢ Treatment of complications:
- o Hematoma
  - Contained, conservative treatment
  - Non contained
    - Selective arterial embolization
    - Exploratory laparotomy with packing
    - Hepatic artery ligation or resection
    - Liver transplantation

➢ Prognosis
- o Mortality rate
  - Mother 20%
  - Fetus 20%
- o Recurs ~ 1/3 of future pregnancies
- o There is an increased risk of recurrence of HELLP in women with severe hypertension, chronic renal

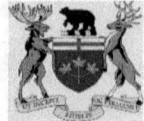

LIVER DISEASES IN PREGNANCY

disease, lupus anticoagulant, or women with a liver transplantation (or other organ transplantation)

Ticks and Treats
- Overlap - questions are often asked of candidates to distinguish between AFLP (acute fatty liver of pregnancy) and HELLP.
- Beware, AFLP is not considered to be a preclamptic liver disease, but about 50% of AFLP may actively have associated pre-eclampsia.
- Both HELLP and AFLP may be associated with inherited defects in the beta oxidation of fatty acids.
- And don't forget: AFLP is associated with severe pericentral microvesicular fat, and HELLP may be associated with fatty liver, albeit not as severe as the pericentral (zone 3) microvesicular fat of AFLP.
- In groups of patients, ALT/AST may be increased in AFLP; although this increase may not be as high as in HELLP, and in the individual patient this relative elevation of differences in ALT/ AST is not useful.
- It is helpful AFLD does not usually have thrombocytopenia.

Acute Fatty Liver of Pregnancy (AFLP)

> Definition:
> - Acute mitochondrial cytopathy characterized by microvesicular fatty liver disease
> - 3rd trimester/post partum

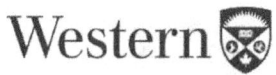

MINI UPDATE

- ➢ Demography
  - o Incidence:
    - About $10/10^5$ pregnancies
    - 1-20% maternal/fetal mortality
  - o Risk factor:
    - Associated with nulliparity, or multiple gestations
  - o AFLP accounts for 16-70% of severe liver disease as well as maternal and fetal deaths during pregnancy
  - o Associated with pre-eclampsia in 30%

- Give the role of deficiency of the mitochondrial fatty acid oxidation enzyme LCHAD (long-chain 3-hydroxyacyl-coenzyme A dehydrogenase) in AFLD.
  - o ↓ ability of fetus to oxidize long-chain fatty acids (LCFA), sometimes from a mutation causing ↓ LCHAD activity.
  - o LCFA from fetus are transferred from fetus to placenta to mother.
  - o If the mother is heterogeneous for LCHAD, she will accumulate LCFA as microvesicular fat, and will develop
    - Hepatic steatosis
    - HE (hepatic encephalopathy)
    - ALF (acute liver failure)
  - o If the newborn child has LCHAD deficiency, she / he has ↑ risk of fatal, fasting non-ketotic hypoglycemia over next several months – must check the newborn for their LCHAD levels.

BEWARE: after AFLD, microvesicular steatosis may progress!

LIVER DISEASES IN PREGNANCY

- o Genetic abnormality in LCHAD (long chain 3-hydroxyacyl-CoA-dehydrogenase) in 20%, possibly other as yet unknown genetic mutations, and the use of drugs such as ASA/ NSAIDs
- o When mother is LCHAD heterozygote but fetus is homozygote, the risk of AFLP is 43%; when the fetus is a heterozygote or normal, the risk of AFLP is 2.7%
- o Pathophysiology: impaired mitochondrial beta-oxidation or oxidative phosphorylation of fatty acids, resulting in mitochondrial damage, reduced ATP production, and destructive of hepatocytes

➢ Pathophysiology
- o Fetal G1528C mutation in long-chain 3-hydroxyacyl-CoA dehydrogenase (LCHAD)
- o This leads to abnormal β oxidation of fatty acids
- o 20x increased risk of HELLP

Danger sign!

A woman in the second trimester of pregnancy with RUQ (right upper quadrant) pain, nausea and vomiting, should be suspected of having HELLP, until proven otherwise.

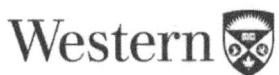

MINI UPDATE

Differential

- Give 6 features which help to distinguish between HELLP and AFLD of pregnancy.

Feature	AFLD	HELLP
o Unique demographic characteristics	+*	+
o Pre-eclampsia	+	+
o Liver failure	+	+**
o Intrahepatic hemorrhage, hematoma, infarction, rupture	-	+
o LCHAD deficiency in mother	+	+/-
o Fatty liver	+	+
o ↑ ALT-AST	+	++
o ↓ platelets	+/-	+

*unique demographic characteristics: first pregnancy, twin pregnancy, male fetus
** from complication of intrahepatic hemorrhages, hepatoma, infarction and rupture

> Swansea diagnostic criteria for diagnosis of acute fatty liver of pregnancy

Six of more of the following features in the absence of another explanation

- o GI tract
  - Vomiting
  - Abdominal pain
- o Liver
  - High bilirubin (>14 µmol/L)

LIVER DISEASES IN PREGNANCY

- Ascites, or bright liver on ultrasound scan
- High AST/ALT (>42 IU/L)
- High ammonia (>47 μmol/L)
- Coagulopathy (PT > 14s or APTT > 34s)
- Microvesicular steatosis on liver biopsy

o Kidney
- Polydipsia/ polyuria
- Renal impairment (creatinine > 150 μmol/L)

o CNS
- Encephalopathy

o Metabolic
- Hypoglycaemia (<4 mmol/L)
- High uric acid (> 340 μmol/L)
- Leucocytosis (>11 × 10^6/L)

Abbreviation: ALT, alanine aminotransferase; AST, aspartate aminotransferase; PT, prothrombin time; APTT, activated partial thromboplastin time.

Adapted from: Joshi D, James A, Quaglia A, et al. Liver disease in pregnancy. *Lancet*. 2010;375:594-605.

o The presentation of that of acute liver failure, including hepatic encephalopathy, coagulopathy, jaundice, ascites, hypoglycemia, renal impairment and pancreatitis

➢ Investigations

o Blood tests
- Abnormal LEs and LFTs
- Hypoglycemia

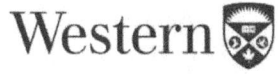

MINI UPDATE

- Lactic acidosis
- ↑ NH3 (encephalopathy)

  o The level of the altered serum transaminases do not reflect the severity of the liver damage and failure. In addition to an elevated INR, anti-thrombin III levels are often increased as well

  o Liver biopsy
  - Not indicated, risk of bleeding due to coagulopathy
  - Microvesicular steatosis

Abbreviation: LEs, liver enzymes; LFTs, liver function tests

Acute Fatty Liver of Pregnancy

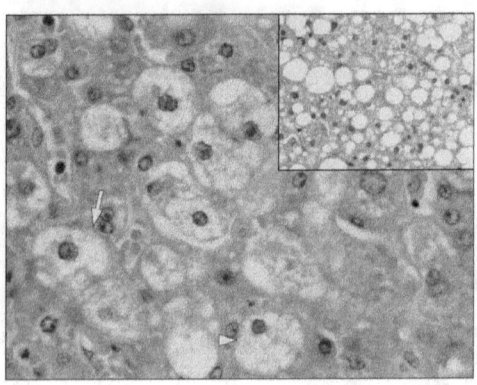

Source: Joshi D, James A, Quaglia A, et al. Liver disease in pregnancy. *Lancet.* 2010;375:594-605.

➢ Fetal testing
  o Chorionic villus sampling for pre-natal genetic testing for LCHAD mutation

- Give the maternal and fetal factors implicated in the pathogenesis of HELLP.

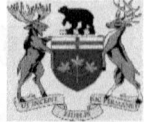

LIVER DISEASES IN PREGNANCY

- o Mother
  - ↑ sFlt1 (soluble fms-like tyrosine kinase 1 (an antagonist of VEGF [vascular endothelial growth factor] and an antagonist of PlGF [placental growth factor])
  - ↑ sEng (soluble endoglin, which reduces the formation of capillaries)
  - ↑ procoagulant (eg, factor V Leiden, anticardiolipin antibody)
  - ↑ systemic vascular resistance
  - ↓ plasma volume
  - ↓ LCHAD (long-chain 3-hydroxyacyl – CoA dehydrogenase, which when reduced leads to ↓ mitochondrial oxidation of fatty acids)
- o Fetus
  - ↓ blood flow of fetus from placenta
  - ↓ trophoblast invasion of wall of uterus
  - Dilation of spiral arteries
  - ↓ uteroplacental perfusion

Abbreviations: H, hemolysis; LP, thrombocytopenia

> Treatment
- o Multidisciplinary, supportive care
- o Prompt delivery
- o Liver transplantation for
  - Liver rupture
  - Severe hepatic encephalopathy
  - Failure to recover post partum
- o Steroids for fetal lung maturity

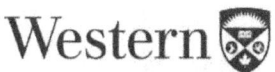

MINI UPDATE

- o Fetal assessment for evidence of defect in β fatty acid oxidation (liver failure, neuropathies, myopathies)
- o Urgent delivery is required; test the mother and infant for LCHAD mutations

➤ Prognosis
- o Usually full recovery post delivery
- o Though full resolution may take up to 4 weeks
- o Intrauterine fetal mortality may be as high as 32%, and maternal mortality rates of 5-26%

➤ Complications of cirrhosis
- o In the pregnant woman with cirrhosis, the maternal mortality rate is 10%, and there is a 3-25% risk of abortion, premature birth and perinatal death (Van Dyke 09)
- o In the pregnant woman with portal hypertension, 18-50% will bleed during pregnancy from esophageal varices

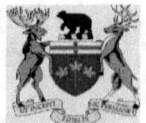

LIVER DISEASES IN PREGNANCY

Liver Diseases Unique to Pregnancy

- Give the trimester of onset and treatment of 4 liver diseases unique to pregnancy.

Liver disease	Onset	Treatment
o Hyperemesis gravidarum	T1	- Supportive care, rehydration
o Intrahepatic cholestasis of pregnancy (ICP)	T2-3	- Ursodeoxycholic acid (UDCA) or cholestyramine
		- Preterm delivery if fetal compromised
o Pre-eclampsia and eclampsia	T2-3	- Antihypertensive drugs, magnesium sulfate
o HELLP syndrome	T3	- Induction of delivery
o Acute fatty liver of pregnancy	T3	- Consider early induction of delivery

HELLP, a syndrome characterized by hemolysis, elevated liver enzymes and a low platelet count; T, trimester

Printed with permission: Keller Jutta, et al. *Nature Clinical Practice Gastroenterology & Hepatology* 2008: 5(8): pg. 437.

Using the presence of elevated serum values of AFP (alpha-fetoprotein) is no longer widely recommended as a screening test for hepatocellular cancer (HCC).

- In the setting of a pregnant woman with cirrhosis or chronic HBV infection who has been found to have an

MINI UPDATE

increased serum AFP, what are the differential possibilities besides HCC?

Mother	Physiological (AFP increases in normal pregnancies)
	Hydatidiform mole
Fetus	Down syndrome
	Neural tube defects

- Give the cautions to be considered when treating the following liver conditions during pregnancy.

➢ Viral hepatitis
  o Hepatitis A and B vaccines are low risk in pregnancy
  o Lamivudine is low risk in pregnancy
  o Adefovir and entecavir have no data in human pregnancy
  o Interferon and ribavirin are <u>contraindicated</u> in pregnancy (use lamivudine, tenofovir)
  o Vaccinate child and give HBIG
  o HCV – don't treat in pregnancy

➢ Wilson disease
  o Maintenance medications for Wilson's disease must be continued during pregnancy.
  o The rate of infant congenital defects is 1.3% when the pregnant mother continues d-penicillamine
  o Switch from D-penicillamine to triampterine or zinc
  o Penicillamine should be avoided, or dose adjusted
  o If necessary, switch to oral zinc

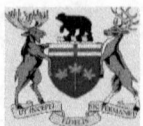

LIVER DISEASES IN PREGNANCY

- PBC/PSC/ICP
  - UDCA low risk after first trimester and effective for cholestasis of pregnancy
- Portal hypertension
  - Propranolol -avoid after first trimester (fetal cardiotoxicity)
  - Nadolol has a long half-life- should be avoided
- Liver transplantation
  - Cyclosporine, tacrolimus- low risk
  - Sirolimus-limited data suggest low risk
  - Mycophenolate mofetil-associated with increased malformations

Abbreviation: ICP, intrahepatic cholestasis of pregnancy

Printed with permission: Mahadevan U. *Best Practice & Research Clinical Gastroenterology* 2007; 21(5): pg. 867.

Intrahepatic cholestasis of pregnancy

- Complications of ICP
  - When serum bile acids > 40 μmol / L, ↑ risk of complications
  - Stillbirth
  - Fetal distress
  - Neconium ileus
  - Vitamin K deficiency
  - Coagulopathy postpartum hemorrhage
- Risk of CD
  - Previous ICP (50% recurrence)
  - Multiple pregnancies

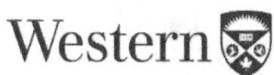

MINI UPDATE

- Multiple gestations
- Descent
- Chilea
- Scandinavian

- ➤ Demography
    - 3rd trimester
    - Present in 2% of pregnancies in America, 6% in Chile and Scandinavia
    - 10-15% of first degree relatives of women with ICP also develop ICP
    - 0.1% to 1.5% of all pregnancies
- ➤ Genetics

- Give the potential genetic basis for cholestasis of pregnancy seen in about 15% of cases
    - About 15% of women with cholestasis of pregnancy have mutations in the MDR3 (ABCB4) gene (a phospholipid flippase that moves PC (phosphatidylcholine) from the inner to the outer surface of the hepatocyte canalicular membrane.
    - More common in women from Chile and Scandinavian countries

- Give the role of SAM (S-adenosyl – L- methoionine) in the treatment of cholestasis of pregnancy.
    - SAM may enhance the benefit of UDCA (ursodeoxycholic acid) in cholestasis of pregnancy.

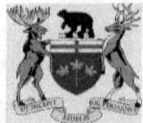

LIVER DISEASES IN PREGNANCY

- ➢ Pathophysiology

- Give 5 changes in bile acid metabolism which occur during pregnancy, and which increase the risk of choletithiasis.
    - cholesterol
    - ↑ supersaturation
    - ↑ bile acid pool
    - ↑ cholic acid
    - ↓ chenic acid (chenodeoxycholic acid)
    - ↑ volume of gallbladder (fasting/ fed states)
    - ↓ gallbladder contraction

    - Due to the usual cholestatic effects of estrogen in pregnancy, plus a genetic predisposition (imitations in canalicular transporters for bile acids, phospholipids and cholesterol [amino phospholipid flippase], as well as FXR, the nuclear regulator of bile acid synthesis)
    - Heterozygous MDR3 mutations responsible for 15% of ICP
    - MDR3 is the main transporter for phospholipids across the hepatic canalicular membrane
    - Possibly related to abnormal bile secretion secondary to female sex hormones

- ➢ Risk factors:
    - Prior history of CP
    - Family history
    - Cholestasis with use of the of oral contraceptive pill (OCP)

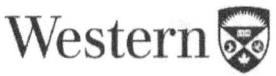

MINI UPDATE

- ➢ Clinical
    - o Painless jaundice (in 10%)
    - o Pruritus of skin on palms & soles
    - o Onset in 2nd or 3rd trimester
    - o Resolves with delivery
    - o Associated steatorrhea, fat soluble vitamin deficiency

- Give the clinical presentation and outcomes from intrahepatic cholestasis of pregnancy (ICP).

Clinical presentation	Maternal outcome	Fetal outcome
o Second or third trimester (T$_2$, T$_3$) o Generalized pruritus with no rash o Marked increases in serum alkaline phosphatase, bilirubin, and serum bile acid levels o Normal or slight increases in GGT levels o Mild increases in serum aminotransferase levels	- Pruritus and abnormal laboratory tests resolve with delivery - Recurs 40-60%)with subsequent gestations - Increased risk for cesarean delivery due to fetal compromise - Can recur with subsequent use of oral contraceptives (OCAs) and hormonal fluctuations	Increase risk for ▪ Prematurity ▪ Still birth ▪ Spontaneous preterm labour and delivery ▪ Fetal compromise ▪ Fetal cardiac dysrhythmias ▪ Meconium stained amniotic fluid ▪ Intrauterine fetal death

Printed with permission: Schutt VA, and Minuk GY. *Best Practice & Research Clinical Gastroenterology* 2007; 21(5): pg. 778.

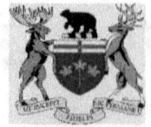

LIVER DISEASES IN PREGNANCY

- Fetal complications
  - Fetal complications usually occur after 32 weeks and include intrauterine growth retardation, fetal disease and premature labour. Fetal death rates in ICP are two-fold increased, usually occur between 37-40 weeks, are associated with much higher concentrations of serum bile acids, and may be sudden and intrauterine; for this reason the fetus should be delivered early (36-37 weeks of pregnancy)

- Laboratory
  - Cholestasis: serum bile acids > 10 μmol/L
  - Fasting bile acid > 10 umol/L
    - >40 umol/L associated with
      - Obstetrical complications placental insufficiency
      - IUGR
      - Prematurity
      - Spontaneous abortion
  - Jaundice in 20%
  - Note: ALT/ AST may be ↑ 20x
  - GGT is usually normal during pregnancy; when GGT is ↑ in CP, suspect mutation in MDR3
  - Pruritus & LE/ LFTs fluctuate

- Liver biopsy
  - Liver biopsy is not necessary, but would show
    - Intrahepatic centralobular cholestasis
    - Bile plugs in cannaliculi and hepatocytes
    - Bland cholestasis

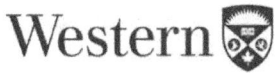

MINI UPDATE

- Treatment
    - Ursodeoxycholic acid (UDCA) 10-15 mg/kg po
        - ↓ pruritus
        - ↓ liver enzyme (ALT, AST, AP, GGT)
        - Well tolerated by mother & fetus
        - Helps steatorrhea, but may worsen vitamin K deficiency
        - Treat fat soluble vitamin deficiency prn
        - Delivery
            - Usually resolves with delivery
            - 60-70% risk of recurrence with subsequent pregnancies

- Give the medical treatment options of cholestatic disorders during pregnancy

Indication/drug	Fetal risk (FDA category)	Use and safety
Immune-mediated disorders		
- UDCA	B	Low risk
- Prednisolone	C	Low risk: increased risk of cleft palate, adrenal insufficiency
- Azathioprine	**D**	Low risk
Bacterial cholangitis		
- Ampicillin	B	Low risk
Sedation and analgesia		
- Fentanyl	C	Use in low doses
- Meperidine	B	Use in low doses

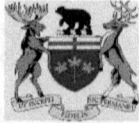

LIVER DISEASES IN PREGNANCY

- Midazolam   D   Use in low doses
- Propofol   B   Avoid in first (and second) trimester

Fetal risk categories (FDA): A – no risk; B – risk in animal studies, but not in humans; C – human risk cannot be excluded; D – risk; X – absolute contraindication.

Printed with permission: European Association for the Study of the Liver. EASL Clinical Practice Guidelines: Management of cholestatic liver diseases. J Hepatol 2009; 51(2), Table 7: 237–267.

Please see: Swan MG. Chapter 58. In: Therapeutic Choices. Grey J, Ed. 6th Edition, Canadian Pharmacists Association: Ottawa, ON, 2011, Table 4: Cholestatic Liver Disease, page 776-777.

➢ Prognosis
  o 2/3 with one episode have recurrence with subsequent pregnancies or
  o Increased risk of cholelithiasis, use of OCAs, cholecystitis, pancreatitis

- Give 4 benefits of UDCA in the management of cholestasis of pregnancy

  o concentration of bile acids in maternal serum and amniotic fluid
  o ↑ transport of bile acids in placenta
  o ↓ cholestatic potential of progesterone during pregnancy

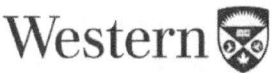

- o ↓ pruritus
- o ↓ fetal distress, premature delivery, stillbirth

- Give 4 factors associated with increased risk of recurrent cholestasis of pregnancy.
    - o Further pregnancies
    - o Use of OCAs
    - o Cholecystectomy for increased risk of cholelithiasis, cholecystitis, pancreatitis
    - o Use of progesterone during subsequent pregnancy
    - o Use of estrogen

References and Suggested Reading

Iryna S. Hepburn. Pregnancy-Associated Liver Disorders. *Digestive Diseases and Sciences* 2008;53:2334-2358.

Joshi D, James A, Quaglia A, et al. Liver disease in pregnancy. *Lancet.* 2010;375:594-605.

Keller, et al. The spectrum and treatment of gastrointestinal disorders during pregnancy. *Nature Clinical Practice Gastroenterology & Hepatology* 2008; 5(8):430-443.

Schutt VA, et al. Liver diseases unique to pregnancy. *Best Practice & Research, Clinical Gastroenterology* 2007;21(5):771-92.

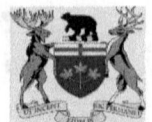

MINI UPDATE

Acute Liver Failure

Aze Wilson

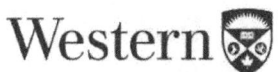

MINI UPDATE

- Definition
  - The rapid development of hepatocellular dysfunction in a patient without pre-existing liver disease.
  - The presence of hepatic encephalopathy is a defining clinical feature.
  - Acute liver failure is defined by an interval between the onset of illness and the appearance of encephalopathy of :
    - 8 weeks or less (Sleisenger & Fordtran's)
    - 26 weeks or less (AASLD Guidelines)
  - ALF is defined as "....the rapid development of hepatocellular dysfunction, specifically coagulopathy and mental status changes (encephalopathy) [and often jaundice] in a patient without prior liver disease".
  - Coagulopathy (INR ≥ 1.5) and encephalopathy in patient without previous cirrhosis and with an illness of < 26 weeks duration
  - ALF is "....a clinical syndrome that represents the final common pathway of severe liver injury resulting from numerous infections, immunologic, metabolic, vascular and infiltrative disorders", leading to severe cellular or mitochondrial dysfunction and hepatocellular necrosis".
  - "Hepatic encephalopathy is a defining criteria" for ALF. (Feldman M., et al. Sleisenger and Fordtran's Gastrointestinal and Liver Disease. 9th Edition. *Saunders/Elsevier* 2010, page 1557).
  - The time interval between the onset of illness and the development of ALF is < 8 weeks, although some authors suggest a range of different time intervals:
    - Hyperacute   ≤ 1 week
    - Acute   1 to 4 weeks
    - Subacute   4 to 24 weeks

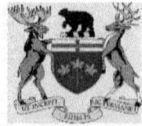

MINI UPDATE

The AASLD Position Paper on ALF defines ALF as coagulopathy and encephalopathy "....... In a patient without pre-existing cirrhosis and with an illness of < 26 weeks duration".

- Mechanism of injury
  - Hepatocellular necrosis
  - Loss of critical hepatocellular function (protein synthesis, intermediary metabolism, detoxification).
  - Severe mitochondrial or cellular dysfunction
- Epidemiology
  - 3.5 deaths/million, USA ($< 1/10^5$)
  - Survival
    - Pre-transplantation era, 15% survival
    - Post-transplantation era, 65%

Worldwide the commonest known causes of ALF are acetaminophen overdose, HBV, HAV, and DILI (drug-induced liver injury) from drugs other than acetaminophen. Other less common drugs and toxins causing ALF are isoniazid, propylthiouracil, phenytoin, valproic acid; and don't forget the mushroom! – Amanita phalloides poisoning). These comprise about 60% of cases.

- Diagnosis
  - Physical exam + supportive lab values
- Main causes
  - Acetaminophen – hepatotoxicity (40%)
  - Idiosyncratic DILI (drug-induced liver injury)
  - Viral hepatitis (HAV, 5%; HBV, 5%)
  - Wilson disease (2%)
  - Autoimmune hepatitis (1%)

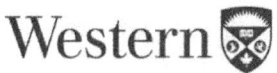

MINI UPDATE

- o AFLP (acute fatty liver of pregnancy [< 1%])
- o Acute ischemic injury (< 1%)
- o Budd-Chiari syndrome (< 1%)
- o Malignant infiltration (< 1%)
- o Ideopathic

- Give a classification of the causes of acute hepatic failure (ALF), and give 15 examples.

➢ Viral
- o Hepatitis A-E
- o Cytomegalovirus (CMV), Epstein-Barr virus (EBV), Herpes simplex (HSV)
- o Parvovirus B19, adenovirus
- o Viral hemorrhagic fever
- o Rarely Herpes zoster, Human herpes virus-6, West Nile virus, coxsackie B virus

➢ Drugs
- o Acetaminophen, isoniazid, NSAIDs, sulfonamides
- o Tetracycline, rifampin, valproic acid, phenytoin, halothane
- o Telithromycin, orlistat, amiodarone

➢ Metabolic causes
- o Wilson's disease, alpha-1 antitrypsin deficiency, galactosemia
- o Tyrosinemia, Reye's syndrome, hereditary fructose intolerance
- o Neonatal iron storage disease

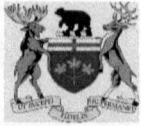

- o Lecithin-cholesterol acyltransferase deficiency
- ➤ Vascular causes
    - o Left heart failure
    - o Shock
    - o Venocclusive disease
    - o Budd-Chiari syndrome
    - o Heat stroke
- ➤ Hematologic/Oncologic causes
    - o Leukemia, lymphoma, metastatic carcinoma
- ➤ Miscellaneous
    - o Acute fatty liver of pregnancy (AFLP), HELLP syndrome (rare)
    - o Syncythial giant cell hepatitis
    - o Primary graft non-function post-liver transplantation

Adapted from: Khashab M, et al. *Curr Gastroenterol Rep* 2007;9(1):66-73.

- Give the 3 hepatic conditions in which often unrecognized pre-existing cirrhosis may be present.
    - o HBV, vertically-acquired
    - o WD (Wilson disease)
    - o AIH (autoimmune hepatitis)

The cause of ALF is not always identified.

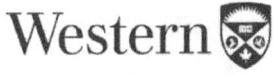

MINI UPDATE

- Give 10 uncommon causes of ALF.
    - Infection
        - EBV (Epstein-Barr virus)
        - HPS (Herpes simplex virus)
        - CMV (cytomegalovirus)
        - HDV (with HBV)
    - Infiltration
        - Lymphoma
        - Hematological malignancy
        - Metastatic lung cancer
        - Metastatic breast cancer
    - Inherited
        - Wilson disease
    - Ischemia
        - Cardiogenic / non-cardiogenic shock
        - Inadvertent occlusion if portal vein at surgery
    - Iatrogenic
        - Uncommon drugs and toxins (see previous questions for examples)
    - Vascular
        - BCS (Budd-Chiari syndrome)
        - SOS (sinusoidal obstruction syndrome)
    - Pregnancy
        - Eclampsia
        - Preeclampsia
        - HELLP
        - AFLP (acute fatty liver of pregnancy)
        - HEV (also seen following organ
    - Post-liver transplantation
        - Primary graft non-function

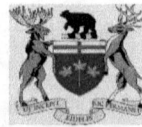

MINI UPDATE

- Give the King's College risk stratification criteria for liver transplantation in ALF.

➢ Acetaminophen
  o INR > 6.5 (PT > 100 sec), serum creatinine > 3.4 mg/dL, stage 3 or 4 encephalopathy
  o Arterial lactate > 3.5 4 hours after resuscitation
  o pH < 7.30 or arterial lactate > 3.0 12 hours after resuscitation; or

➢ Non-acetaminophen
  o INR > 6.5 (PT > 100 sec); or
  o Any 3 of the following:
  o INR > 3.5 (PT > 50 sec)
  o Age < 10 or > 40 years
  o Bilirubin > 17.5 mg/dl
  o Duration of jaundice > 7 days
  o Etiology: drug reaction

Printed with permission: Fontana RJ, and Chung RT. *AGA Institute 2007 Spring Postgraduate Course Syllabus*: 636.

➢ Differential
  o Previous chronic liver disease
    - Decompensation
    - Flares of Chronic Viral Hepatitis
    - Sepsis
    - SLE
    - TTP-HUS
    - Alcoholic hepatitis
  o New
    - Primary graft non-function after L-Tx

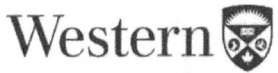

MINI UPDATE

- Give the 7 important hepatic and non-hepatic conditions which may mimic the clinical presentation of ALF.
    - The diagnosis of ALF is based on clinical findings, and must be differentiated from conditions with similar clinical findings:
    - Acute decompensation of chronic liver disease
    - Acute HBV
    - Acute flares of chronic HCV
    - Alcoholic hepatitis
    - Sepsis (low factor VIII; normal factor VIII in ALF)
    - SLE (systemic lupus erythematosus)
    - TTP (thrombotic thrombocytopenic purpura)

Abbreviation: L-Tx, liver transplantation; HAV, hepatitis A virus infection; HBV, hepatitis B virus infection

➤ Clinical
    - Major complications of ALF include HE, coagulopathy, jaundice, GI bleeding, and hypoglycemia.

- Give 5 other major complications of ALF.

    - Coagulopathy — Clinically significant bleeding in 10% to 20%
    - Bacterial and fungal infections — Bacterial infections in 80% of ALF patients (Staphylococcus gram-negative aerobes)
      - Bacteremia in 25%

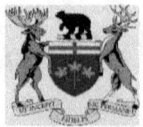

MINI UPDATE

- Fungal infections (Candida albicans, Aspergillus) in ~30%

- o MOFS (multiple Organ Failure Syndrome)
  - Hypertension (↓ MAP [mean arterial pressure] from peripheral vasodilation)
  - Pulmonary edema
  - Renal failure
  - DIC

- o Acute pancreatitis
  - Seen in 44% of patients dying from ALF, especially from acetaminophen overdose
- o Acute respiratory failure
  - Pulmonary edema
  - ARDS (acute respiratory distress syndrome); DAD, diffuse alveolar damage)
- o Acute renal failure
  - Acute renal failure in 50% of ALF, from HRS (hepatorenal syndrome) and ATN (acute tubular necrosis)
  - Intermittent hemodialysis, continuous hemofiltration, hemodiadsorption, MARS (albumin dialysis using the molecular adsorbent recirculating system)

> Prognosis
  - o Etiology of ALF is an indicator of prognosis, dictates specific management options. (AASLD, 2005)

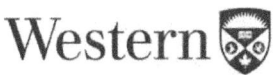

MINI UPDATE

King's College Criteria for Liver Transplantation in ALF

- Acetaminophen cases
  - Arterial pH < 7.3
    or
  - Arterial lactate
    - >3.5 at 4 hrs, or
    - >3 at 12 hrs or
  - INR>6.5 & Cr>3.4 & Stage 3 or HE

- Non-acetaminophen cases
  - INR>6.5
    or
  - Any 3 of the followings:
    - Age<10 or >40 yrs
    - Duration of jaundice>7 d
    - Total Bilirubin >17.5
    - INR>3.5
    - Etiology: idiosyncratic drug, halothane, idiopathic, non-A non-B hepatitis

- Acetaminophen hepatotoxicity
  - Dose-dependent (usually > 10 gm/day)
  - Overdose
    - Intentional
    - Non-intentional
  - Very high aminotransferases may be seen
  - Low or absent serum acetaminophen concentrations do not rule out acetaminophen poisoning

- Treatment
  - ABCs
  - Supportive care

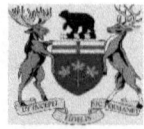

MINI UPDATE

- Access for possible liver transplantation
- Administration of activated charcoal (standard dose 1g/kg orally, in a slurry), for GI decontamination just prior to administration of N-acetylcysteine (NAC)
- NAC is the antidote for acetaminophen poisoning.

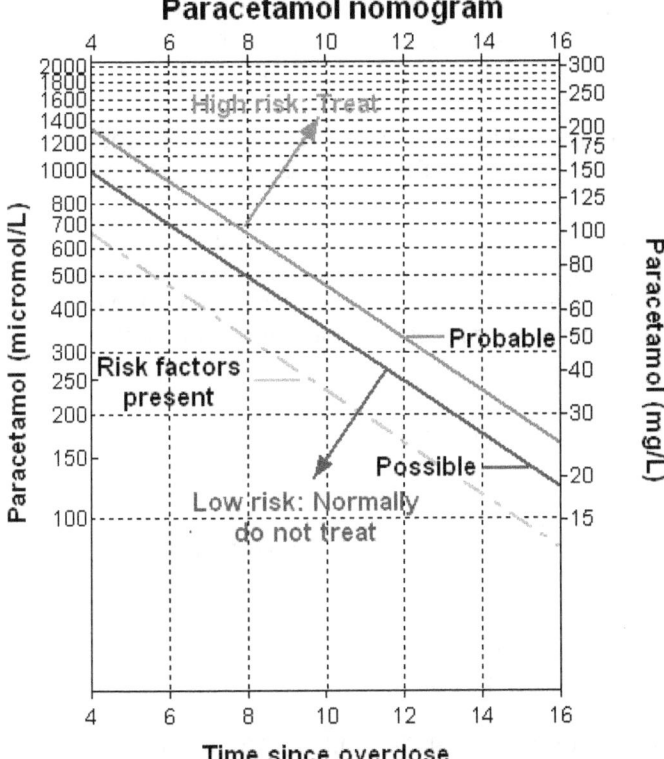

- Administration of NAC is recommended in any case of ALF in which acetaminophen overdose is even just suspected.
- NAC should be given as early as possible, but may still be of value 48 hours or more after ingestion.
- NAC may be given:

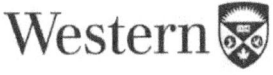

MINI UPDATE

- Orally
  - 140mg/kg by mouth or nasogastric tube, diluted to 5% solution, followed by 70 mg//kg by mouth q 4 h for 17 doses
- Intravenously
  - loading dose of 150 mg/kg in 5% dextrose over 15 minutes
  - maintenance dose of 50 mg/kg given over 4 h, followed by 100 mg/kg over 16 h

  o Liver transplantation may be needed in the patient with ALF secondary to EHS (exertional heat shock)

  o About 2/3 of patients with ALF have adrenal insufficiency, so the patient may either be given a treat of IV steroids, or adrenal insufficiency may be formally tested with a cosyntropin stimulation test.

Drug Induced Liver Injury (DILI)

➤ Causes

  o Numerous prescription drugs have been implicated in ALF - the "Anti's":
  - Antibiotic
    - isoniazid (16%)
    - dapsone
    - septra
  - Non-steroidal anti-inflammatory drugs especially diclofenac
  - Anti-seizure Rx
    - valproic acid (7%)
    - dilantin (7%)
  - OTCs Kava kava, chaparral, skullcap, rattleweed

Abbreviation: OTCs, over – the – counter

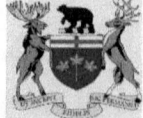

MINI UPDATE

- Epidemiology
    - Incidence $1/10^5$ – not dose-dependent

- Management
    - No specific antidotes
    - Corticosteroids are <u>not</u> indicated (unless a drug hypersensitivity reaction is suspected).
    - Stop offending agents should be stopped immediately.
    - L-Tx may be life-saving

Viral Hepatitis

- Epidemiology
    - HAV and HBV more common cause of ALF in developing countries
    - HEV: a leading cause of ALF in India and other tropical countries.
    - Pregnant women at increased risk for developing ALF with acute HEV infection.

- Treatment
    - Mainly supportive - fluids, blood, FFP
    - Reactive of HBV
        - HBsAg⁺ patients who are to begin chemotherapy or immunosuppression should be treated with a nucleoside analog (continued 6mos post-tx) to prevent reactivation of HBV, and ALF *AASLD*
    - Acute HBV - Lamivudine

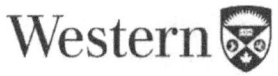

MINI UPDATE

Wilson Disease
- Demography
  - An uncommon cause of ALF: 2-3% in US
  - Early recognition is critical, because ALF in Wilson disease is fatal without L-Tx.
  - Typically presents
    - In young people (2nd-3rd decade)
    - Abrupt onset of hemolytic anemia and bilirubin > 342 mmol/l.
    - Kayser-Fleischer rings are present in about 50% of patients presenting with ALF due to Wilson disease.

- Lab' diagnosis
  - ↑ serum ceruloplasmin, ↑ serum/ urinary copper (Cu) levels.
  - ↓↓ ALP or uric acid levels.

- Treatment
  - Acute lowering of Cu using direct plasma reduction techniques:
    - Albumin dialysis,
    - Continuous hemofiltration,
    - Plasmapheresis
    - Plasma exchange.
  - Initiation of treatment with penicillamine is not recommended in ALF, since there is a risk of drug hypersensitivity.
  - Recovery is infrequent without transplantation

Autoimmune Hepatitis (AIH)
- When AIH is suspected as the cause of ALF, liver biopsy should be performed to establish this diagnosis.

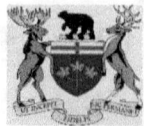

MINI UPDATE

- ALF in AIH is treated with prednisone po 40-60 mg/day
- Even while corticosteroids are being administered, patients should be placed on the list for transplantation.

Acute Fatty Liver of Pregnancy (AFLP)

> Epidemiology

- A small number of women will develop ALF from AFLP in the 3rd trimester of pregnancy (0.0008% of all pregnancies)
    - Associated with increased fetal and maternal mortality.
- Usually presents with
    - Jaundice
    - Coagulopathy
    - Low platelets
    - Features pre-eclampsia (hypertension, proteinuria) are common.
- Recovery is rapid after delivery of child
- Supportive care is the only treatment required.
- Keep in mind that ALF in pregnant women may also be caused by entities not necessarily related to the pregnant state.

Acute Ischemic Injury

- Syndrome of "shock liver" after
    - Cardiac arrest
    - Prolonged hypovolemia
    - In the setting of CHF.
- ↑↑ ALT/ AST, which fall with stabilization of the circulatory problem.

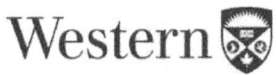

MINI UPDATE

- o Simultaneous onset of renal dysfunction and muscle necrosis may be noted.
- o Outcome is determined by management of underlying cause
- o L-Tx is seldom indicated.

Budd-Chiari Syndrome (B-CS)

- o Acute hepatic vein thrombosis can present as ALF.
- o Abdominal pain, ascites and hepatomegaly are often present.
- o Confirmed diagnosis of B-CS with hepatic imaging studies
    - Doppler ultrasonography
    - Computed tomography
    - Venography
    - MR venography
- o Venous decompression is necessary for B-CS, except in the presence of ALF where L-Tx may be required.
- o Prior to L-Tx for B-CS, rule out underlying cancer as a cause of the hypercoagulability leading to B-CS.

Malignant Infiltration

- o Rare cause of ALF.
- o Massive hepatic enlargement may be seen.
- o Acute, severe hepatic infiltration occurs with
    - breast cancer
    - small cell lung cancers
    - lymphoma
    - melanoma

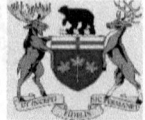

MINI UPDATE

- o Diagnosis should be made by imaging and biopsy, and treatment appropriate for the underlying malignant condition is indicated.
- o L-Tx is not an option.

Hepatic encephalopathy (HE)

➢ Grading

- o Stage 1:
  - Subtle changes in affect
  - Altered sleep patterns
  - ↓ Concentration
- o Stage 2:
  - Drowsiness
  - Disorientation
  - Confusion

➢ Asterixis or tremor
  - o ICU monitoring
  - o CT head
  - o Avoid sedating-hypnotic Rx
  - o Treat precipitants

- o Stage 3:
  - Somnolence
  - Incoherence

- o Stage 4:
  - Coma with minimal or no response to noxious stimuli

Abbreviation: ICP, intracranial pressure

➢ Hyperreflexia, clonus, muscular rigidity
  - o Intubation & ventilation
  - o Recognize/ treat ↑ ICP & cerebral edema
    - Early recognition of cerebral edema cannot reliably be made clinically
    - The clinical signs of hypertension, bradycardia and irregular respirations (Cushing's triad) are not uniformly present;
    - These and other neurological changes such as pupillary dilatation or signs of decerebration are typically evident only late in the course.
    - Treatment:
      - Position - with the head elevated at 30°.

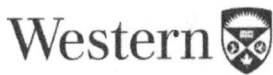

MINI UPDATE

- Stimulation avoid patien stimulation that may increase ICP.
- Osmotherapy - 1st line, short term, requires intact renal function
- Barbiturates - 2nd line, (renal dysfunction, refractory)
    o Manage CVS, renal, metabolic disorders ('lytes, blood sugar, acid-base status)

o Hyperventilation - no role for prophylactic hyperventilation

o Hypertonic saline
 - Administration of hypertonic saline to maintain serum Na^+ levels of 145-155 may be used to prevent the rise in ICP values, but no survival benefit demonstrated

o Corticosteroids - no benefit

o HE is defining criterion of ALF

o Caused by
 - Cerebral edema and resulting ↑ intracranial pressure

o It is likely multifactorial:
 - Gut-derived neurotoxins escape hepatic clearance and are released into the systemic circulation.
 - Increased brain glutamine levels causing cytotoxic edema with swelling of endothelial and astroglial cells.
 - Disruption of the BBB vacuolization of the basement membranes of capillaries, causing vasogenic edema.
 - Inflammation/ infection, may also contribute

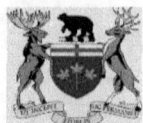

MINI UPDATE

- Portosystemic shunting of toxins
- Other contributors to development of HE
  - Sepsis
  - Hypoglycemia
  - Hypoxia
  - Hypotension
  - Hypokalemia
  - Renal failure
  - GI bleeding

Coagulopathy and Bleeding

➢ Epidemiology

- Clinically significant bleeding occurs in 20% of ALF cases
- Most common sources of bleeding
  - GI tract
  - Nasopharynx
  - Skin puncture sites

➢ Mechanism

- ↓ platelet
- ↓ synthesis:
- ↑ consumption

➢ Treatment

- Platelet (plt) transfusion when plt
  - < 10, 000, with no active bleeding
  - < 50,000 with active bleeding
  - require an invasive procedure

➢ FFP:

- INR > 1.5, with active bleeding

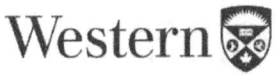

Infection

In ALF, High level of suspicion for infection and a low threshold for starting treatment are required.

- Bacterial

- Demography
    - Bacterial infections may develop in as many as 80% of patients with ALF.
    - Most likely organisms
        - Staphylococcus
        - Gram-negative aerobes
    - Uncontrolled infection accounts for exclusion of ~25% of patients from L-Tx.

- Etiology
    - Factors increasing risk for infection in ALF:
        - Gut-derived organisms may enter the systemic circulation from portal venous blood as a result of damaged Kupffer cells.
        - ↓ PMN function may result from ↓ hepatocellular synthesis of acute phase reactants
        - Patients are subjected to more frequent invasive procedures.
    - Treatment
        - For active infection
            - Choice of abx should be based on the spectrum of most likely organism: Staphylococcus, gram-negative aerobes
            - Empiric tx with vancomycin and a 3rd generation cephalosporin or fluoroquinolone.
        - Prophylaxis:

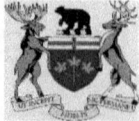

MINI UPDATE

- A small RCT (1993) showed a significant reduction in infection and a small survival benefit in ALF patients treated with prophylactic cefuroxime.
- Other studies have shown a reduction in infection with NO survival benefit (AASLD guidelines)
- Requires further investigaton

- Fungal
    - Develop in up to 1/3 of patients with ALF.
    - Candida albicans (majority)
    - Risk factors
        - Renal failure
        - Prolonged antibiotic therapy
        - Use of invasive monitoring devices

Multiple Organ Failure

- Clinically
    - Manifests as
        - Peripheral vasodilatation
        - Hypotension
        - Pulmonary edema
        - Renal failure
        - DIC

- Mechanisms
    - Liver failure may trigger the microcirculatory derangements via:
        - Platelet activation in the capillary lumen causing endothelial injury
        - Impaired clearance with accumulation of vasoactive substances in the systemic circulation.

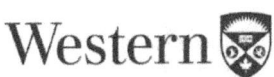

MINI UPDATE

- Therapy
  - Optimize
    - Mean arterial pressure > 60 mm Hg
    - Tissue oxygenation.
    - Intravascular volume depletion (using blood and colloids)
  - Avoid volume overload given propensity for ARDS
  - Have a
    - Low threshold for initiating venovenous hemofiltration
  - Avoid nephrotoxic medications

- Predictors of outcome

- Prognosis
  - 2 categories
    - Those in whom intensive medical care enables recovery of hepatic function
    - Those who require L-Tx to survive.
  - Patients with acetaminophen toxicity have a better prognosis than those with ALF - indeterminate (see King's College Criteria)
  - Liver histology in ALF is associated with sampling artifact and does not reliably predict outcome.

- Treatment
  - Liver transplantation (L-Tx)
    - The only definitive therapy for patients who are unable to achieve regeneration of sufficient hepatocyte mass to sustain life
    - Survival from ALF
      - No L-Tx less than 30% of patients with ALF survived.
      - L-Tx
        - 1-year: 70%
    - Due to donor shortages, patients with ALF are more likely to receive:

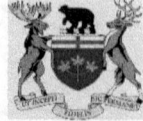

MINI UPDATE

- An ABO-incompatible graft
- Marginal donor grafts
- These contribute to higher rate of primary graft non-fct and rejection.
- Contraindications:
  - Irreversible brain damage (ICP>50 mmHg)
  - Active extrahepatic infection
  - Multiple organ failure syndrome
  - Malignancy
  - Advanced pulmonary or cardiac disease

- Investigational Approaches
  - Auxillary Liver Transplantation
    - Donor graft is implanted beside or below resected diseased liver allowing it to regenerate
  - Extracorporeal Liver Support
    - "liver dialysis" vs bioartificial livers
  - Hepatocyte transplantation
    - Bridge to transplantation or regeneration

Acetaminophen

For persons with ALF thought to be due to acetaminophen overdose,

- Immediately give activated charcoal (1gm/kg body weight [BW] po in a slurry (does not reduce the effect of NAC [N-acetylcysteine]).
- NAC should be given within 4 hours of overdose, but may still be of value 48 or more hours after ingestion.
- For causes of ALF other than acetaminophen, and in patients with stages I or II encephalopathy, NAC may improve outcomes.

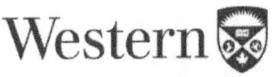

MINI UPDATE

- Suspect acetaminophen overdose if the transaminases are > 1000 IU/mL, and if the serum bilirubin concentrations are normal (in the absence of possible ischemic hepatitis, i.e. hypertension or CV collapse).
- Give
  - NAC IV

    150 mg/kg BW IV loading dose in 5% dextrose over 15 min, followed by 500 mg/kg over 4 hours, then 100 mg/kg over 16 hours or 6 mg/kg/hr

Mg/kg	Frequency (hr)
150	0.25
50	4
100	16

  - Oral administration also possible

    140 mg/kg po / NG tube, followed by 70 mg/kg po q 4 hr for 17 doses

- Stopping rules after 72 hours, or when liver chemistry improves

- Outline the management of the patient with acetaminophen (ACM) overdose.

➤ Initial measures
  - ABC`s
  - Rule out other co-ingestions
  - Contact liver centre
  - Serum ACM level, urine toxicology screen, LFT's, INR, arterial lactate

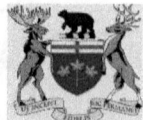

MINI UPDATE

- o Determine likelihood of hepatotoxicity from nomogram (except in non-intentional cases)
- o Lavage stomach if presenting within 12 hours of ingestion or narcotic/anticholinergic ingestion
- o 60 grams of activated charcoal if within 12 hours of ingestion

➢ Oral N-Acetylcysteine (NAC)
- o Loading dose: 140 mg/kg po/NG x 1
- o 70 mg/kg q 4 hours x 17 doses
- o Compazine/raglan for nausea prn
- o Cimetidine (P450 inducer)

➢ IV N-Acetylcysteine (NAC)
- o Dose 1. Loading dose: 140 mg/kg NAC in 200 mL D5W over 1 hour
- o Dose 2. 50 mg/kg NAC in 500 ml D5W over 4 hours
- o Dose 3. 125 mg/kg NAC in 1000 mL D5W over 19 hours
- o Dose 4. 150 mg/kg NAC in 1000 mLD5W over 24 hours
- o Dose 5. 150 mg/kg NAC in 1000 ml D5W over 24 hours

➢ Caution:
- o Do not administer NAC to patients with known sulfa allergy
- o Administer IV formulation of oral NAC through a leukopore filter in a monitored setting after consent obtained from patient/family.
- o IV infusion of NAC leads to anaphylactoid/hypersensitivity reactions in 3 to 5% most commonly during loading dose.

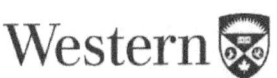

MINI UPDATE

- Hold and reduce infusion rate by 50% if rash/nausea occurs. Administer fluids, IV benadryl, IV steroids as needed.

➢ Psychological assessment

➢ Treat complications if ALF present

Adapted from: Chun LJ, et al. *J Clin Gastroenterol* 2009;43(4):342-9.

A toxic nomogram is available to predict how long after ingestion NAC remains effective. Because of the relative safety of the use of NAC, and that it may be efficacious even 48 hours after overdose, or in persons with non-acetaminophen ALF, the nomogram is not always strictly followed. In addition, the nomogram may have limitations.

- Give 3 examples of when the standard acetaminophen toxicity nomogram may not correctly reflect possible severe liver disease.
    - Multiple doses of acetaminophen taken, rather > 4 g at once
    - Unknown time of overdose ingestion
    - Alcoholic patient
    - Fasting patient

MINI UPDATE

- Give the use of NAC (N-acetylcysteine) in non-acetaminophen ALF.

End point	NAC	No-NAC
➢ Adults		
○ Liver transplantation-free survival		
- All patients	40%	27%
- Stages ½ at entry	52%	31%
○ MOFS		
↑ tissue oxygenation		
➢ Children		
○ ↓ LOS (length of hospital stay)		
○ ↑ rate of spontaneous recovery		

Abbreviation: MOFS, multiple organ failure syndrome

- Give the reason why drinking alcohol and fasting lower the threshold of acetaminophen hepatotoxicity.

Alcohol and fasting →↑ CYP2E1 expression → ↑ NAPQI (the toxic metabolite) ↓ glutathione stores below a critical level, thereby allowing NAPQI to cause hepatic damage

- Give the reason why NAC has to be given PO or IV within 12 to 16 hours of an acetaminophen overdose.

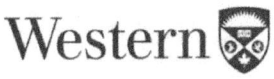

MINI UPDATE

- o NAC provides the cysteine substance to stimulate the hepatocytes to synthesize glutathione and to protect against NAPQI
- o After 12 to 16 hours, the NAPQI-associated hepatocyte damage and the cell death pathways cannot be reversed.
- o Further, as the hepatocytes are destroyed, there are not enough metabolically healthy cells to convert the cysteine from NAC to glutathione.
- o If this is true, give the reason why is NAC given for acetaminophen toxicity even 36 hours after poisoning.
- o NAC will stabilize vascular reactivity in persons with liver failure, so it may have some benefit beyond the mechanisms of glutathione and NADPQI.

With the extent of international travel, it remains mindful for us to recall the countries where HEV is endemic, and therefore should be suspected as cause of ALF, especially in a pregnant woman.

➤ Mushroom poisoning (Amanita phalloides)

- o NAC, in IV or po doses as per acetaminophen toxicity, plus
- o Penicillin G IV 1 million units / kg BW / day, plus
- o Silibinin (silymarin, milk thistle) IV / po 30-40 mg / kg BW / day for 3-4 days.

➤ Drug-induced liver injury (DILI)

- o Glucocorticosteroids, only for DRESS syndrome:
  - Drug rash
  - Eosinophilia
  - Systemic symptoms

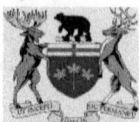

MINI UPDATE

- o NAC, at doses suggested above

- Give the cause of ALF in which there is marked increase in both ALT and LDH.
  - o Acute ischemic injury of the liver

- Give what must be excluded in the patient with Budd-Chiari Syndrome before considering LT?
  - o Associated malignancy

- Give the factors which increase the children's suspicion that the patient's ALF is due to malignant infiltration of the liver.

  - o Massive hepatomegaly

  - o History of cancer
    - Breast
    - Lung (small cell)
      Lymphoma
      Melanoma
      Myeloma

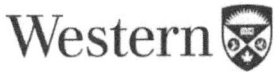

References and Suggested Reading

Alba L, et al. Lactulose therapy in acute liver failure. *J Hepatol* 2002;36:33A

Blei AT, et al. Ammonia-induced brain edema and intracranial hypertension in rats after portacaval anastomosis. *Hepatology* 1994;19:1437-1444.

Clemmesen JO, et al. Cerebral herniation in patients with acute liver failure is correlated with arterial ammonia concentration. HEPATOLOGY 1999;29:648-653.

Feldman M, et al. Sleisenger GI and Liver Disease. *Saunders Elsevier.* 8th Edition. 2:1 993-2006.

Hoofnagle JH, et al. Fulminant hepatic failure: summary of a workshop. *Hepatology* 1995;21(1):240

Lee WC, et al. Lamivudine is effective for the treatment of reactivation of hepatitis B virus and fulminant hepatic failure in renal transplant recipients. *Am J Kidney Dis* 2001;38(5):1074-81.

Polsen J, et al. AASLD Position Paper: The Management of ALF. *Hepatology* 2005. 41: 1179-97.

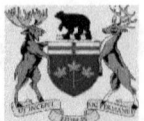

Liver Transplantation

Natasha Chandok

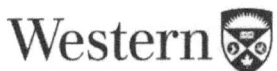

LIVER TRANSPLANTATION

Take Home Message
- Think about the need for liver transplantation n each of your liver patients
- If you aren't certain if your liver patient is "sick enough", call us please.

Indications for LT
- Referrals can be considered for any patient with acute or chronic liver failure of any cause
- Two Important Considerations:
  - Does the patient need a transplant now?
  - Survival benefit?
  - Have all appropriate treatments been attempted?
    - Is anti-HCV/HBV/HIV therapy appropriate?
    - Has AIH / PBC been optimally managed?

Natural History of Chronic Liver Disease

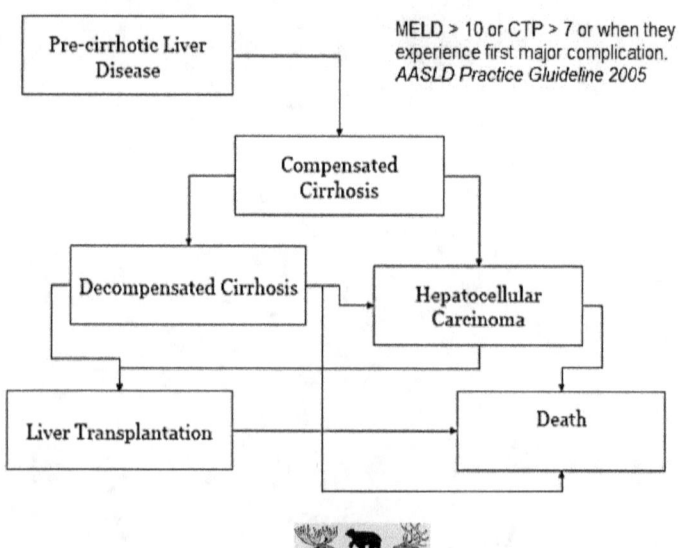

MELD > 10 or CTP > 7 or when they experience first major complication.
AASLD Practice Gluideline 2005

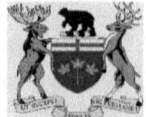

LIVER TRANSPLANTATION
Hepatic Decompensation

- Usual definition
  - Ascites
  - Variceal bleeding
  - Encephalopathy
  - Jaundice
- Ascites: Most common first event (~50%)
- Occurrence of decompensation: 5–7% per year

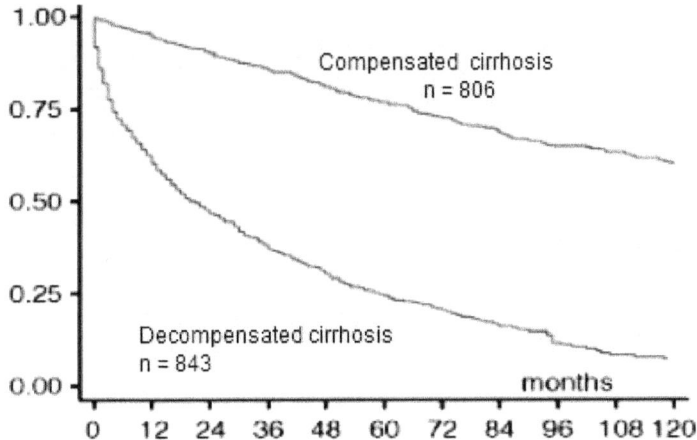

Printed with permission: D'Amico G, et al. J Hepatol. 2006;44(1):217-31.

LIVER TRANSPLANTATION

Four Stages of Cirrhosis

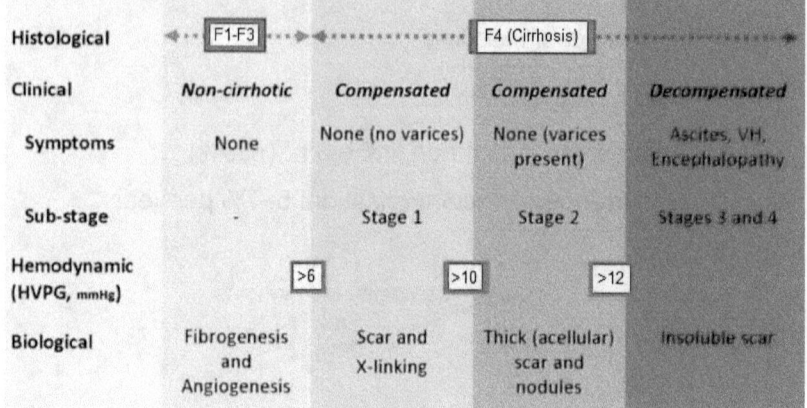

Printed with permission: Garcia-Tsao G, et al. Hepatology. 2010;51(4):1445-9.

Four Stages of Cirrhosis and the Natural History

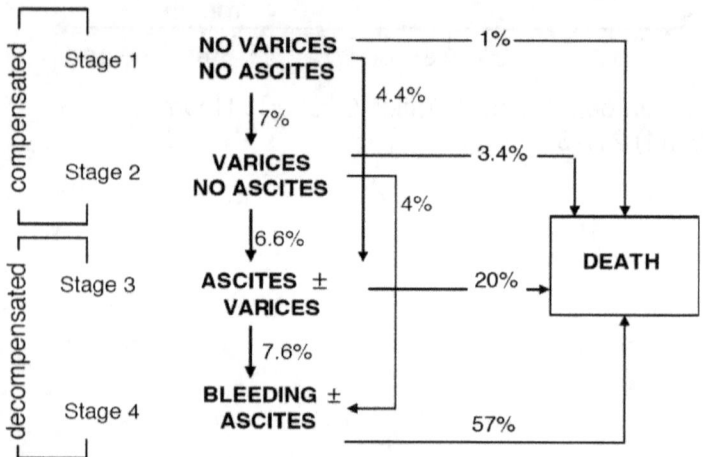

Printed with permission: D'Amico G, et al. J Hepatol. 2006;44(1):217-31.

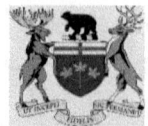

LIVER TRANSPLANTATION

Referral Tips

- Refer early
    - The decompensated phase of cirrhosis
    - HCC with cirrhosis
- Send most recent labs, medical history (including vaccinations and list/dose of medication), endoscopy reports, imaging and anything else that might be relevant to their operative risk or candidacy
- Counsel on
    - Smoking cessation
    - Complete alcohol abstinence

Special Consideration – Alcoholic Cirrhosis

- Minimum of 6 months of abstinence, demonstration of insight, and completion of an alcohol rehabilitation program
- Patient may undergo random alcohol screens
- Time frame of abstinence ensures that patients who may not need LT do not undergo the surgery

Special Consideration – Acute Liver Failure

- Call our service pager or LHSC "One Number"; contact us in the early phase of evaluation
- Admit and monitor regularly (preferably in ICU)
- Patients should be transferred here if they have a high likelihood of death from liver failure; we can make this determination with you
- Where possible, find the cause to guide further management
- Start NAC promptly in all patients with suspected or confirmed acetaminophen

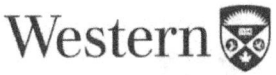

LIVER TRANSPLANTATION

- o Consider prophylactic
  - Antibiotics
  - Anti-fungals
  - PPIs
- o Call our program if you have any questions or concerns – we are here to help your patients!

The Transplant Assessment

- o History & Physical exam
- o Cardiopulmonary assessment
  - Nuclear stress test
  - Pulmonary function
  - Echocardiogram, etc.
- o Laboratory studies, Creatinine clearance
- o Abdominal images to determine
  - Hepatic artery
  - Portal vein anatomy
  - Stage of any HCC
- o Hepatologist, Transplant surgeon, Coordinator, Social Worker, Physical Therapist, Anesthesia

Miscellaneous Considerations

- o Body Mass Index ideally ≤ 35 kg/m2
- o Some patients with liver disease as well as chronic renal disease might require combined kidney transplantation
- o Screen for extrahepatic malignancies
- o Bone density screening/treatment may prevent pathologic fractures before and after LT

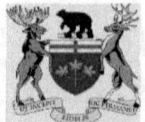

LIVER TRANSPLANTATION

- At the time of assessment, our surgeon will discuss deceased versus live-donor donation
- LT for patients with HIV is possible

Outcomes Post LT

- Short-term survival has had the greatest improvement because of advancements in
  - Surgical technique
  - Intensive care
  - Immunosuppression
- Long-term survival has been at a stagnant because of comorbidities after LT, e.g.
  - Metabolic syndrome
  - Malignancy

Outcomes: Recipient Survival at London Health Sciences Center (LHSC), Canada 2000 – 2010

> Deceased donor

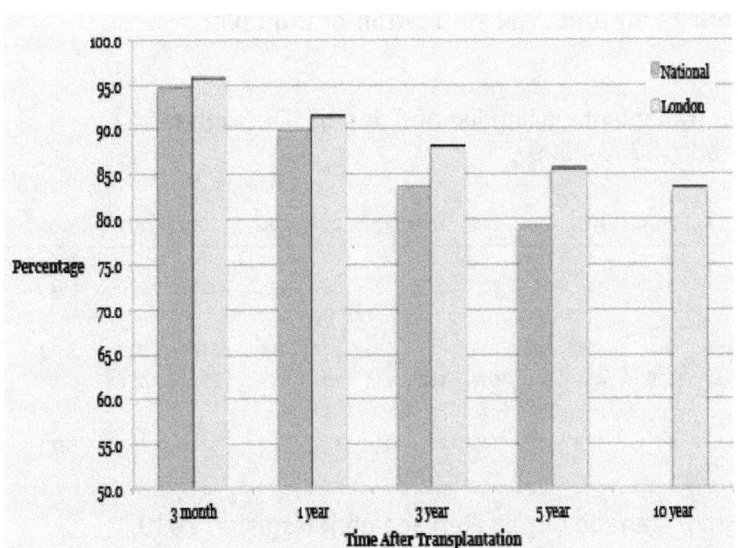

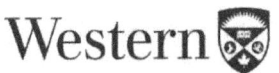

LIVER TRANSPLANTATION

> Living related donor

Outcomes: LDLT at LHSC

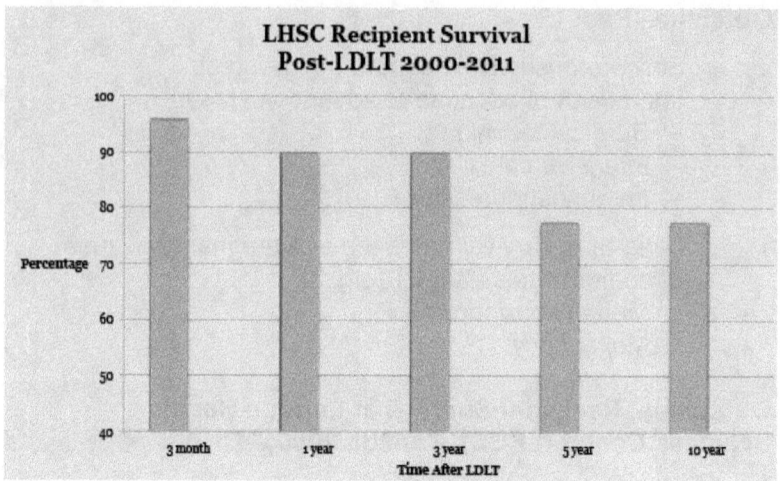

Toward Fair and Just Allocation of the Liver

Liver transplant waiting list and deaths, December 31, Canada, 2000-2009

	2000	2001	2002	2003	2004	2005	2006	2007	2008	2009	Total
o Age 0-17	27	36	31	30	37	32	36	19	17	19	284
o Age 18+	311	418	528	539	630	681	687	616	570	532	5512
- Total	338	454	559	569	667	713	723	635	587	551	5796
o Deaths on waiting list	51	57	82	100	96	141	120	77	92	91	907

Source: Canada Organ Replacement Register, 2010, Canadian Institute for Health Information

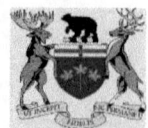

LIVER TRANSPLANTATION
Allocation Based on CTP (Child-Turcotte-Pugh) Score

- 1955: Drs. Child and Turcotte (U of Mi)
  - Risk of open portal systemic shunt
  - Class A-C: ascites, encephalopathy, nutrition, bilirubin and albumin
- 1972: Pugh (London)
  - Risk of esophageal transection for variceal bleeding

Variable	Score 1	Score 2	Score 3
Ascites	None	Mild	Moderate+
Encephalopathy	None	Grade 1-2	Grade 3-4
Bilirubin	< 2	2-3	> 3
Albumin	< 2.8	2.8-3.2	> 3.2
Prothrombin time	< 4 s	4-7 s	> 7 S

Overview of MELD (model for end-stage liver disease)

- MELD is based on bilirubin, creatinine and INR
  - Objective; no ambiguity like is present in the Child-Pugh classification
  - MELD = 3.78[Ln serum bilirubin (mg/dL)] + 11.2[Ln INR] +9.57[Ln serum creatinine (mg/dL)] + 6.43 Score is 6 to 40
- Prospectively developed and validated in chronic liver disease and acute liver failure
- Excellent predictor of 3 month mortality

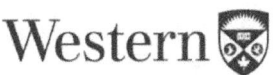

LIVER TRANSPLANTATION

Model for End-stage Liver Disease (MELD)

MELD=
11.2 LN (INR)
+3.78 LN (Bilirubin)
+9.57 LN (Creatinine)
+6.4

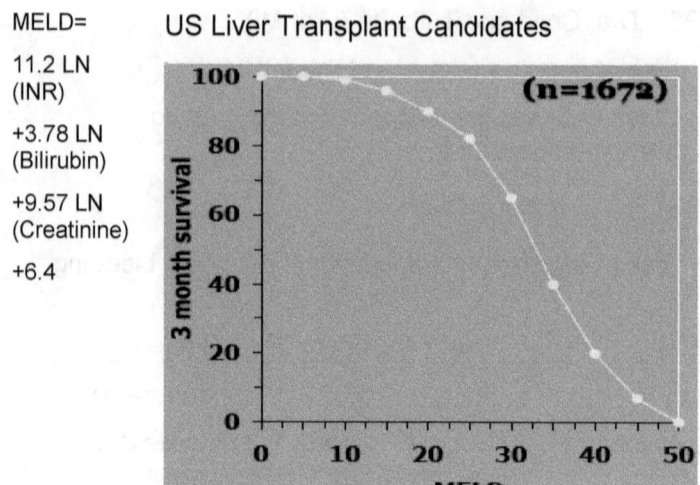

Printed with permission: Freeman RB Jr, et al. Liver Transpl. 2002 ;8(9):851-8.

Predictive value of MELD Score

MELD Score	Survival rate, %	
	Waiting list	1 year post-LT
10	90	83
15	81	80
20	63	78
25	42	74
30	31	71

- For a MELD Score < 15, the survival for standard of Care (`waiting list`) is as good as LT, so LT is not of added value
- When MELD > 15, the benefit of LT becomes clear

LIVER TRANSPLANTATION

MELD Allocation System

- MELD reduces mortality on the waitlist
- De-emphasizes wait times as a factor in prioritizing patients
- High-risk deceased donors are used in patients with lower MELD scores
- Might result in a reduction in health care disparities
- But MELD is not perfect:: it under estimates mortality with
  - Hyponatremis and ascites
  - HCC (hepatocellular cancer)
  - ALF (acute [fulminant] liver failure)
- Additional points need to be added to the MELD score (such as MELDNa to improve its performance characteristics)

MELDNa

- MELDNa = MELD − Na − [0.025 X MELD X (140-Na)] +140
- Hyponatremia is associated with
  - Hepatorenal syndrome
  - Ascites
  - Lliver-related death
- Hyponatremia is associated with increased morbidity post-LT (e.g. central pontine myelinolysis)
- MELDNa provides better calibration and discrimination of the risk of death among candidates for LT

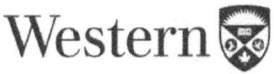

LIVER TRANSPLANTATION

- Thus, MELDNa may reduce mortality among patients on the waitlist; reduction in waiting list deaths may be as high as 7%
- Frequency of need to determine MELD score

Source: Kim WR et al. NEJM 359;10: 2008

Frequency of MELD Score Testing

- MELD score greater than or equal to 25; Labs needed every 7 days
- MELD score 24-19; Labs needed every 30 days
- MELD score 18-11; Labs needed every 90 days
- MELD score less than or equal to 10; Labs needed every year

MELD Exceptions UNOS

Points Awarded	Points NOT awarded
- Hepatopulmonary syndrome	- Portopulmonary hypertension
- Primary hyperoxaluria	- Budd Chiari syndrome
- Familial amyloid polyneuropathy	- Polycystic liver disease
- Small for size syndrome	- Any "quality of life" appeal; e.g.

- HCC within accepted criteria*	– Itch
	   – Ascites
	   – Variceal bleed

- Rare metabolic disorders (case by case basis only)	- Non-HCC tumor

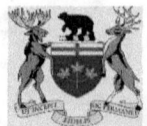

LIVER TRANSPLANTATION

- Cholangiocarcinoma (exception points only if Mayo Clinic-Like Protocol)
- Cystic fibrosis
- Down-staged HCC not granted exception points

Source: Freeman RB, Gish RG, Harper A, et al. Liver Transplantation 2006.
*Milano, UCSF or TTV (total tumor volume) <115 cm^3 and AFP (alpha-fetoprotein) < 400 u/L.

Accepted Criteria for LT for HCC

- Treatment of choice for any patient with HCC who is not a surgical candidate and in whom the HCC is confined to the liver and fits within validated criteria
  - Milan: Single lesion 2 to 5 cm; or ≤ 3 lesions, the largest of which is <3cm, with no extrahepatic disease
  - UCSF: Single lesion ≤6.5 cm; or ≤3 lesion, largest ≤ 4.5 cm and total diameter ≤ 8 cm
  - Alberta: Total tumor volume ≤ 115 cm3 and AFP < 400 U/L

Stage 2 HCC Current UNOS policy

- Prioritization, extension at 3 month intervals
  - Listing score of 22 (15% mortality)
  - First extension 25 (25% mortality)
  - Second extension 28 (35% mortality)
  - Third extension 29 (45% mortality)
  - Fourth extension 31 (55% mortality)
  - Fifth extension 33 (65% mortality)

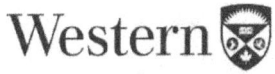

Outcomes: Recipient Survival in Canada

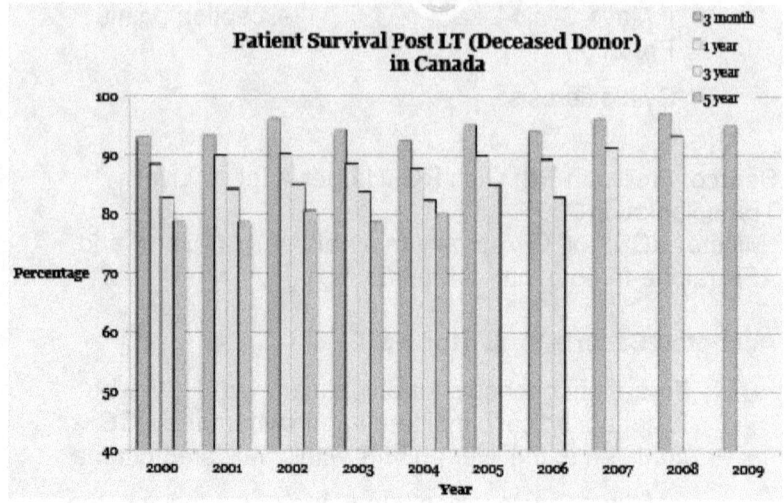

- LT survival rate (SR)
  - 92% 5 yr SR
  - 80% 10 yr SR

- Causes of death Post-LT
  - "natural" causes
  - Malignancy 21% organ cancers } - 2X ↑ Risk non-skin solid
    - -30X ↑ lymphoproliferative disorders
  - Infection
  - Recurrent liver disease
  - "de-novo malignancy post liver transplant (L-Tx)"

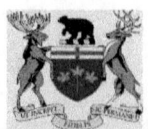

LIVER TRANSPLANTATION

- PTLD (post-transplant lymphoproliferative disorder)
  - Most commonly first 18 month post LT
  - EBV-associated latent infection in B-cells
  - Extranodal, high grade, poor prognosis
  - B cells originate from recipient, not from donor cells
  - May occur in GI tract (e.g. colon)
  - ↑ LDH, ↑ EBV viral load
  - More immune suppression in heart Tx patients, so more PTLD.
  - 5 year SR, 50%
- Management
  - Short-term, 70% effective
  - ↓ immune suppression (↓ by 25% to 50%)
  - EBV treatment
  - Multi-gent chemo (CHOP), radiation, surgery, rituximab
  - Rituximab 50% remission rate (for CD20+ PTLD)
  - Sometimes even used for CD20+
- Non-skin solid organ tumors
  - 10% per year
  - Risk 2x > general population
    - Esophageal Ca
    - Head/neck Ca
    - Karposi sarcoma
- Non-melanoma skin cancer (NMSC)

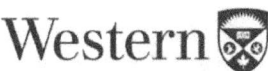

LIVER TRANSPLANTATION

- o Alcohol L-Tx for ALD ↑ risk
- o CRC
- o IBD/PSC
  - 10% at 10 yrs
  - 22% at 20 yrs

➢ Sirolimus - m TOR inhibitor (anti-proliferative properties)

No ↓ non-lymphoproliferative cancers

Non-IBD / PSC post L-Tx – no ↑ risk CRC

- Post Liver transplantation (L-Tx)

➢ Biliary obstruction 1 month post L-Tx
  - o CBD
    - Stone
    - Stricture
    - Bile duct injury and cholestasis in both post-LT HCV and with acute rejection cholestatic syndrome has a serious prognosis.
  - o Ischemic stricture of CBD post L-Tx, above anastomosis
  - o Chronic rejection
  - o Post L-Tx, can see anastomosis on ERCP

➢ Primary non-function of graft
  - o More likely to occur if donor had marked steatosis

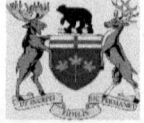

LIVER TRANSPLANTATION

- Give 4 medical methods introduced recently to increase the availability or to extend the fair allocation of livers for transplantation.

    - MELD (Model for End-Stage Liver Disease)
        - Equitable organ allocation
    - Modified MELD
        - Hyponatremia (dilutional)
        - HCC
        - HPC (hepatopulmonary syndrome)
    - LDLT (liver-donor liver transplantation)
    - Split decreased-donor grafts
    - Marginal / extended criteria grafts

> Definition of the word "Contraindications"

    - Definition: Absolute contraindication – "…a clinical circumstance in which the likelihood of a successful outcome is so remove that liver transplantation should not be offered (Feldman M., et al. Sleisenger and Fordtran's Gastrointestinal and Liver Disease. 9th Edition. *Saunders/Elsevier* 2010, page 1596),
    - While there are many "absolute" contraindications to LT (please see (Feldman M., et al. Sleisenger and Fordtran's Gastrointestinal and Liver Disease. 9th Edition. *Saunders/Elsevier* 2010, Table 95.2, page 1596), there are many shades of grey" which will not be discussed further here.

Please see, Feldman M., et al. Sleisenger and Fordtran's Gastrointestinal and Liver Disease. 9th Edition. Saunders/Elsevier 2010, Table 95.4, page 1600, regarding Factors Associated with Severe Hepatitis C Virus Recurrence Following Liver Transplantation.

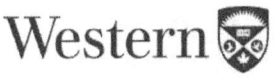

LIVER TRANSPLANTATION

There are many indications for liver transplantation (LT) (Please see, Feldman M., et al. Sleisenger and Fordtran's Gastrointestinal and Liver Disease. 9th Edition. Saunders/Elsevier 2010, Table 95.1, page 1594, Indications for Liver Transplantation). In adults,

- In adults, give the commonest diseases of the liver for which transplantation is performed include
    o HCV, 33%
    o Cholestatic disorders, 14%
    o ALD (alcoholic liver disease), 12%
    o NASH, 9%
    o HCC, 6%
    o HBV, 4%

- Give the major indications for L in children.
    o Biliary atresia
    o Failed portoenterostomy (Kasai procedure) for biliary atresia.

- Give the success rate of insertion of a permanent chest tube to drain hepatic hydrothorax.
    o Bad question! – hepatic hydrothorax is corrected only by a reduction in portal pressure.

- Give the prognostic significance of a person requiring hemodialysis before LT.
    o "…return of adequate renal function is unlikely after transplantation of dialysis has been required for more than one month prior to liver transplantation"

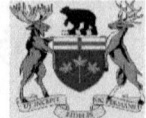

LIVER TRANSPLANTATION

(Feldman M., et al. Sleisenger and Fordtran's Gastrointestinal and Liver Disease. 9th Edition. Saunders/Elsevier 2010, page 1597); combined liver-kidney transplantation may need to be considered.

- Give the pathological features of acute cellular rejection after Liver Transplantation (LT).

Acute cellular rejection after LT is characterized by

- Portal tract — Inflammation, with lymphocytes eosinophils and plasma cell; Extension of inflammation into periportal area
- Bile ducts — Extension of inflammation into bile ducts
- Central vein — Lymphocytic infiltration around central vein, representing endothelitis

➤ MELD score and retransplantation

- The MELD score has helped to equitably allocate donor livers for transplantation, with the sick patients with higher MELD scores moving to "...the head of the line [waiting list]". When patients undergo retransplantation, then probability of survival is about 20% lower than their outcome expected following the initial transplantation.
- Maximal utility is achieved with MELD score for
    - HCV   21
    - Non-HCV   24

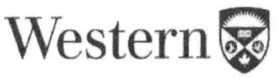

LIVER TRANSPLANTATION

- Give the 6 most common primary liver diseases in North America representing indications for liver transplantation.
  - Chronic HCV
  - Alcoholic liver disease (ALD)
  - Cryptogenic cirrhosis (NASH)
  - PSC
  - PBC
  - Chronic HBV
  - ALD + HCV
  - Hepatoma
  - AIH
  - α, AT deficiency
  - Drug induced liver disease
  - Hemochromatosis, Budd-Chiari syndrome, Wilson's disease

Adapted from: Martin P, et al. *Sleisenger & Fordtran's gastrointestinal and liver disease: Pathophysiology/Diagnosis/Management* 2006: pg. 2037; and 2010, pg. 1594.

- Give the indications for liver transplantation.
  - Acute liver failure (ALF; fulminant hepatic failure; King's College criteria)
  - Complications of cirrhosis
    - Ascites
    - Encephalopathy
    - Synthetic dysfunction
    - Liver cancer

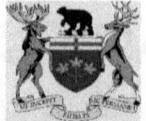

LIVER TRANSPLANTATION

- Refractory variceal hemorrhage
- Chronic gastrointestinal blood loss due to portal hypertensive gastropathy
- INR
- Na
- HCC
- DILI
- Cr
- MELD >13
- PSE
- Ascites
- Hepatorenal syndrome
- Vascular
- Weber Rendir (intractable bleed)
- GAVE; Budd-Chiari

o Systemic complications of chronic liver disease
  - Hepatopulmonary syndrome
  - Portopulmonary hypertension

o Liver-based metabolic conditions causing systemic disease, and which may also cause liver disease
  - Primary oxaluria
  - Familial Amyloidosis
  - $α_1$-antitrypsin deficiency
  - Wilson's disease
  - Urea cycle enzyme deficiencies
  - Glycogen storage disease
  - Tyrosemia

Adapted from: Lilly LB, Girgrah N, and Levy GA. *First Principles of Gastroenterology* 2005: pg. 634.

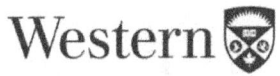

LIVER TRANSPLANTATION

- Give 15 possible contraindications to liver transplantation.
  - Patient
    - Ongoing alcohol or drug abuse
    - Non-adherence
    - Lack of social support
    - Serious underlying symptomatic illness
    - Advanced cardio-pulmonary disease
    - Sepsis
    - Marked psychiatric impairment
    - HIV/ AIDS
    - Diabetes mellitus
    - Advanced age
    - Obesity
    - Multi-organ failure
    - Increased intracranial pressure
    - Jehovah Witness
    - Non-adherence
  - Anatomy
    - Metastatic cancer
    - Anatomical abnormalities
    - PV thrombosis (large size)
    - Outside Milan criteria for HCC (1 lesion <5 cm, 3 lesions <3 cm)
    - Cholangiocarcinoma
  - Liver
    - Mild liver disease (Child <7, or MELD <9)
  - Co-morbidity
    - Pulmonary hypertension
    - Right heart dysfunction
    - Extrahepatic cancer

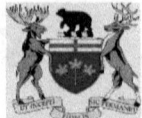

LIVER TRANSPLANTATION

Adapted from: Hay J. *Mayo Clinic Gastroenterology and Hepatology Board Review* 2008: pg. 433.

- Outline the protocol for evaluation of potential living-related liver donors.

Stage 1   Complete history and physical examination

                Laboratory blood tests: liver biochemical test, blood chemistry, hematology, coagulation profile, urinalysis, alpha-fetoprotein, carcinoembryonic antigen, and serologic tests for hepatitis A, B, and C, cytomegalorvirus, Epstein-Barr virus, and human immunodeficiency virus

                Imaging studies: abdominal ultrasound examination, chest x-ray

Stage 2   Complete psychiatric and social evaluation

                Imaging studies: computed tomography scan of the abdomen

                Other studies: pulmonary function tests, echocardiography

Stage 3   Histology: liver biopsy

                Imaging studies: celiac and superior mesenteric angiography with portal phase

Stage 4   Imaging studies: magnetic resonance cholangiogram Informed consent

Printed with permission: Ghobrial RM, et al. *Clin Liver Dis* 2000; 4: 553.

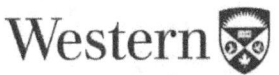

LIVER TRANSPLANTATION

- Give 20 early and/or late complications arising after liver transplantation.

    o Surgery-related
    - Non-specific
    - Cannot get off of ventilator
    - Dehiscence
    - Ileus
    - DVT
    - Atelectasis

    o Metabolic
    - Hypertension
    - Hypercholesterolemia
    - Diabetes mellitus
    - Obesity

    o Abdominal bleeding
    - Anastomoses (immediate)
    - Site of implantation (immediate)

    o Vascular complications
    - Suprahepatic/infrahepatic vena caval obstruction (immediate)
    - Hepatic artery thrombosis (early)
    - Portal vein thrombosis (early)
    - Hepatic artery stenosis (late)

    o Biliary complications
    - T-tube insertion (early)
    - Anastomosis (early)
    - Stenosis of papilla vateri (early)
    - T-tube removal (late)
    - Anastomosis, extrahepatic (late)
    - Multiple strictures, intra-hepatic, abscesses

    o Renal failure (adverse effects of treatment)

    o Vascular
    - Coronary artery disease (dyslipoproteinemia)

LIVER TRANSPLANTATION

- Cerebrovascular
- Peripheral vascular

o CNS/PNS
- Depression
- Neuropathy
- Seizures

o Malignancy
- Lymphoma
- EBV-PTLD (Ebstein-Barr virus – post transplant lymphoproliferative disorder)
- Pre-existing malignancies (within 5 years)
- Acquired donor malignancy
- Skin cancers (non melanoma)
- Cervical cancer (HPV), as per usual standard of care
- Prostate cancer, as per usual standard of care
- Pharyngeal cancer
- Lung cancer
- Increased risk of all malignancies

o Infections
- Viral (HSV, CMV, EBV)
- Bacterial (lines, wound)
- Fungal (PCP, Candida - catheters)

o Drug reactions

o 1° graft failure

o Rejection

o Recurrence of disease

o Death

Adapted from: Mueller AR, Platz KP, and Kremer B. *Best Practice & Research Clinical Gastroenterology* 2004;18(5): 882.

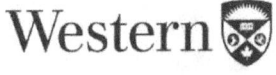

LIVER TRANSPLANTATION

- Give 5 hereditary liver diseases, and outline their diet therapy (always avoid alcohol).

Disorder	Dietary intervention
o Hemochromatosis	- Avoidance of excess dietary iron, selection of foods containing phytates or tannins to reduce iron absorption (together with appropriate phlebotomy treatment)
o Wilson disease	- Low-copper diet - Zinc supplementation (together with chelating agent) - Green tea
o Cystic fibrosis	- High-fat diet, pancreatic enzyme supplements, fat-soluble vitamin supplements, medium chain triglycerides (MCT)
o Hereditary fructose intolerance	- Low fructose, low sucrose diet
o Galactosemia	- Galactose-free diet
o Tyrosinemia	- Low phenylaline and tyrosine diet
o Glycogen storage disease	- Continuous glucose feeding

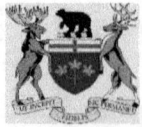

LIVER TRANSPLANTATION

- o Cerebrotendinous xanthomatosis - Deoxycholic acid supplementation

Adapted from: Thapa BR. *Indian J Pediatr.* 1999; 66(1 Suppl): S110-9.

- Give 8 inherited disorders that involve the liver.
  - o Alagille syndrome
  - o Benign intrahepatic cholestasis
  - o Cholesterol ester storage disease
  - o Cystic fibrosis
  - o Dubin-Johnson syndrome
  - o Gilbert syndrome
  - o Hemochromatosis
  - o Pharmacogenetics/pharmacogenomics
  - o Progressive familial intrahepatic cholestasis
  - o Wilson disease
  - o Wolman disease
  - o Zellweger syndrome

Printed with permission: Wright TL. *2007 AGA Institute Postgraduate Course.* pg. 44.

- Give 7 examples of liver disorders which may recur in the liver following liver transplant (recurrence rates in brackets).
  - o HBV (100%)
  - o HCV (more virulent; cholestatic type often fatal)
  - o Alcoholic liver disease (~50% in yr, but may be mild)
  - o NASH

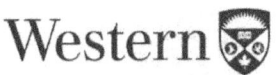

LIVER TRANSPLANTATION

- o PBC, AIH, PSC (20%)
- o Hemochromatosis (late)
- o 2° amyloid
- o HCC

Adapted from: Lilly LB, Girgrah N, and Levy G.A. *First Principles of Gastroenterology* 2005: pg. 642.

Useful background: The UNOS listing criteria for status 1, 2A, 2B and 3 for liver transplantation.

➢ Status 1

- o Fulminant hepatic failure. Onset within 8 weeks of initial symptoms and one of the following:
    - Stage 2 encephalopathy
    - Bilirubin > 15 mg/dl
    - INR > 2.5
    - Hypoglycemia (glucose level < 50 mg/dl)
- o Primary non-function of graft transplanted within 7 days
- o Hepatic artery thrombosis occurring within 7 days of transplantation
- o Acute decompensated Wilson's disease

➢ Status 2A

- o Patient with chronic liver failure and a Child-Pugh score ≥10, in the critical care unit, with a life expectancy without a liver transplant of less than 7 days, with at least one of the following criteria:
    - Unresponsiveness active variceal hemorrhage with failure or contraindication of surgical or transjugular intra-hepatic shunt
    - Hepatorenal syndrome

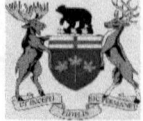

LIVER TRANSPLANTATION

- Refractory ascites/hepatorenal syndrome (hydrothorax)
- Stage 3-4 encephalopathy unresponsive to therapy

o Contraindications to status 2A listing:
  - Extrahepatic sepsis unresponsive to antimicrobial therapy
  - Requirement for high dose or two or more pressor agents to maintain an adequate blood pressure
  - Severe, irreversible multi-organ failure

➢ Status 2B

o Patients with chronic liver disease and a Child-Pugh score ≥ 10, or ≥ 7 and one or more of the following clinical considerations:
  - Unresponsive variceal hemorrhage
  - Hepatorenal syndrome
  - Spontaneous bacterial peritonitis
  - Refractory ascites/hepatorenal syndrome (hydrothorax)

o Liver transplant candidates with hepatocellular carcinoma can be registered as status 2B if they meet the following criteria:
  - Thorough assessment has excluded metastatic disease
  - Recipient has one nodule ≤ 5 cm or three or fewer nodules all ≤ 3cm
  - Patient is not a resection candidate

➢ Status 3
o Patients with chronic liver disease and a Child-Pugh score ≥ 7

Adapted from: United Network Organ Sharing. *UNOS policy 3.6* June 23, 2009.

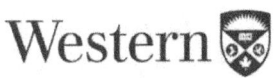

LIVER TRANSPLANTATION

Rejection
Allograft dysfunction

- Acute early cellular rejection of graft occurs in the first few weeks after liver transplantation, especially for REC and AH
- Chronic rejection occurs in 10% of liver transplant recipients, especially in HCV or AH
- Chronic hepatitis of graft develops in 5-10% of liver transplanted patients, and may lead to cirrhosis in the allograft
- Liver diseases that may recur in the transplanted graft include PBC, DSC and AH
- Strictures of biliary tree occur in 20-35% of patients post liver transplantation, especially at the duct-to-duct anastamosis, or at the Roux-en-Y
- Post transplant biliary strictures result from hepatic artery occlusion, chronic allograft rejection, or prolonged cold ischemia time

➤ Hyperacute rejection

- Hyperacute rejection (also known as massive hemorrhagic necrosis) seldom occurs, but when it does it results in rapid graft destruction with coagulative parenchymal necrosis owing to widespread endothelial dysfunction.
- Endothelial cells are primarily targeted by a pre-existing anti-donor humoral immune response that leads to the deposition of antibodies, platelets, fibrin and erythrocytes within the portal venules and hepatic sinusoids.
- Lymphocytes are usually absent and bile ducts unaffected.
- This form of rejection is seen more commonly in recipients with ABO incompatible grafts.

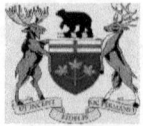

LIVER TRANSPLANTATION

- Acute rejection
  - Acute rejection (also known as cellular rejection) is more common than hyperacute rejection, and usually occurs in the first 3 months post-transplantation.
  - It is characterized by portal tracts that are heavily infiltrated with lymphocytes, bile duct damage and venular inflammation.
  - Early acute rejection (within the first 3 months post-transplantation) generally responds well to increased doses of immunosuppressive agents, with resolution of biliary inflammation and stable long-term allograft function.
  - The degree of inflammation and graft damage does not correlate with either the response to increased immunosuppression or with long-term outcome.
  - By contrast, late acute rejection, recurrent rejection and steroid-resistant rejection are more likely to develop into chronic rejection.

- Chronic rejection
  - Chronic rejection (also known as ductopenic rejection or vanishing bile duct syndrome) affects a small minority of liver allograft patients and may lead to graft loss.
  - A central late feature of chronic rejection is a loss of bile ducts (ductopenia), and pruning of the distal branches of the portal venous system owing to persistent inflammation and arterial foam cell infiltration and the presence of arterial foam cells.
  - Vanishing bile duct syndrome eventually ensues, with progressive cholestasis and liver dysfunction and, ultimately, graft failure.

Printed with permission: Eksteen and Neuberger. *Nature Clinical Practice Gastroenterology & Hepatology* April 2008;5(4): pg 210.

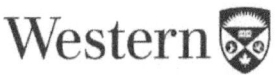

LIVER TRANSPLANTATION

- Give 10 gastrointestinal complications of transplant immunosuppression.
  - Infections
    - Viral: CMV (especially for MMF), HSV
    - Fungal: Candida albicans, candida tropicalis
    - Bacterial: versinia enterocolitica, Clostridium difficile
    - Parasites: microspordia, Strongyloides, *H. pylori* (70% in renal transplant recipients, and 60% in hemodialysis patients)
  - Mucosal injury and ulceration
    - Diarrhea, constipation dyspepsia (especially tacrolimus and MMF)
    - Ulcerations: stress/NSAID ulcers
      - Giant gastric ulcers (>3cm, lung transplant recipients)
    - Diverticular disease: complicated diverticulitis (perforation, abscess, Phlegmon, fistula); especially with polycystic kidney disease
    - Perforations: early, late (especially from diverticulitis or CMV colitis)
  - Biliary tract disease
    - Cholecystectomy (often as an emergency, high mortality [MR])
    - Cholelithiasis
  - Pancreatitis
    - 5% in liver, Tx, MR 64%
  - GI malignancy
    - Lymphomas, Kaposi sarcomas, skin cancer

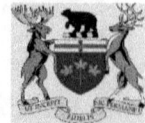

LIVER TRANSPLANTATION

- o Gastric MALT lymphomas; may be associated with *H. pylori*
- o Colorectal cancer (liver Tx, RR, CRC 12.5)
- o Post transplantation Lymphoproliferative disorder (PTLD) (10% of Tx pts; acute perforation, obstruction, bleeding; associated with EBV)

Printed with permission: Helderman JH, and Goral S. *J Am Soc Nephrol* 2002; 13: 277-287.

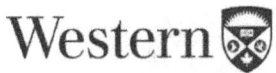

LIVER TRANSPLANTATION

- Give the most common adverse effects of immune-suppressive drugs frequently used after orthotopic liver transplantation.

Adverse effect	Cyclo-sporin	Tacro-limus	Gluco-Corticoids	Azathio-prine	Myco-phenolate Mofetil	mTOR Inhibitors
o Alopecia	-	+	-	+	+	-
o Arterial hypertension	+++	++	+++	-	-	+
o Bone marrow suppression	+	+	-	+++	+++	++
o Dermatitis	-	+ (rash, pruritus)	+	-	-	++ (oral ulcers, acne)
o Gastrointestinal Toxicity	+	+	+	+ pancreatitis	+++ (gastritis and/or diarrhea)	++
o Hirsutism and/or gingival hyperplasia	+	-	-	-	-	-
o Hyperglycemia and diabetes mellitus	-(?)	+	+++	-	-	-
o Hyperlipidemia	++	+	++	-	-	+++
o Impaired wound healing	-	-	+	+	+	++
o Lymphoma or malignancy	++	++	-	?	?	-
o Myalgia and/or arthralgia	-	-	+	+	-	++
o Nephrotoxicity	+++ (K$^+$, Mg^{2+})	+++ (K$^+$, Mg^{2+})	-	-	-	+ proteinuria
o Neurotoxicity[a]	++[a]	++[a]	+ psychiatric	-	+ headache	-

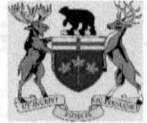

LIVER TRANSPLANTATION

- o Osteoporosis +   +   +++   -   -   -
- o Pneumonitis   -   -   -   -   -   +

- It should be noted that each agent has other specific adverse effects in addition to those listed in the table.

[a]Neurotoxicity includes mainly peripheral neuropathy, headaches, tremor, convulsions, akinetic mutism, and insomnia.

?, Incidence unknown; - not reported; + rarely reported; ++ commonly reported; +++ very frequently reported adverse effect limiting usage of the drug.

Printed with permission: Benten D, et al. *Nature Clinical Practice Gastroenterology and Hepatology* 2009;6:1:23-36.

Longterm considerations after liver transplantation

- ➤ Post-transplant diabetes and cardiovascular disease
    - o Early after liver transplantation, transient hyperglycemia occurs in 40% of patients, and 9-21% have persistent hyperglycemia (new onset diabetes)
    - o Hyperlipidemia occurs in 20-50% of liver transplant patient, with a 2.6 fold higher risk of coronary artery disease (CAD) and 20% of deaths occurring 3 years after liver transplantation coming from CAD
    - o Squamous cell and basal cell skin cancer is 12-90 times more common in transplanted patient
    - o There is a 10-fold increased risk of non-Hodgkins lymphoma (B-cell related to EBV) after liver transplantation, giving a relative risk of 3%

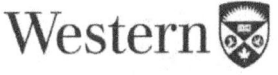

LIVER TRANSPLANTATION

- In patients given a liver transplant for PSC in the settling of associated UC, the incidence of CRC is 1% per year, with a cumulative risk of colonic mucosal dysplasia of 15% at 5 years and 21% at 8 years

Abbreviation: CAD, coronary artery disease

➢ Steatosis
  - Steatosis occurs in as many as a third of persons following a liver transplantation (LT), with a histological diagnosis of NASH occurring in about 10% of these persons.
  - Multivariant analysis has shown that seven factors predict the risk for post-LT steatosis: post-LT obesity, diabetes mellitus, hyperlipidemia, arterial hypertension, a tacrolimus-based immunosuppression regimen, and alcoholic cirrhosis as the primary indication for LT (Dumortier et al., AJG 2010; 105: 613-620). The more of these risk factors that are present, the higher their rate for steatosis: for example; 3 factors, 30% risk; 4-66%; 5-82%; 6 risk factors, 100% ped LT steatosis.

➢ Sexual function and pregnancy
  - Decreased libido in 25% of men and women after liver transplantation
  - Erectile dysfunction in 30% of men after liver transplantation
  - Post-transplant, pregnancy is associated with increased fetal loss (18%), low birth weight (31%), and premature delivery (39%), pre-eclampsia (21%), and the need for caesarian section (47%)

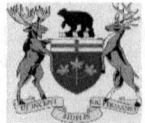

LIVER TRANSPLANTATION

- Allograft rejection occurs in 10-20% of women during pregnancy, with increased risk of miscarriages and premature labour

References and Suggested Reading

Benten D, et al. Orthotopic liver transplantation and what to do during follow-up: recommendations for the practitioner. *Nature Clinical Practice Gastroenterology & Hepatology* 2009;6(1):23-36.

Cholongitas E, et al. Prioritization for liver transplantation. *Nature Reviews Gastroenterology and Hepatology* 2010;7:659-668.

Clark NM, et al. Infectious complications in liver transplantation. UptoDate; www.uptodate.com 2014

Cotler SJ, et al. Diagnosis of acute cellular rejection in liver transplantation. UpToDate online Journal. www.uptodate.com 2014

Cotler SJ, et al. Living Donor Liver transplantation. UpToDate online Journal. www.uptodate.com 2014

Croome KP, et al. Should a lower quality organ go to the least sick patient? Model for end-stage liver disease score and donor risk index as predictors of early allograft dysfunction. *Transplant Proc.* 2012;44(5):1303-1306.

Dove LM. Et al. Patient selection for liver transplantation. UptoDate; www.uptodate.com 2014

DuBay D, et al. Liver transplantation for advanced hepatocellular carcinoma using poor tumour differentiation on biopsy as an exclusion criterion. *Annals of Surgery* 2011;253:166-172.

Dufy JP, et al. Long term patient outcome and quality of life after liver transplantation: analysis of 20 year survivors. *Annals of Surgery* 2010;252:652-661.

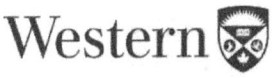

Lesurtel M, et al. 2010 International consensus conference on liver transplantation for hepatocellular carcinoma. *Liver Transplantation* 2011;17 (suppl 2):S1-5.

Mathur AK, et al. Racial and ethnic disparities in access to liver transplantation. *Liver Transplantation* 2010;16:1033-1040.

Merion RM. Current status and future of liver transplantation. *Seminars in Liver Disease* 2010;30:411-421.

Michael R, et al. Frequency and Outcomes of Liver Transplantation for Nonalcoholic Steatohepatitis in the United States. *Gastroenterology* 2011;141:1249-1253.

Mukherjee S, et al. Immediate listing for liver transplantation for alcoholic cirrhosis: Curbing our enthusiasm. *Annals of Internal Medicine* 2009;150(3):216-217.

Pastor CM, et al.Therapy insight: hepatopulmonary syndrome and orthotopic liver transplantation. *Nature Clinical Practice Gastroenterology & Hepatology* 2007;4(11):614-621.

Schaubel D, et al. Survival benefit-based deceased-donor liver allocation. *American Journal of Transplantation* 2009;9:970-981.

Sorrell MF, et al. Immediate listing for liver transplantation for alcoholic cirrhosis: Curbing our enthusiasm. *Annals of Internal Medicine* 2009;150(3):216-7.

Vanlemmens C, et al. Immediate listing for liver transplantation versus standard care for child-Pugh stage B Alcoholic cirrhosis: A Randomized Trial. *Annals of Internal Medicine* 2009;150(3):153-161.

Waki K, et al. Outcome of Liver Transplantation for Recipients With Hepatitis B and Hepatitis C Virus Coinfection: Analysis of UNOS Data. *Transplantation* 2011;92:809-814.

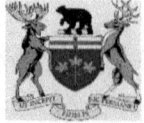

Zarrinpar A, et al. Liver Transplantation: Toward a unified allocation system *Nature Reviews Gastroenterology and Hepatology* 2011;8:542-543.

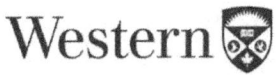

MINI UPDATE

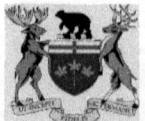

De Novo Malignancy in the Liver Transplantation Recipient

Natasha Chandok

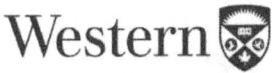

Outline and Aims

1. Background
2. Incidence and risk factors
3. Post-transplant lymphoproliferative disorder (PTLD) pathogenesis, management
4. Screening and preventive measures for non-lymphoproliferative cancers
5. Future directions

Background

- Overall mortality rates following liver transplantation have dropped incrementally in the last decades
- Recipient survival ~ 92% at 1 year and ~ 80% at 5 years in Canada in 2010
- Survival rates beyond one year have been more stagnant

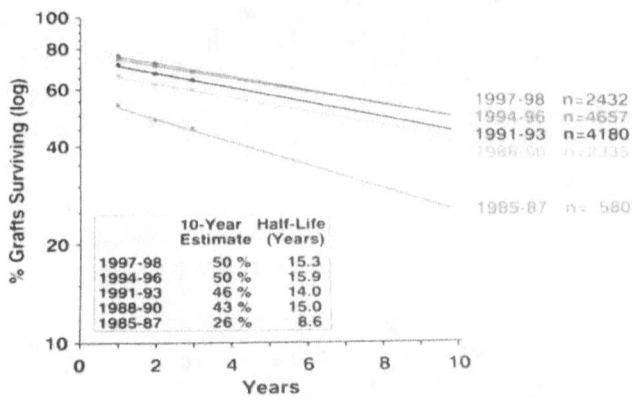

Source: United network for organ sharing, 2012; European liver transplant registry. 2011; Gelson W, et al. *Transplantation.* 2011;91(11):1240-4; Lodhi SA, et al. *Am J Transplant.* 2011;11(6):1226-35.

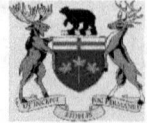

LIVER TRANSPLANTATION

- o Have long-term recipient survival rates after LT reached a plateau, or is there room to improve further
- o Post-transplant morbidity and mortality statistics are difficult to gather
- o Geography, patient privacy/ laws, lack of centralized electronic medical records, etc.
- o What is the London story?

- o Maintains Exceptional long-term follow-up data
- o Why?
  - Complexity of care mandates periodic assessments
  - Limited transplant centers in Canada
  - Shortage of subspecialized care in largely rural catchment area
  - Referring provider preference
  - Emotional attachment of the recipient to the center

> "You don't have to see the whole staircase, just take the first step."
>
> Unknown

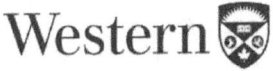

134 consecutive deaths

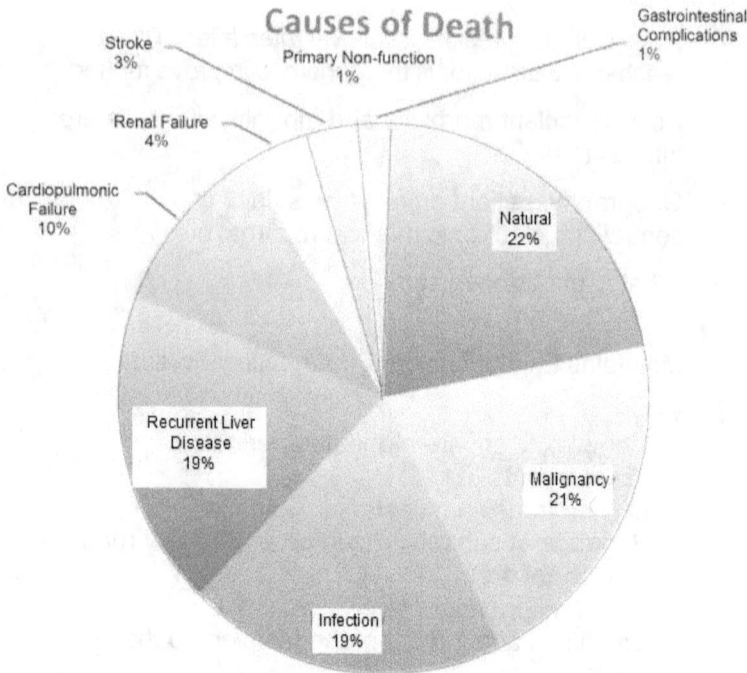

- De Novo cancer
  - Among the top 3 causes of death post-LT
  - 2 x risk for non-skin solid organ; 30x risk for lymphoproliferative
- Why?
  - Recipients are older
  - Calcineurin inhibition
  - Environmental exposures
  - Infectious exposures

Vogt DP, et al. The long-term survival and causes of death in patients who survive at least 1 year after liver transplantation. *Surgery*. 2002;132(4):775-80

Haagsma EB, et al. Increased cancer risk after liver transplantation: a population-based study. *J Hepatol*. 2001 Jan;34(1):84-91.

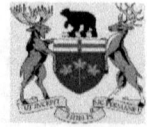

LIVER TRANSPLANTATION

Magnitude of the Problem

- Non-lymphoproliferative: Cumulative incidence 10% in 10 years
- Lymphoproliferative: 1-5% of adult recipients; 5-15% of pediatric recipients
- 3 of the top 10 causes of death in developed countries are some kind of malignancy (WHO), so do recipients really have a higher risk of solid organ cancer?
- Problems with the literature: Mono-centric, retrospective, registry based studies rely on voluntary disclosure
- Nevertheless ... countless single center studies, and a handful of high quality population based studies, that definitively demonstrate de novo cancer as a frequent cause of late death

WHO 2011
Pisani P, Bray F, Parkin DM. Estimates of the world-wide prevalence of cancer for 25 sites in the adult population. *Int J Cancer.* 2002;97(1):72-81.
Aberg F, et al. Risk of malignant neoplasms after liver transplantation: a population-based study. *Liver Transpl.* 2008;14(10):1428-36.

Post-transplant lymphoproliferative disorder (PTLD)

- Uncontrolled lymphoproliferation in an immunocompromised patients after solid organ transplant
- Incidence 1-2% (incidence incrementally higher in renal, heart, lung, intestine or multi-organ recipients paralleling greater degree of immunosuppression)
- Most likely time to onset: the first 12-18 months after

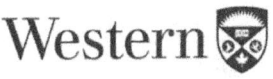

Abbreviation: PTLD, post-transplant lymphoproliferative disorder

Kremers WK, et al. Post-transplant lymphoproliferative disorders following liver transplantation: incidence, risk factors and survival. *Am J Transplant.* 2006;6(5 Pt 1):1017-24.

Opelz G, Henderson R. Incidence of non-Hodgkin lymphoma in kidney and heart transplant recipients. Lancet. 1993;342(8886-8887):1514-6.

Newell KA, et al. Comparison of pancreas transplantation with portal venous and enteric exocrine drainage to the standard technique utilizing bladder drainage of exocrine secretions. *Transplantation.* 1996 Nov 15;62(9):1353-6.

➢ Risk factors PTLD

Variable	Comment
o Recipient age	- Pediatric incidence is ≥ 3X vs adults
o EBV serostatus	- Higher risk statuses include mismatch, primary infection or reactivation. - Incidence rate ratios > 70X higher with EBV seropositivity.
o Degree of immunosuppression	- No effect with type of CNI or retransplantation status. - Higher rates in non-liver recipients.

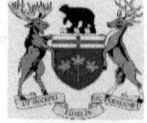

LIVER TRANSPLANTATION

- 3-fold higher rates in those exposed to OKT3.

o Time from LT < 18 months
- Most likely to occur within the first year
- Occurs earlier in children than adults.

Nelson BP, et al. Epstein-Barr virus-negative post-transplant lymphoproliferative disorders: a distinct entity? *Am J Surg Pathol.* 2000;24(3):375-85.

Parker A, et al. Management of post-transplant lymphoproliferative disorder in adult solid organ transplant recipients - BCSH and BTS Guidelines. *Br J Haematol.* 2010;149(5):693-705. Epub 2010 Apr 16.

➢ Pathogenesis

o EBV establishes latent infection in B cells

o Immunosuppression → weakened surveillance capacity of T cells → propagation of EBV – infected B cells → lymphoma

o EBV-negative and/ or T cell PTLD has poorly understood pathogenesis and dire prognosis

o 85% are B-cell origin (80% of these are EBV associated)

o Compared with lymphoma in non-transplant patients, PTLD is associated with
- Extranodal involvement
- High grade, poor clinical outcome

Saha A, Robertson ES. Epstein-Barr virus-associated B-cell lymphomas: pathogenesis and clinical outcomes. *Clin Cancer Res.* 2011;17(10):3056-63.

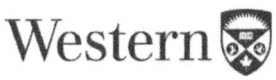

Nelson BP, et al. Epstein-Barr virus-negative post-transplant lymphoproliferative disorders: a distinct entity? *Am J Surg Pathol.* 2000;24(3):375-85.

- Negative prognostic factors
    - High grade/ stage
    - T-cell disease
    - CNS or bone marrow involvement
    - Poor performance status
    - EBV negativity
    - Graft involvement
- Clinical manifestations
    - Correlate to disease location and stage
    - Often nonspecific/ constitutionalCommonest sites of involvement: lymphatic system, GI system (especially the hepatic graft), kidneys
    - Must have high index of suspicion

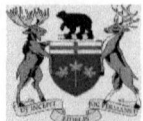

LIVER TRANSPLANTATION

PTLD of skin

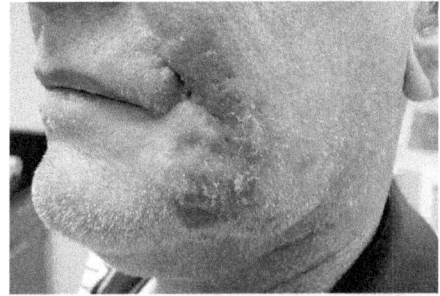

PTLD of colon

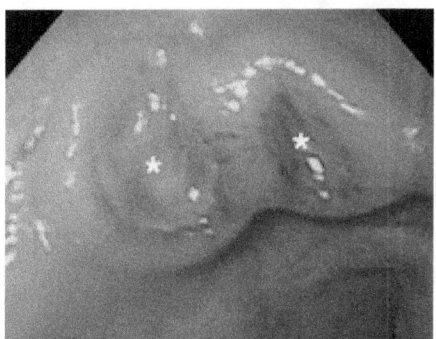

PTLD of brain

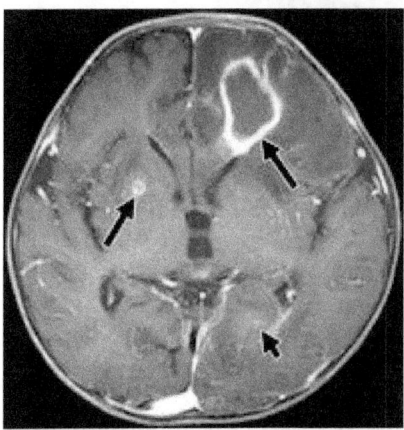

Parker A, et al. Management of post-transplant lymphoproliferative disorder in adult solid organ transplant recipients - BCSH and BTS Guidelines. *Br J Haematol.* 2010;149(5): 693-705.

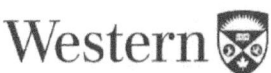

- Diagnosis
    - Elevated lactate dehydrogenase (LDH), high/ rising EBV viral load, and characteristic diagnostic imaging findings
    - Routine EBV monitoring to facilitate early diagnosis is postulated but unproven to be of use.
    - Tissue diagnosis (with excisional or needle core liver biopsy) and comprehensive staging
    - Various grading systems, e.g. Society for hematopathology, European American lymphoma group

PLTD of liver

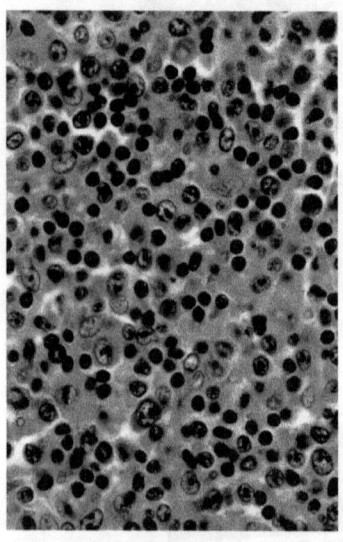

Paya CV, et al. Epstein-Barr virus-induced posttransplant lymphoproliferative disorders. ASTS/ASTP EBV-PTLD Task Force and The Mayo Clinic Organized International Consensus Development Meeting. *Transplantation.* 1999;68(10):1517-25.

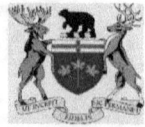

Parker A, et al. Management of post-transplant lymphoproliferative disorder in adult solid organ transplant recipients - BCSH and BTS Guidelines. *Br J Haematol.* 2010;149(5):693-705.

Allen U, et al. Epstein-Barr virus infection in transplant recipients: Summary of a workshop on surveillance, prevention and treatment. *Can J Infect Dis.* 2002;13(2):89-99.

> **Prognosis**
>   - Historically, mortality rates are 50%
>   - Large U of Michigan series: median overall survival 8.23 years, 95% confidence internal 2.28 – 30.0 years
>   - Actuarial patient survival rates at 1, 5, 10 years post-diagnosis: 85%, 49%, 55%

Richendollar BG, et al. Predictors of outcome in post-transplant lymphoproliferative disorder: an evaluation of tumor infiltrating lymphocytes in the context of clinical factors. *Leuk Lymphoma.* 2009;50(12):2005-12.

Harris NL, Ferry JA, Swerdlow SH. Posttransplant lymphoproliferative disorders: summary of Society for Hematopathology Workshop. *Semin Diagn Pathol.* 1997;14(1):8-14.

Trofe J, et al. Analysis of factors that influence survival with post-transplant lymphoproliferative disorder in renal transplant recipients: the Israel Penn International Transplant Tumor Registry experience. *Am J Transplant.* 2005;5(4 Pt 1):775-80.

> **Management**
>   - Immunosuppression reduction (start with 25 to 50% reduction)
>   - Likely to work in patients with

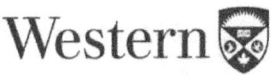

- Early polymorphic disease
- Without high LDH, organ dysfunction or multi-organ involvement
- 90% response rate usually seen within 4 weeks

  o Overall effectiveness of this strategy: 70%

  o Antiviral therapy (acyclovir, ganciclovir) is unproven

  o Chemotherapy

  o Biologics therapy (rituximab)

  o Radiation therapy } Localized disease / Rx - CNS

> Surgery

Buell JF, et al. Skin cancer following transplantation: the Israel Penn International Transplant Tumor Registry experience. *Transplant Proc.* 2005;37(2):962-3.

Tsai DE, et al. Reduction in immunosuppression as initial therapy for posttransplant lymphoproliferative disorder: analysis of prognostic variables and long-term follow-up of 42 adult patients. *Transplantation.* 2001;71(8):1076-88.

- Chemotherapy

  o E.g. cyclophosphamide, doxorubicin, vincristine, prednisone (CHOP)

  o Multi-agent > single-agent; No "superior" regimen

  o Response rate ~ 65%

  o Inadequate response to other Rx, High-grade; organ compromise

Choquet S, et al. CHOP-21 for the treatment of post-transplant lymphoproliferative disorders (PTLD)

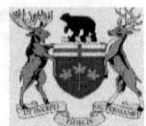

LIVER TRANSPLANTATION

following solid organ transplantation. *Haematologica.* 2007;92(2):273-4.

- Biologics therapy
  - Rituximab – monoclonal antibody to CD 20
  - Majority of PTLD – CD20 +ve
  - Remission rate 44-65%
  - Well-tolerated (many centers use rituximab as 2nd line treatment for CD20+ PTLD)

Blaes AH, et al. Rituximab therapy is effective for posttransplant lymphoproliferative disorders after solid organ transplantation: results of a phase II trial. *Cancer.* 2005;104(8):1661-7.
Choquet S, et al. CHOP-21 for the treatment of post-transplant lymphoproliferative disorders (PTLD) following solid organ transplantation. *Haematologica.* 2007;92(2):273-4.

Non-Lymphoproliferative - De Novo Malignancy post liver transplantation after L-Tx

➢ Risk factors
  - Recipient age
  - Immunosuppression
  - Underlying ALD or PSC
  - Sun exposure
  - Smoking

Abbreviation: ALD, alcoholic liver disease; PSC, primary sclerosing cholangitis; L-Tx, liver transplantation

Non-melanoma Skin Cancer (NMSC)

  - Most common malignancy after L-Tx
  - Standardized incidence ratio > 30

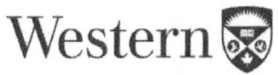

- UNOS study of 8049 L-Tx recipients followed for 5 years: 104 cases (1.29%) of NMSC; these patients had a lower risk of dying within 5 years (adjusted for era, CNI agent, +/- induction Rx)
- ? higher immunosuppression = less allograft failure = Better recipient surviaal & NMSC is rarely fatal
- Level I evidence that skin checks and sun screen prevent NMSC

Abbreviation: L-Tx, liver transplantation

Ulrich C, et al. Prevention of non-melanoma skin cancer in organ transplant patients by regular use of a sunscreen: a 24 months, prospective, case-control study. *Br J Dermatol.* 2009;161 Suppl 3:78-84.

Non-skin solid organ cancers in liver transplantation (L-Tx) recipients
- 1% per annum; overall incidence is 3-15%
- More common after the 1st year
- Associated with increasing age of recipient
- Skin cancer and sarcoma is more common
- Liver cancer more common in L-tx recipients who had
    - ALD (alcoholic liver disease)
    - IBD – associated PSC

Abbreviation: IBD, inflammatory bowel disease; PSC, primary sclerosing cholangitis

Watt KD, et al. Long-term probability of and mortality from de novo malignancy after liver transplantation. *Gastroenterology.* 2009 Dec;137(6):2010-7.

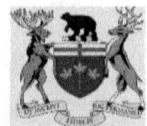

LIVER TRANSPLANTATION

Solid organ cancers
- Less common but impose notable threat on recipient survival
- Overall risk is 2X higher than general population
- Non-skin cancers at the highest frequencies: Kaposi sarcoma (SIR 212), esophagus (SIR 18.7), H&N (SIR 4.6)
- Prospective study of L-Tx database of NIDDK from 1990-2003: 95 of 798 (11.9%) of adult recipients

Watt KD, et al. Long-term probability of and mortality from de novo malignancy after liver transplantation. *Gastroenterology.* 2009;137(6):2010-7.

Alcohol
- Risk factor for many cancers
  - Oropharyngeal
  - Laryngeal
  - Esophageal
  - Liver
  - Colon
- No high level evidence to quantify this risk in L-Tx reciepients
- Adults transplanted for ALD have a 2-fold higher rate of non-skin cancer development in 10 years compared with adults transplanted for other conditions (except PSC)
- 18% at 10 years vs 10% at 10 years

Abbreviation: ALD, alcoholic liver disease; PSC, primary sclerosing cholangitis

Watt KD, et al. Long-term probability of and mortality from de novo malignancy after liver transplantation. *Gastroenterology.* 2009;137(6):2010-7.

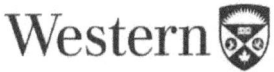

Primary Sclerosing Cholangitis (PSC)
- PSC has the highest cumulative incidence of de novo malignancy as compared with all other liver disease groups
- 22% at 10 years vs 10% at 10 years (non-EtOH)
- Estimated hazard ratio for the development of colorectal cancer (CRC) in IBD-PSC post L-Tx is 3.51 (p=0.005)
- No evidence that L-Tx recipients without IBD-PSC have higher rates of CRC
- However, given epidemiologic associations between immunosuppression and several cancers, aggressive screening is advised

Abbreviation: CRC, colorectal cancer; IBD-PSC, inflammatory bowel disease – associated primary biliary cirrhosis; L-Tx, liver transplantation

Watt KD, et al. Long-term probability of and mortality from de novo malignancy after liver transplantation. *Gastroenterology*. 2009;137(6):2010-7.

Other cancers
- Prostate, lung and breast cancer do not appear to occur at increased frequency in L-Tx recipients compared with the general population

Herrero JI. De novo malignancies following liver transplantation: impact and recommendations. *Liver Transpl*. 2009;15 Suppl 2:S90-4.

➢ Management
- Select recipients and donors carefully

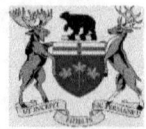

LIVER TRANSPLANTATION

- Many risk factors are non-modifiable
  - Recipient age
  - Viral exposures
  - Underlying liver disease
- o Minimize immunosuppression
- o Counselling on
  - Smoking cessation
  - Excess alcohol abstinence
  - Sun protection and avoidance
  - Adherence to guidelines for screening for breast, prostate, colon
- o Multidisciplinary care pathways with screening protocols may improve detection rates
- o Excellent communication with general providers

Herrero JI. De novo malignancies following liver transplantation: impact and recommendations. *Liver Transpl.* 2009;15 Suppl 2:S90-4.

- o Sirolimus – inhibitor of the mammalian target of rapamycin (m TOR) with anti-proliferative properties

  - mTOR is a member of the phosphoinositide 3-kinase related kinase (PIKK) family that is the principal mediator of cell proliferation

  - Complex between FKBP12 (FK506 binding protein 12, site of binding of sirolimus) and mTOR
    - Prevents cyclin-dependent kinase activation
    - Blocks retinoblastoma protein phosphorylation
    - Accelerates turnover of cyclin DI that causes deficiency of active CD-k4-cyclin DI

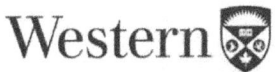

- Complexes → inhibits mTOR → blocks phosphorylation of key effector molecules (p70 S6 kinase; eukaryotic initiation factor 4E) → anti-proliferation

    o No evidence of a reduction in non-skin cancer

- Summary
    o De novo malignancy is a leading cause of morbidity and mortality in L-Tx recipients
    o Survival rates after 1 year form L-Tx have been stagnant, and targeted efforts to reduce the burden of post-transplant cancers may improve long-term outcomes on an otherwise successful surgery
    o Risk factors – recipient characteristics, underlying liver disease, immunosuppression, environmental exposures
    o Multicenter consortiums to facilitate research (e.g. immunosuppression optimization, protocolized screening)

References and Suggested Reading

Aberg F, et al. Risk of malignant neoplasms after liver transplantation: a population-based study. *Liver Transpl.* 2008;14(10):1428-36.

Gelson W, et al. The pattern of late mortality in liver transplant recipients in the United Kingdom. *Transplantation.* 2011;91(11):1240-4.

Herrero JI. De novo malignancies following liver transplantation: impact and recommendations. *Liver Transpl.* 2009;15 Suppl 2:S90-4.

Lodhi SA, et al. Solid organ allograft survival improvement in the United States: the long-term does not mirror the

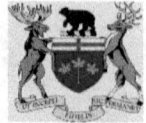

dramatic short-term success. *Am J Transplant.* 2011;11(6):1226-35.

Parker A, et al. Management of post-transplant lymphoproliferative disorder in adult solid organ transplant recipients - BCSH and BTS Guidelines. *Br J Haematol.* 2010;149(5):693-705.

Paya CV, et al. Epstein-Barr virus-induced posttransplant lymphoproliferative disorders. ASTS/ASTP EBV-PTLD Task Force and The Mayo Clinic Organized International Consensus Development Meeting. *Transplantation.* 1999;68(10):1517-25.

Pisani P, Bray F, Parkin DM. Estimates of the world-wide prevalence of cancer for 25 sites in the adult population. *Int J Cancer.* 2002;97(1):72-81.

Richendollar BG, et al. Predictors of outcome in post-transplant lymphoproliferative disorder: an evaluation of tumor infiltrating lymphocytes in the context of clinical factors. *Leuk Lymphoma.* 2009;50(12):2005-12.

Saha A, Robertson ES. Epstein-Barr virus-associated B-cell lymphomas: pathogenesis and clinical outcomes. *Clin Cancer Res.* 2011;17(10):3056-63.

Trofe J, et al. Analysis of factors that influence survival with post-transplant lymphoproliferative disorder in renal transplant recipients: the Israel Penn International Transplant Tumor Registry experience. *Am J Transplant.* 2005;5(4 Pt 1):775-80.

Tsai DE, et al. Reduction in immunosuppression as initial therapy for posttransplant lymphoproliferative disorder: analysis of prognostic variables and long-term follow-up of 42 adult patients. *Transplantation.* 2001;71(8):1076-88.

Ulrich C, et al. Prevention of non-melanoma skin cancer in organ transplant patients by regular use of a sunscreen: a 24 months, prospective, case-control study. *Br J Dermatol.* 2009;161 Suppl 3:78-84.

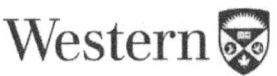

United network for organ sharing, 2012

Vogt DP, et al. The long-term survival and causes of death in patients who survive at least 1 year after liver transplantation. *Surgery*. 2002;132(4):775-80

Watt KD, et al. Long-term probability of and mortality from de novo malignancy after liver transplantation. *Gastroenterology*. 2009;137(6):2010-7.

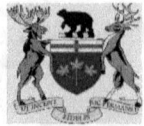

MINI UPDATE

Minimal Hepatic Encephalopathy

Malcolm Wells

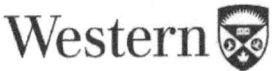

INTERESTING ERCP CASES

Starting with Hepatic Encephalopathy (HE)

- Demography
  - HE occurs in ½ to ¾ of cirrhotics
  - Effects of HE non-transplanted mortality rate > 50% in 3 year

- Pathophysiology

- Outline the contribution of the small and large intestine, liver, skeletal muscle, kidney and brain in patients with liver failure and HE.

  - Small bowel and large intestine
    - Dietary amino acids and urease-positive bacteria → glutamine

    $$\text{glutamine} \quad \xrightarrow{\text{glutaminase (deamination)}} \quad \text{glutamate} + NH_3$$
    $$\xleftarrow{\text{glutamine synthetase (amination)}}$$

    - Activity of gut glutaminase increased in liver disease
    - Uptake of glutamine

  - Liver
    - Portosystemic shunting, by-passing portovenous system with less hepatic detoxification of ammonia via the urea cycle
    - NH_3 → urea, periportal hepatocytes → glutamine, perivenous hepatocytes

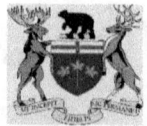

MINI UPDATE

- In presence of hyponatremia, myoinositol falls, with less compensation for ↑ intracellular glutamine

o Skeletal muscle
  - Normally responsible for uptake of 50% of NH_3
  - In cirrhosis, atrophy of skeletal muscles → ↓ muscle synthesis of glutamine

o Kidney
  - ↑ NH_3 production in presence of hypokalemia

o Brain
  - NH_3 and glutamate are normally converted and detoxified to glutamine by glutamine synthetase in astrocytes
  - In cirrhosis
    - ↑ brain blood flow
    - ↑ blood brain barrier permeability → ↑ brain NH_3 and glutamate → asteocyte swelling
  - In presence of hypokalemia and metabolic alkalosis, NH_4 → NH_3, which crosses BBB
  - Plasma NH_3 > 150 µmol is associated with brain herniation
  - Abnormal form and function of astrocytes, with reduced glutamine synthetase and peripheral type benzodiazepine receptors (PTBR)
    - ↑ mitochondrial permeability → ↑ astrocyte swelling → ↑ brain edema
  - ↑ NH_3 activates N-methyl-D-aspartate-nitric oxide-C-guanylate cyclase (NMDA-NO-C6MP) signal transduction pathway → impairment of
    - Memory
    - Learning

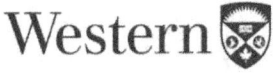

- Sleep

Neurotransmitter system	Findings in HE
o Glutamate (neuro-excitation)	- ↓ receptors → ↓ uptake of glutamate → - ↓ glutamatergic neurotransmitter function
o GABA/BZ (neuro-inhibition)	- ↑ endogenous BZs
o Dopamine/Noradrenaline (motor/cognitive)	- ↓false neurotransmitters
o Serotonin (arousal)	- ↑ serotonin turnover, synaptic defect

Abbreviations: BZ, benzodiazepine; GABA-γ-aminobutyric acid

- o Brain
  - ↑ BB permeability → ↑ NH$_3$ uptake
  - ↑ NH$_3$ taken uptake into
    - Cerebellum
    - Basal ganglia
    - ↑ brain edema
    - ↑ swelling of astrocytes - ↑ neurosteroids → ↑ activity of GABA-benzodiazepine system
    - ↑ benzodiazepine system
    - ↑ production of glutamine by astrocytes

➢ Pathology

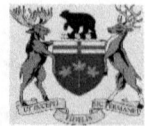

MINI UPDATE

SO YOU WANT TO BE A HEPATOLOGIST!

- Give the pathological changes in the brain of persons dying from hepatic encephalopathy (HE).

    - Capillaries — Vacuolization of basement membranes (↑ permeability of blood-brain barrier)
    - Edema — Brain
      - Endothelial cells
      - Astroglial cell
    - Herniation — Brainstem

> Clinical

- Give a grading of the mental state of persons with HE.

    - Stage 0 — No clinical findings, but abnormal psychometric tests may progress to higher stages of HE

    - Stage 1 — Minor changes in
      - Affect
      - Sleep
      - Concentration
      - Trivial lack of awareness
      - Euphoria or anxiety
      - Shortened attention span
      - Impaired performance of addition; sleep-wake disorder; tremor

    - Stage 2 — Dowiness
      - Disorientation
      - Confusion

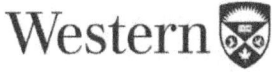

- Lethargy or apathy
- Minimal disorientation of time or place
- Subtle personality changes
- Inappropriate behavior
- Impaired performance of subtraction

- Stage 3
  - Somnolence
  - Incoherence
  - Somnolence to semi-stupor, but responsive to verbal stimuli
  - Confusion
  - Gross disorientation

- Stage 4
  - Coma (unresponsiveness to verbal or noxious stimuli), with
    - Minimal response (4a)
    - No response (4b)

Adapted from: Fitz GJ. *Sleisenger & Fordtran's Gastrointestinal and Liver Disease: Pathophysiology/Diagnosis/Management* 2006: pg. 1966.; and 2010, pg. 1545.

Patients with stage 0 to 2 HE and who can co-orperate with the physical examination will have tremor and asterixis. Patients with stage 3 or 4 may not be able to corporate for the clinical testing for these signs.

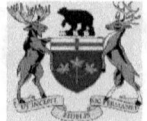

MINI UPDATE

- Give the 3 upper motor neuron signs in stage 3 or 4 HE which can be demonstrated without the patient's co-orporation.
  - Hyperreflexia
  - Clonus
  - Hyperigidity
  - Positive Babinski sign

Minimal Encephalopathy (MHE)

- Definition: Minimal Encephalopathy (MHE) is detected on psychometric testing, and not by the standard clinical examination

- Pathophysiology
  - Ammonia (NH_3) acting with other toxins may lead to changes in
    - Blood-to-brain transport of neurotransmitter precursors
    - Changes in the metabolism of amino acid neurotransmitters
    - Cerebral glucose oxidation.
  - These changes may lead to
    - Activation of inhibitory (GABA, serotonin)
    - Impairment of excitatory (glutamate, catecholamines) neurotransmitter systems

- Clinical
  - Overt Hepatic Encephalopathy (OHE, Stages 1-4)
    - Patients had decreased survival even with one episode
    - Range of deficits
  - Minimal Hepatic encephalopathy

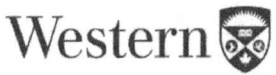

- Leading cause of cognitive dysfunction in cirrhotics
- Marked impairment in QoL and job performance
- Increased risk of developing overt HE
- Increase in overall mortality
- Impaired Driving
  - Lower driving scores on simulations and standardized on-road tests
  - Impaired navigation skills, more traffic violations and more accidents
  o Rule Out other causes of confusion/↓ LOC in OHE and MHE
  - Gastrointestinal bleeding
  - Infection (including spontaneous bacterial peritonitis and urinary tract infections)
  - Hypokalemia and/or metabolic alkalosis
  - Renal failure
  - Hypovolemia
  - Hypoxia
  - Sedatives or tranquilizers
  - Hypoglycemia
  - Constipation
  - Hepatocellular carcinoma
  - Vascular occlusion (hepatic vein or portal vein thrombosis)

Abbreviations: OHE, overt hepatic encephalopathy; MHE, minimal hepatic encephalopathy; LOC, level of consciousness

➢ Blood
  o Venous Ammonia concentration
    - Not useful
    - Correlated with OHE to 2X ULN
    - Any further increase in venous [NH_3] doesn't confer additional risk of OHE

  o Partial pressure of gaseous ammonia (pNH3)

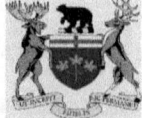

MINI UPDATE

- The grade of HE is more closely related to pNH3 than the total arterial ammonia concentration, since gaseous ammonia readily enters the brain
- Rarely measured outside clinical trials

o Other potential markers
  - Serum 3-nitrotyrosine may be elevated in patients with MHE
  - a cutoff of 14 nM, was 93 percent sensitive and 89 percent specific for detecting MHE

Source: Am J Gastroenterol. 2011;106(9):1629.

"Challenges are what make life interesting and overcoming them is what makes life meaningful."

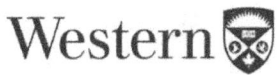

INTERESTING ERCP CASES

> Diagnostic Algorithm

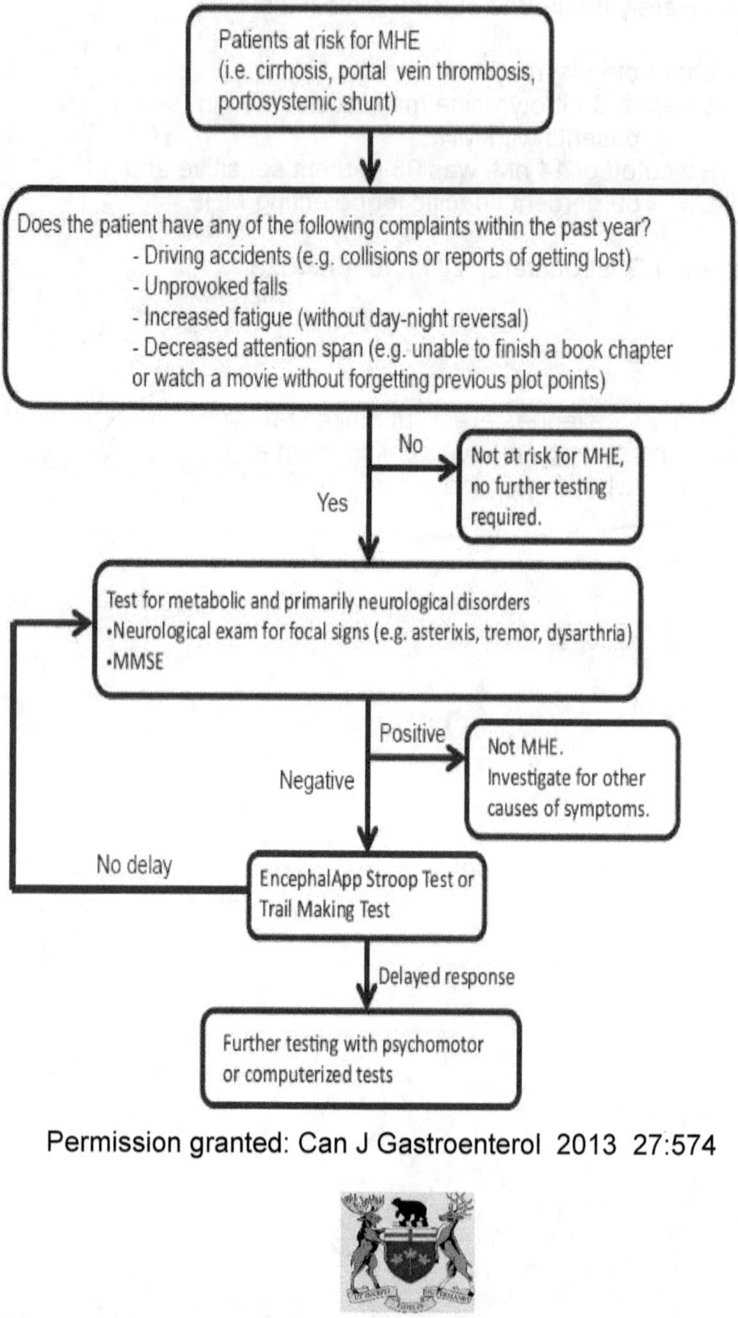

```
┌─────────────────────────────────────┐
│ Patients at risk for MHE            │
│ (i.e. cirrhosis, portal vein        │
│ thrombosis, portosystemic shunt)    │
└─────────────────────────────────────┘
                 │
                 ▼
```

Does the patient have any of the following complaints within the past year?
- Driving accidents (e.g. collisions or reports of getting lost)
- Unprovoked falls
- Increased fatigue (without day-night reversal)
- Decreased attention span (e.g. unable to finish a book chapter or watch a movie without forgetting previous plot points)

→ **No**: Not at risk for MHE, no further testing required.

↓ **Yes**

Test for metabolic and primarily neurological disorders
- Neurological exam for focal signs (e.g. asterixis, tremor, dysarthria)
- MMSE

→ **Positive**: Not MHE. Investigate for other causes of symptoms.

↓ **Negative**

EncephalApp Stroop Test or Trail Making Test

← **No delay** (loops back)

↓ **Delayed response**

Further testing with psychomotor or computerized tests

Permission granted: Can J Gastroenterol 2013 27:574

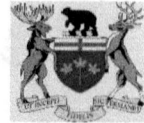

MINI UPDATE

- Psychometric testing

  - Number connection test (NCT, aka Reitan Test)
    - The most frequently used psychometric test
    - A timed connect-the-numbers test.
    - Finish in a number of seconds less than or equal to their age
    - The test traditionally has two parts, but often only the first part of the test can be confusing and often does not add additional clinical information
    - Wasn't designed specifically for MHE, but has some validation for it

  - Psychometric Hepatic Encephalopathy Score (PHES)
    - Designed specifically for MHE
    - Combination of five paper and pencil tests
      - Line tracing test
      - Digit symbol test
      - Serial dotting test
      - Both parts of the NCT (Reitan number connection test)
    - Performed in 10-20 min
    - Possible PHES scores range from -18 to +6 points.
    - PHES score ≤ -4 has a high sensitivity and specificity for detecting MHE
    - Recommended by panel of international experts, though in practice it is rarely used

  - Other test
    - Inhibitory Control Test
      - Attention and response test designed for ADHD and psychosis
      - Patient responds when targets are alternating
    - Cognitive Drug Research Battery
      - Computerized testing
      - Doesn't rely as heavily on motor function
      - Compares well to PHES

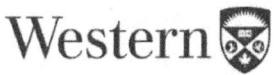

- Repeatable Battery for the Assessment of Neuropsychological Status (RBANS)
  - Not yet compared to PHES
- Stroop test
  - Outcomes included time to complete five correct runs as well as number of trials needed in on (Ontime) and off (Offtime) states
  - A cutoff of >274.9 seconds (Ontime plus Offtime) had an area under the curve of 0.89 in all patients and 0.84 in patients without previous OHE
  - Compared to standard psychometric tests (SPTs; 2 of 4 abnormal is MHE, gold standard), psychometric hepatic encephalopathy score (PHES), and inhibitory control tests (ICTs)
  - Stroop score performance:
    - Correlated with MELD
    - Worse in those with previous OHE

Source: Hepatology 2013 58:1122-1132.

- EEG
  - Psychometric tests are more sensitive than EEG for the detection of MHE

> Treatment

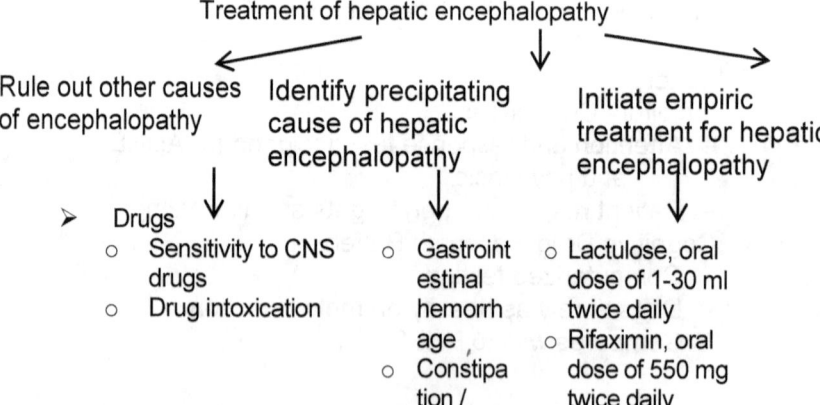

> Drugs
  - Sensitivity to CNS drugs
  - Drug intoxication
  - Gastrointestinal hemorrhage
  - Constipation /
  - Lactulose, oral dose of 1-30 ml twice daily
  - Rifaximin, oral dose of 550 mg twice daily

MINI UPDATE

- CNS
  - Prior seizure or stroke (postictal confusion)
  - Delirium tremens
  - Wernicke-Korsakoff syndrome
  - Intracerebral hemorrhage
  - CNS sepsis
  - Cerebral edema and/or intracranial hypertension*

- Lung
  - Hypoxia
  - Hypercapnia
  - Acidosis

- Kidney
  - Gross electrolyte changes
  - Uremia

- dietary protein overload
- Poor compliance with lactulose therap
- Recent anesthesia
- Bowel obstruction or ileus

- Liver
  - Prior portal decompression procedure (eg. TIPS)*
  - Superimposed hepatic injury*
  - Development of hepatocellular carcinoma

- Dehydration
- Hypokalemia / alkalosis
- Uremia

- Neomycin, oral dose of 500 mg four times daily (use high doses with caution)
- Metronidazole, oral dose of 250 mg four times daily
- Vancomycin, oral dose of 250 mg four times daily
- Sodium benzoate, oral dose 5 g twice daily (not approved for use in the USA)
- Flumazenil, intravenous injection of 1-3 mg (potentially effective, but very short duration of action)

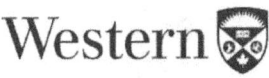

- Endocrine
  - Hypoglycemia*
  - Pancreatic encephalopathy
- CNS
  - CNS active drugs
  - Sepsis

Abbreviation: AB, acid base

* predominantly observed in patients with acute liver failure

- Give 5 reasons to treat MHE.
  - ↑ cognitive function
  - ↑ quality of life
  - ↑ driving performance
  - ↑ performance in workplace
  - ↑ sleep
  - ↑ survival
  - ↓ development of overt clinically evident HE

Adapted from: Ortiz M, et al. *J Hepatol* 2005;42 Suppl(1):S45-53.

- Give 5 management options for MHE.
  - Reverse any precipitants
  - Cathartics: Lactulose
  - Antibiotics: Flagyl, vanesmycin, ampicillin, rifamycin
  - Probiotics
  - High calorie, high protein diet

Adapted from: Holstege A, et al. *Best Practice & Research Clinical Gastroenterology* 2007; 21(3): pg. 541.

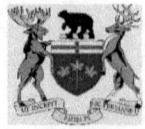

MINI UPDATE

- o Lifestyle
  - Altering lifestyle to avoid situations that lead to accidents
  - Driving: "Patients with symptomatic HE should not be allowed to drive
  - CMA's Determining Medical Fitness to Operate Motor Vehicles 2006

- o Correct reversible causes
  - Treat infections (e.g. spontaneous bacterial peritonitis [SBP], GI bleeding

- o Medications
  - Unlike overt HE, few trials on the treatment of MHE
  - Lactulose
    - Non-absorbable disaccharide
    - Catabolized by the bacterial flora to short chain fatty acids [SCFAs] (eg, lactic acid and acetic acid), which lower the colonic pH to about 5.0.
    - ↓ pH favors the formation of the nonabsorbable NH_4^+ from NH_3, trapping NH_4^+ in the colon and thus ↓ plasma NH_3 concentrations.
    - Meta-analysis shows significant improvement in psychometric and neurophysiologic testing (Aliment Pharmacol Ther 2011;33:662-671)
    - Improves QoL and psychometric testing in patients with MHE
    - Decreases MVAs during a 5-year follow-up period
  - Lactitol
    - Non-absorbable disaccharide
    - No trials in MHE, but class effect postulated

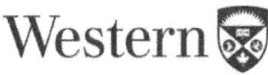

- Rifaximin
    - Non-absorbable gut-specific antibiotic
    - Improves symtoms of overt HE
    - In MHE
        - ↑ HRQoL (health-related quality of life) in double-bind placebo-controlled study (Aliment Pharmacol Ther 2011;34:853-861)
        - Significantly improves driving simulator performance (Gastroenterology 2011;140:478-87)
            - ↓ speeding tickets
            - ↓ illegal turns
            - ↓ total errors
    - Only available in Canada through special access

- Other antibiotics
    - Neomycin
        - Similarly efficacy to rifaximin
        - Beware of totoxicity and nephrotoxicity
    - Metronidazole
        - Some efficacy
        - neurotoxicity
    - Vancomycin
        - Concerns about bacterial resistance
- Probiotics
    - ↓ MHE (Aliment Pharmacol Ther 2011;33:662-671)
- L-ornithine
- L-aspartate (LOLA)
    - Oral LOLA is frequently used for the treatment of hepatic encephalopathy outside of North America
    - ↓ plasma ammonia concentrations by enhancing the metabolism of ammonia to glutamine.
    - 2 RCT's show benefit in MHE

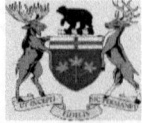

MINI UPDATE

- Give the mechanisms of action in HE / MHE of 5 treatments in ME / HE.
  - Lactulose (beta-galactosidofructose), lacitol beta-galactosidosorbitol (traps NH_3)
    - Enters colon, broken down by colonic bacteria to lactic acid and acetic acid, with acidification of stool pH < 5

pH < 5
$NH_3 \rightarrow NH_4^+$ (non-absorbable)

    - Lactulose enemas (300 mL in 1L of water) in patients who are unable to take lactulose po
    - Lactulose 30 mL p.o every 1-2 h until bowel evacuation, then adjust to a dosage that will result in 2-3 formed bowel movements per day (usually 15-30 mL po bid)
    - Lactulose can be discontinued once the precipitating factor has resolved
  - Hyperosmolar purgation (including lactulose)
    - ↑ stool volume
    - ↑ loss of nitrogen compounds
  - Acarbose
    - α-glucosidic inhibitor → ↓ glucose absorption → ↑ SAC charolytic bacteria and ↓ proteolytic urea producing luminal microbiotica → ↓ NH_3
  - Antibiotics (pre-, pro- and synbiotics)
    - ↑ lactobacillus spp., ↓ urease-containing bacteria → ↓ NH_3 production

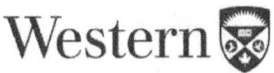

- ↑ bacterial NH_3 utilization
- ↓ pro-inflammatory response
- ↓ gut permeability
- ↓ bacterial translocation
- LOLA (L-ornithine-L-aspartate)
  - Activate the urea cycle → ↑ NH_3 clearance
  - Improves grade 3 or 4 HE in ~ 25% of patients
- Neurotransmitters: flumazenil (a competitive GABA-benzodiazepine receptor antagonist) or bromocriptine

> Nutrition
- ↓ bacterial translocatioTreat malnutrition, including EN, TPN
- Treat associated zinc deficiency
- Branched chain amino acids
- Short term (<72h) protein restriction may be considered in severe HE, but is not used for mild to moderate HE
- No long term protein restriction

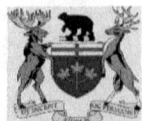

MINI UPDATE

Benign and Malignant Liver Mass Lesions

Mahmoud H Mosli

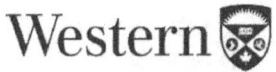

BENIGN AND MALIGNANT LIVER MASS LESIONS

Overview

- Benign liver lesions are found in more than 20% of the general population
- The most common benign liver lesion is hemangioma
- The most common malignant liver lesion is metastasis.
- Liver lesions arise from
  - Hepatocytes
  - Biliary epithelium
  - Mesenchymal tissue
  - Metastasis from extrahepatic tumors
- Most incidentally noted liver masses are benign.
- It may be difficult to differentiate benign hepatic lesions.
- Benign lesions have malignant potential
- Lesions < 1 cm are commonly benign incidental findings, representing
  - Cysts
  - Hemangiomas
  - Biliary hamartomas

Suggested reading: Choi BY, Nguyen MH. The diagnosis and management of benign hepatic tumors. J Clin Gastroenterol. 2005;39:401-412; Mayo clinic GI review, 3rd edition.

Differential Diagnosis of Hepatic Masses

➢ Benign:
  - Hepatocellular
    - Hepatic Adenoma (HA)*,
    - Nodular regenerative hyperplasia (NRH)*,

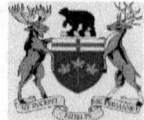

BENIGN AND MALIGNANT LIVER MASS LESIONS

- Focal nodular hyperplasia (FNH)*
- o Cholangiocellular
  - Bile duct adenoma
  - Biliary cystadenoma
- o Mesenchymal
  - Hemangioma*,
  - Angiolipoma (hamartomas)
- o Heterotopic
  - Adrenal
  - Pancreatic

➢ Malignant:
- o Hepatocellular
  - Hepatocellular carcinoma (HCC)
  - Fibrolamellar carcinoma
  - Hepatoblastoma

- o Cholangiocellular
  - Cholangiocarcinoma
  - Cystadenocarcinoma
- o Mesenchymal
  - Angiosarcoma,
  - Primary lymphoma
- o Heterotopic
  - Metastasis

Imaging
- o The imaging studies most frequently helpful in the differential diagnosis of liver mass lesions include
  - Abdominal ultrasonography
    - Useful to determine if lesion is "cystic"
  - Cross-sectional modalities
    - CT/MRI +- feridex/multihance "solid lesion"
    - CT-angiography "vascular lesions"
  - Nuclear imaging studies

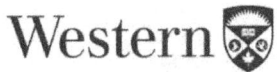

- Tagged RBC studies "haemangiomas"
  - Technetium 99m sulfur colloid imaging "FNH (focal nodular hyperplasia) vs. HA (hepatic adenoma)"
- Positron emission tomography (PET scan) and fused PET/CT
  - Useful to detect metastatic disease

Hepatic Adenomas (HA)

> Demography
  - Usually solitary (70%-80%) and hypervascular.
  - More often in the right lobe {2}
  - HA occur predominantly in women of child-bearing age.

> Causes
  - Strongly associated with use of oral contraceptive pill (OCP).
  - Although they can regress or completely disappear after withdrawal of OCP, they may continue to enlarge despite discontinuation the drug.
  - HA was extremely rare before the introduction of OCP in the 1960s
  - OCP (oral contraceptive pill) and anabolic steroids are implicated as a cause, especially meth-androstenolone and methyltestosterone.
  - Patients with glycogen storage disease (type 1A and type 3) are at ↑ risk of developing multiple adenomas.

> Clinical
  - 48% of cases of HA are detected incidentally

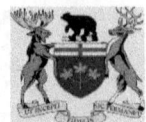

BENIGN AND MALIGNANT LIVER MASS LESIONS

- 44% of patients with HA have symptoms that depend on the size of the lesion, as well as the location.
- Can undergo malignant transformation in 10% of cases
- Tendency to undergo spontaneous hemorrhage
- Benign primary hepatic neoplasm

➢ Pathology
- Sheets of normal appearing hepatocytes separated by dilated sinusoids but lacking the normal acinar architecture of the surrounding hepatic parenchyma
- Hepatocytes may be rich in lipid or glycogen, and kupffer cells are occasionally present
- Bile ducts and portal tracts are absent.
- Lesion may be surrounded by a fibrous capsule (pseudo-capsule) with or without calcifications.

Hepatic Adenoma

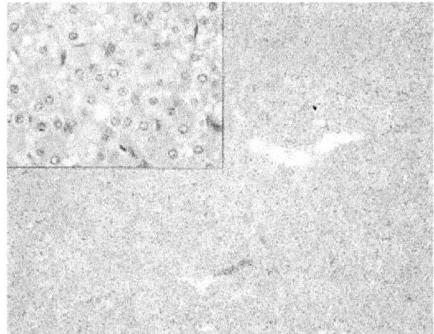

BENIGN AND MALIGNANT LIVER MASS LESIONS

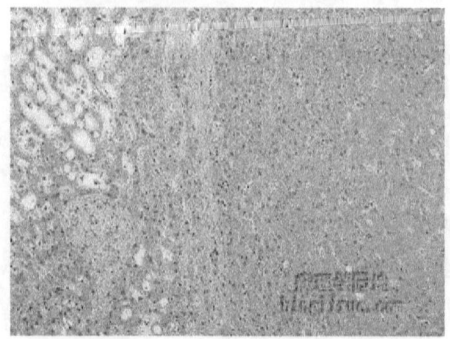

- Diagnostic imaging
  - HA have non-specific radiological appearance in general
  - US
    - Heterogenous
    - Hyper echoic
    - Periphery anechoic centre (if hemorrhagic)
    - Variable flow with Doppler US
  - CT scan (Tri-phasic)
    - Homogenous>heterogenous
    - Peripheral feeders filling in from periphery
  - MRI
    - Capsule
    - Hyperintense in T1 (intra-lesional fat)
  - PET scan
    - No uptake (unless degenerates to HCC)
  - CT-angiography
    - Hyper-vascular
    - Large peripheral vessel
    - Central scar if hemorrhagic

BENIGN AND MALIGNANT LIVER MASS LESIONS

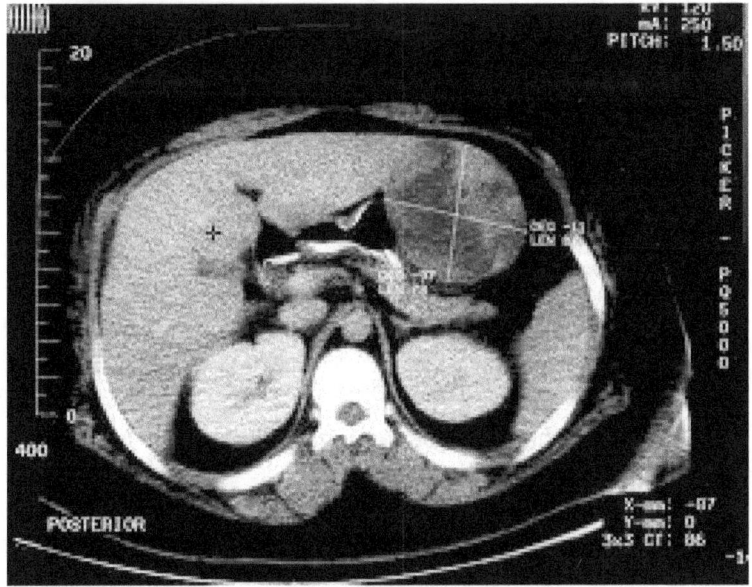

CT Scan of Hepatic adenoma (HA)

- Treatment
  - Lesions <5 cm
    - Stopping OCP/steroids
    - Surveillance repeated periodic imaging and
  - Lesion >5 cm or rapidly enlarging lesions despite stopping OCP/anabolic steroids
    - Surgical enucleation or resection
  - Patients are advised against pregnancy

Nodular Regenerative Hyperplasia (NRH)

- Synonyms
  - Nodular transformation
  - Non-cirrhotic nodulation
  - Partial nodular transformation

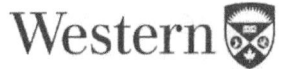

BENIGN AND MALIGNANT LIVER MASS LESIONS

- Demography
  - The prevalence of NRH per autopsy studies is approximately 2 %
- Causees / Associations
  - Behcet disease
  - Rheumatic diseases
  - Myeloproliferative disorders
  - Chronic venous congestion
  - Metastatic neuroendocrine tumors
  - Budd-Chiari syndrome
  - Drugs
    - Steroids
    - Contraceptives
    - Antineoplastics
    - Anticonvulsives
    - Immunosuppressives
- Clinical
  - Most NRH patients are asymptomatic
  - Lesions are usually discovered incidentally during surgery or imaging studies.
  - Some patients present with portal hypertension on cholestasis.
  - Rarely, hepatic failure, rupture of the liver or malignant transformation can occur.
- Pathology
  - Multiple bulging regenerative nodules in clusters of 1 to 40 mm.

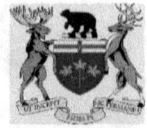

- o Diffuse involvement of the liver with nodules composed of hyperplastic hepatocytes
- o Hyperplastic hepatocytes
  - Multi-nucleated
  - Thickened with centri-lobular atrophy)
  - No fibrosis
  - Reticulin characteristic

Nodular regenerative hyperplasia (NRH)

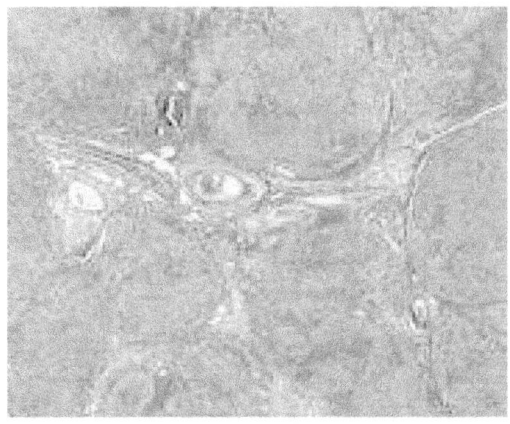

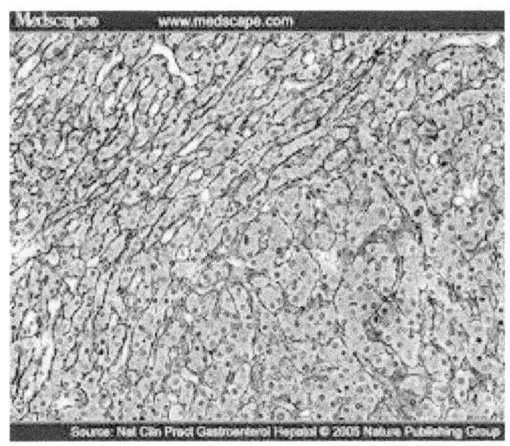

BENIGN AND MALIGNANT LIVER MASS LESIONS

- Speculated pathogenesis
  - Primary vascular process → obliteration of the portal vein → ischemia → atrophy of hepatocytes in the central zone, and the proliferation of hepatocytes in portal zone; or
  - Para-neoplastic process → hepatocyte dysplasia (20%-42%) → HCC

Source: Choi BY, Nguyen MH. The diagnosis and management of benign hepatic tumors. J Clin Gastroenterol. 2005;39:401-412; Assy N, Nasser G, Djibre A, Beniashvili Z, Elias S, Zidan J. Characteristics of common solid liver lesions and recommendations for diagnostic workup. World J Gastroenterol. 2009;15:3217-3227.

- Diagnostic imaging
  - US
    - Usually normal hepatic parenchyma
    - Rarely well delineated hyperechoic or isoechoic nodules
  - CT (tri-phasic)
    - Usually normal finding
    - Rarely hypoattenuating nodules
    - Hyperattenuating portion of a nodule may represent
      - Hemorrhage
      - Arterioportal shunting
  - MRI: hyperintense on T1
  - Iso- or hypointense to normal liver on T2
  - Accurate diagnosis should be confirmed with biopsy.

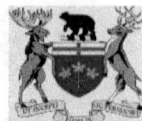

BENIGN AND MALIGNANT LIVER MASS LESIONS

- Treatment
    - Management depends on the clinical status
    - Asymptomatic
        - Surveillance for rare transformation into HCC
    - Portal hypertension: appropriate management including
        - Drug therapy
        - Endoscopic therapy
        - Vaccination
    - Liver failure
        - Liver transplantation

Focal Nodular Hyperplasia (FNH)

- Useful background
    - FNH is the 2nd most common benign solid liver tumor of the liver, with an estimated prevalence of 2.5-8%.
    - Usually solitary (80%), and 3-5 cm in size.
    - Usually detected incidentally (on imaging or autopsy)
    - Associated with vascular anomalies such as hereditary hemorrhagic telangiectasia.
    - No etiological association with use of OCP
    - The usual course of FNH is benign and the incidence of complications like hemorrhage or infection is rare.
    - Rare complications include hepatic vein thrombosis and Kasabach-Merritt syndrome.
    - There is no reported malignant transformation in FNH.

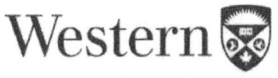

BENIGN AND MALIGNANT LIVER MASS LESIONS

- Diagnostic imaging
  - US
    - Periphery homogenous iso-, hypo- or hyper-echoic
    - Central hyperechoic area
    - Central arterial signal
    - High flow on doppler US with spectral broadening
  - Tri-phasic CT
    - Homogenous
    - Enhances strongly with hepatic arterial phase
    - Central low density scar
  - MRI
    - Homogenous
    - Hypervascular with Gd
    - Isodense on T1
    - Hyperintense scar on T2 (SS > 95%/SP > 95%)

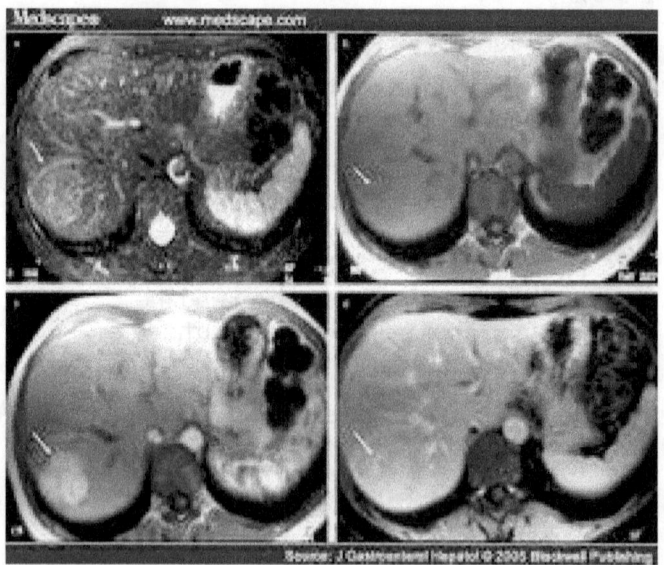

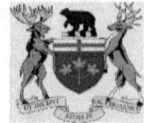

- Hepatic scintigraphy with technetium-99m-labeled sulfur colloid (useful in confirming diagnosis)
    - FNH contains Kupffer cells and it concentrates sulfur colloid.
    - In approximately one-half of cases the degree of radiotracer accumulation is similar to that of the normal hepatic parenchyma
    - In 10% of cases increased concentration of colloid is seen.
    - In the remaining 40% of FNH patients shows a photopenic defect (indicating that the Kupffer cells in the lesion have concentrated the sulfur colloid to a lesser degree than the surrounding liver).
    - Regenerative nodules, focal hepatic steatosis, and HA may also concentrate sulfur colloid
- Hepatobiliary scanning with technetium-99m diethyl-iminodiacetic acid.
    - The abnormal biliary drainage of FNH results in uptake and delayed excretion of the agent, revealing the lesion as a hot spot within the liver on delayed images.
- PET: no uptake
- CT-angiography
    - Hypervascular (70%) centrifugal supply

➢ Pathology
- Resembles inactive cirrhosis with proliferating hepatocytes around a normal prominent
- Central artery with central fibrous scar

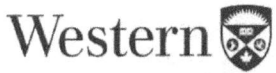

BENIGN AND MALIGNANT LIVER MASS LESIONS

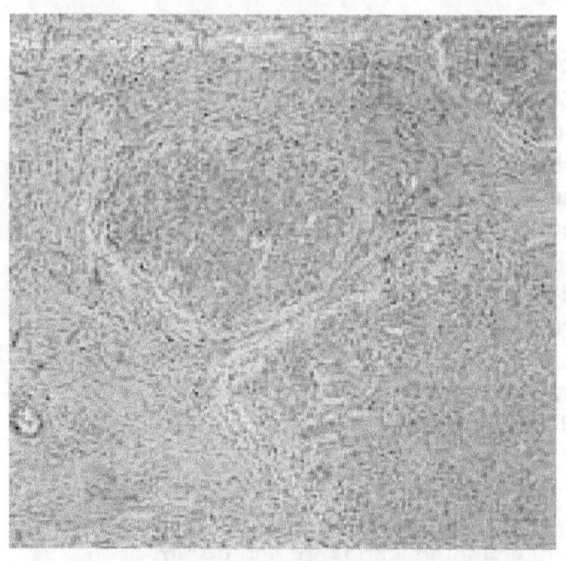

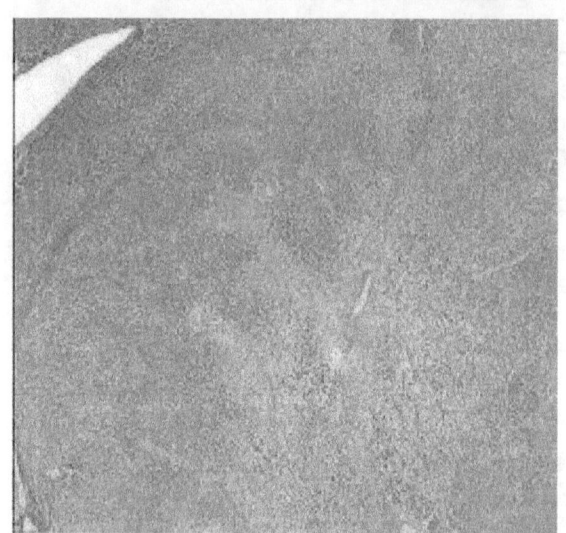

- ➢ Treatment
    - ○ Surgery
        - For the rare symptomatic FNH lesion

BENIGN AND MALIGNANT LIVER MASS LESIONS

- For those in which the diagnosis is still uncertain despite multiple imaging modalities

Hemangioma

- Demography
  - Most common benign hepatic tumor.
  - Prevalence ranges on autopsy from 3% to 20% and it is mostly seen in middle-aged women.

- Pathology
  - Pathology usually located in the sub-scapular region of the right lobe
    - Ranging from < 1 cm to > 20
    - Well-circumscribed and compressible tumor with dark color
    - Microscopically arises from the endothelial cells
    - Multiple, large vascular channels lined by a single layer of endothelial cells and supported by collagenous
    - Blood supply that arises from the hepatic artery

- Pathology

Hepatic hemangiomas

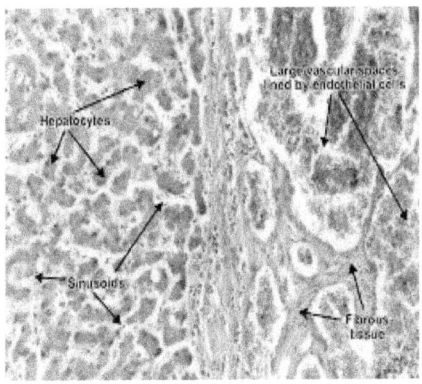

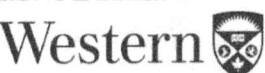

BENIGN AND MALIGNANT LIVER MASS LESIONS

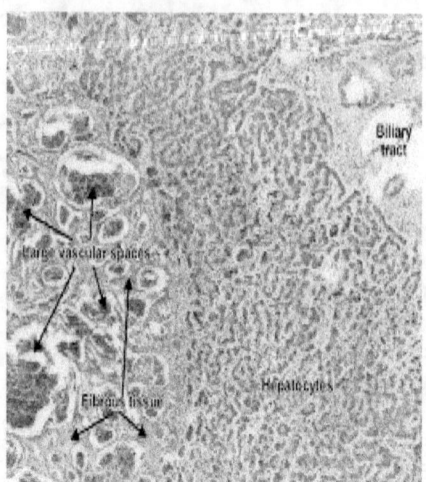

- ➢ Pathophysiology
  - Some hemangiomas have estrogen receptors
  - Accelerated growth has been observed with high estrogen states such as those associated with
    - Puberty
    - Pregnancy
    - Oral contraceptives
    - Androgen treatment
  - Growth due to ectasia, rather than hypertrophy or hyperplasia

- ➢ Clinical
  - Usually asymptomatic, and
  - Rare complications include
    - Spontaneous hemorrhage
    - Kasabach-Merritt syndrome (thrombocytopenia and DIC [disseminated intravascular coagulation])

- ➢ Diagnostic imaging
  - US

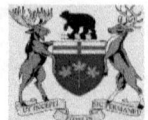

BENIGN AND MALIGNANT LIVER MASS LESIONS

- Hyperechoic
- Low flow/index on doppler
- No spectral broadening

o Tri-phasic CT
- Peripheral puddles, fill in from periphery
- Enhancement in delayed scan

o MRI
- Peripheral enhancement
- Centripetal progression
- Hyperintense on T2
- Hypointense on T1 (SS > 95%/SP 95%)

o PET
- No uptake.

o CT-angiography
- Cotton-wool pooling of contrast
- Normal vessels without AV shunt
- Persistent enhancement

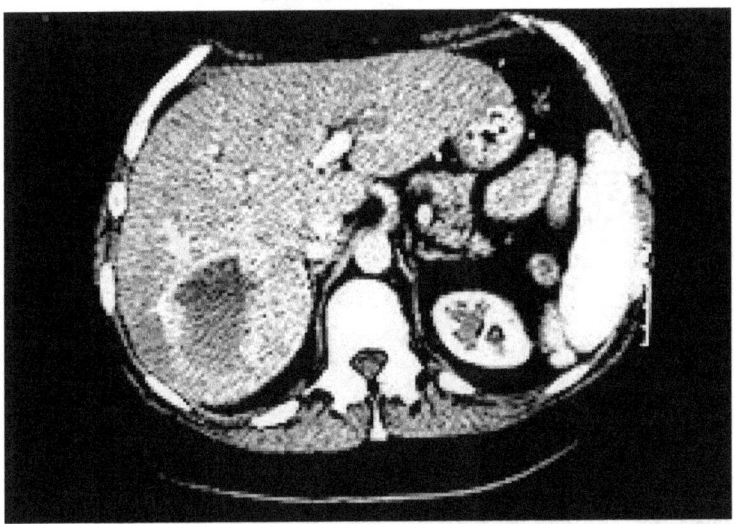

- Hepatic Tc-99m RBC scan
  - Diagnoses hemangiomas > 2.5 cm

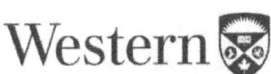

BENIGN AND MALIGNANT LIVER MASS LESIONS

- Treatment
    - Asymptomatic lesions, or < 5 cm in diameter
        - No follow-up or treatment
    - Symptomatic lesions, > 15 cm diameter, or and rapidly enlarging
        - Surgical intervention
            - Resection
            - Enucleation
            - Hepatic ligation
            - Liver

Hepatocellular Cancer (HCC)

- Demography
    - Ranks eighth in frequency among cancers worldwide
        - Sixth among men and eleventh among women
    - Distribution varies widely worldwide
        - Men are affected at least twice as often as women

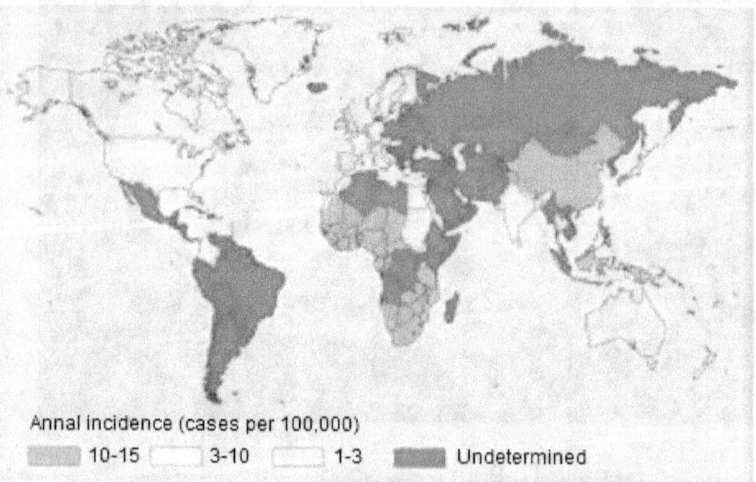

Annal incidence (cases per 100,000)
10-15   3-10   1-3   Undetermined

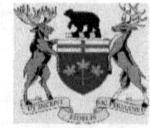

BENIGN AND MALIGNANT LIVER MASS LESIONS

- ➢ Risk factors
    - o Liver cirrhosis (80-90% of HCC cases)
    - o HBV
    - o HCV
    - o Alcoholic liver disease
    - o Hemochromatosis
    - o Tyrosinemia
    - o OCP/Anabolic steroids
    - o Alpha-one anti-trypsin deficiency
    - o Primary biliary cirrhosis
    - o Fungal aflatoxins
- ➢ Histopathology

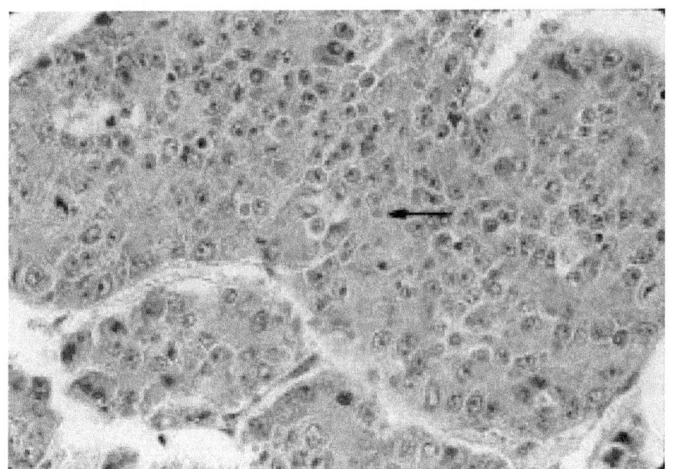

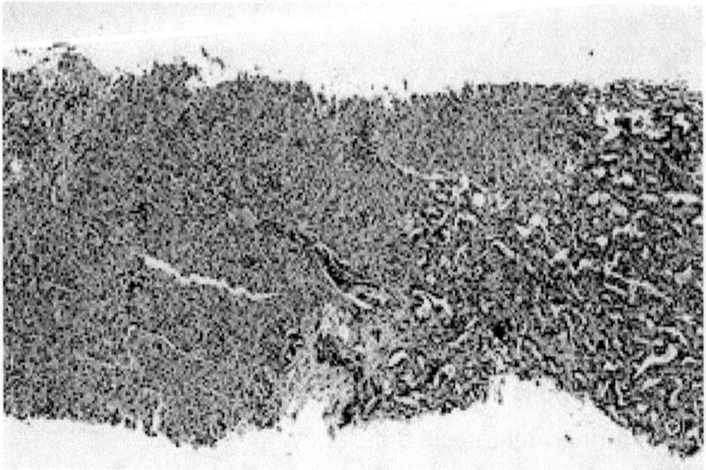

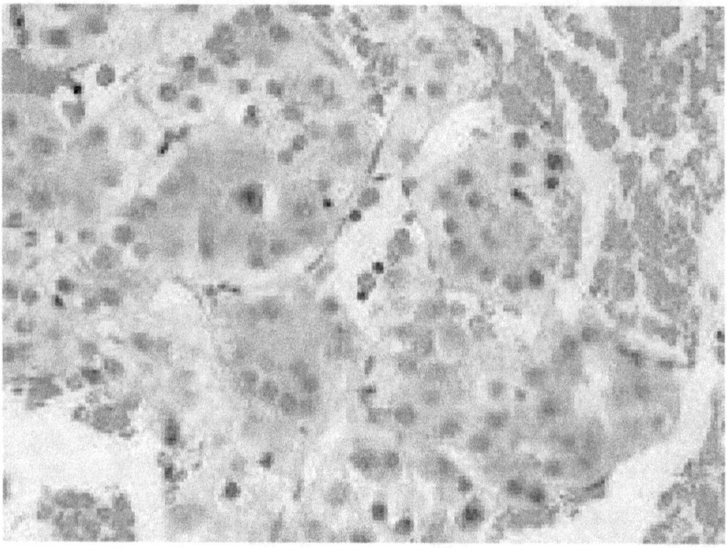

BENIGN AND MALIGNANT LIVER MASS LESIONS

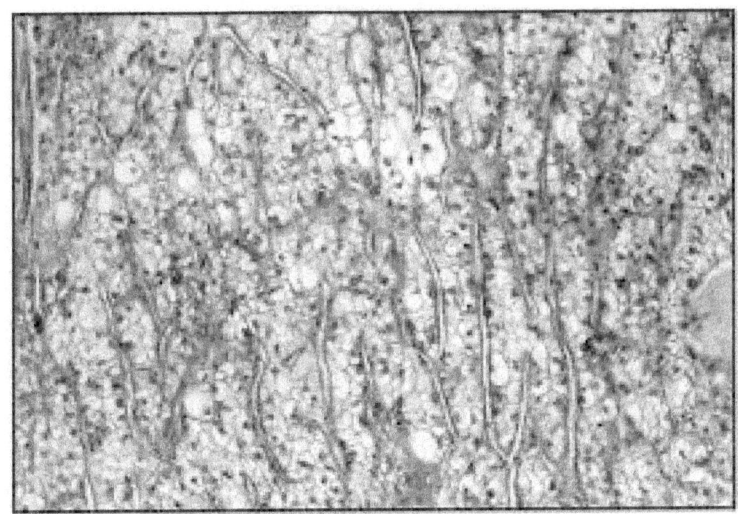

- ➢ Variants of HCC
  - o Clear-cell type ("classic")
  - o Fibro-lamellar HCC
    - Better prognosis
    - Not associated with cirrhosis or hepatitis
  - o Sclerosing HCC
  - o Sarcomatoid HCC
    - Poor prognosis"
  - o Combined HCC-Cholangiocarcinoma
    - Poor prognosis"

- ➢ Clinical Manifestations
  - o Asymptomatic (incidental finding vs. surveillance)
  - o Symptoms
    - RUQ pain
    - Jaundice
    - Fever
    - Anorexia
    - Weight loss

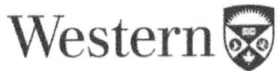

BENIGN AND MALIGNANT LIVER MASS LESIONS

- Fatigue
- Signs
  - RUQ mass
- Deterioration of stable compensated liver cirrhosis
- Portal hypertension
- Para-neoplastic syndrome
  - Erythrocytosis,
  - Hypercalcemia
  - Hypoglycemia
  - Dysfibroginemia

➤ Diagnostic imaging
  - US
    - Hypoechoic or hyperechoic
    - Hypervascular + spectral broadening/elevated indexflow with dopplers
  - CT (tri-phasic)
    - Hypervascular irregular borders
    - Heterogenous > homogenous
    - Abnormal internal vessel
    - Hallmark is early arterial enhancement, with venous washout (SS 22-54%)
    - Lesions > 2 cm with radiological appearance characteristic of HCC (early arterial enhancement with wash-out in the portal venous phase)
    - Lesions 1-2 cm with radiological appearance characteristic of HCC on both contrast enhanced CT and MRI.
    - Lesions smaller than 1 cm are unlikely to be HCC
  - MRI
    - Hypervascular
    - Poor differentiation is hypointense in T1 and hyper-intense on T2, well differentiate is hyper-

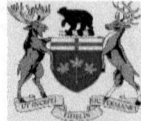

intense on T1 and iso-intense on T2 (SS 53-78%)
- PET
  - No uptake, or increased uptake
- CTA arteriogram
  - Hyper-vascular
  - AV shunting
  - Angiogenesis

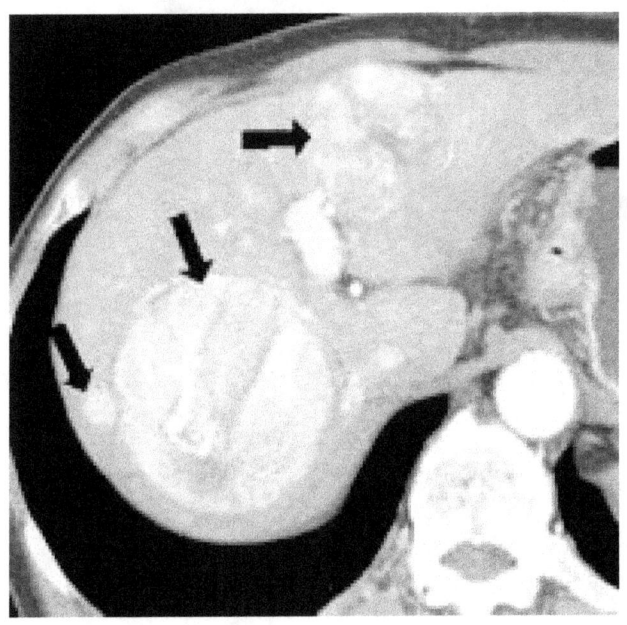

BENIGN AND MALIGNANT LIVER MASS LESIONS

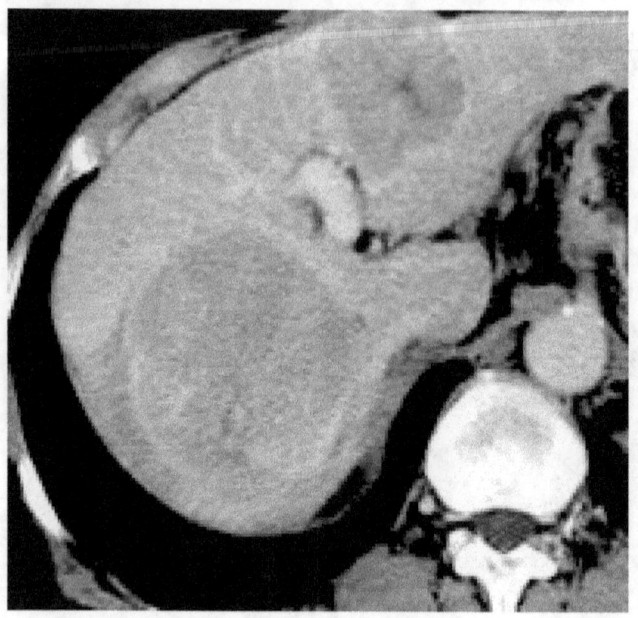

- ➢ Surveillance of persons at risk
  - ○ Guidelines for surveillance of patients with liver cirrhosis recommend U/S every 6 months to screen for HCC
  - ○ Persons with chronic HBV infection without cirrhosis should start screening at:
    - Age 20 for Africans
    - Age 40 for Asian men
    - Age 50 for Asian women
    - Age 50 for whites

- ➢ Treatment
  - ○ Liver resection
    - Patients with well-preserved function and little or no cirrhosis
    - 5 year survival rate 30-50%

- Liver transplantation
  - One tumor < 5 cm or up to three tumors < 3 cm, with no vascular involvement (Milan Criteria)
    - 5 year survival rate is 70-80%, recurrence rate is 15% ""
- Local modalities
  - Radio-frequency ablation
  - Endoscopic therapies percutaneous ethanol injection
- Loco-regional therapies
  - Transarterial chemoembolization (TACE)
  - Transarterial radio-embolization (TARE)
  - Conformal beam radiotherapy
- Chemotherapy: Sorafenib (tyrosine kinase inhibitor)

Cholangiocarcinoma

➤ Demography

- $8/10^6$ per year, representing 10-15% of hepatobiliary malignancies and 3% of all GI malignancies.
- The second most common primary liver cancer after hepatocellular carcinoma (HCC)
- 5-year survival rate; 5%

➤ Risk factors

- Usually no known risk factor
- Risk factors : {10,11}
- PSC (main risk factor in western countries)
- Liver flukes (main risk factor in several countries in Asia)
- Choledochal cysts
- Caroli disease

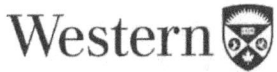

BENIGN AND MALIGNANT LIVER MASS LESIONS

- o HCV cirrhosis
- o Typhoid carrier
- o Thorotrast (antiquated radiocontrast agent used in the 1930's)

➤ Pathology
- o Arise from bile duct epithelium
- o Histologically, cholangiocarcinomas are adenocarcinomas.
- o Classified into three types:
  - Klatskin tumors (60-70%)
  - Cholangiocarcinomas at the bifurcation of the right and left hepatic ducts
  - Intra-hepatic biliary tree (5-15%)
    - Usually presents with pain & jaundice
    - Typically a large intra-hepatic mass +/- intrahepatic or regional lymph node metastasis
  - Extra-hepatic biliary tree (20-30%)
    - Painless
    - Obstructive jaundice

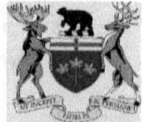

BENIGN AND MALIGNANT LIVER MASS LESIONS

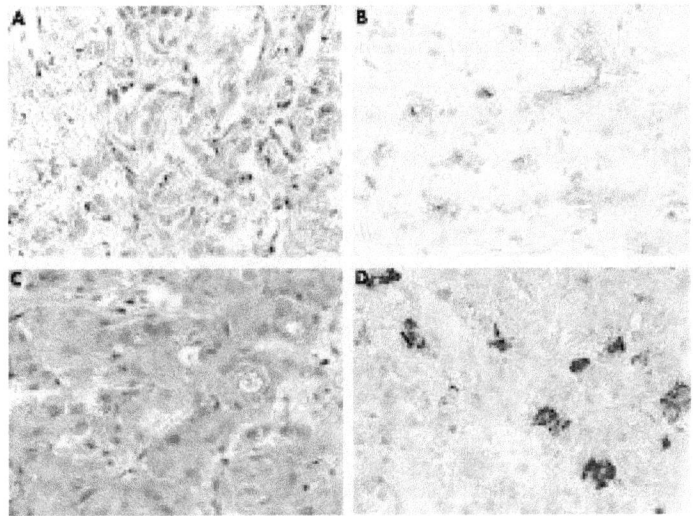

- Predictors of good outcome
    - Single lesion
    - No positive lymph nodes
    - Clear resection margin (> 1 cm)
    - No vascular invasion
- Diagnostic imaging
    - US
        - Bile duct dilatation if major ducts are involved (usually no bile duct dilatation with intrahepatic CC)
    - CT (tri-phasic)
        - Hypodense lesion
        - Delayed enhancement
    - MRI
        - Hypointense in T1 and hyper-intense on T2
        - MRCP is useful
    - CTA
        - Angiogram hypervascular

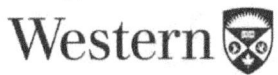

BENIGN AND MALIGNANT LIVER MASS LESIONS

- o PET
  - ↑ uptake (sensitivity 93%)

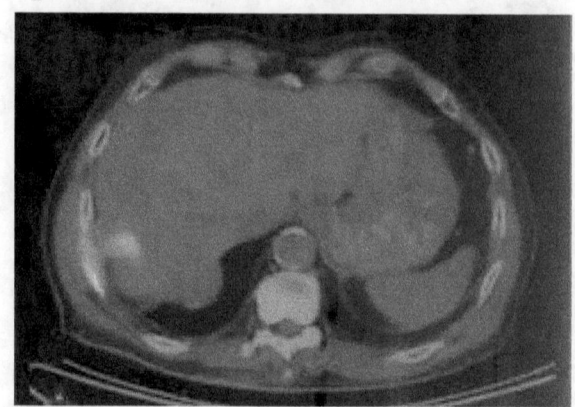

- ➤ Other diagnostic tests
  - o EUS +/- FAN (fine needle aspiration)
    - Mother / daughter scopes
  - o Tumor markers: CA19-9
    - \> 100 ng/ml is 60-65% sensitivity and 80-85% specificity
    - \>1000 ng/ml is predictive of extrahepatic metastasis
  - o Endoscopy
    - ERCP ± brushings for cytology
  - o Biopsy

- ➤ Treatment
  - o Surgical resection: 5-year survival rate is only 20-45%
  - o Liver transplantation
  - o Chemotherapy
  - o Radiotherapy
  - o Palliation

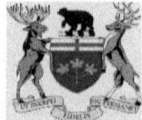

- Decompression using
  - Percutaneous
  - Surgical
  - Endoscopic approaches

References and Suggested Reading

Assy N, Nasser G, Djibre A, Beniashvili Z, Elias S, Zidan J. Characteristics of common solid liver lesions and recommendations for diagnostic workup. World J Gastroenterol. 2009;15:3217-3227.

Bahirwani R, Reddy KR. Review article: the evaluation of solitary liver masses. Aliment Pharmacol Ther. 2008;28:953-965.

Chung YE, Park MS, Park YN et al. Hepatocellular carcinoma variants: radiologic-pathologic correlation. AJR Am J Roentgenol. 2009;193:W7-13.

Trotter JF, Everson GT. Benign focal lesions of the liver. Clin Liver Dis. 2001;5:17-42, v.

Ustundag Y, Bayraktar Y. Cholangiocarcinoma: a compact review of the literature. World J Gastroenterol. 2008;14:6458-6466

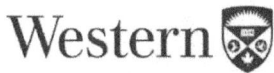

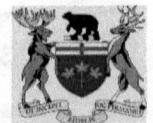

INDEX

A

Abdomen
    CT scanning of, 4–26. *See also individual organs*
        anatomy self-test and answers, 26–32
        recurrent pain in adolescents, *H. pylori* infection and, 237

Acanthosis nigricans, 273–274, 274f
Acarbose, in MHE management, 525
Acetaminophen hepatotoxicity, 428–429
    liver transplantation and, 425, 428
    threshold for, alcohol and fasting and, 445
    treatment and management of, 428–430, 429f, 441–444

Acetylcholine (Ach), gastric acid secretion and, 116

N-Acetylcysteine (NAC)
    for acetaminophen hepatotoxicity, 441–442, 443, 444, 445–446
    for non-acetaminophen hepatotoxicity, 445

Activated charcoal, for acetaminophen hepatotoxicity, 441

Acute appendix, 25, 26f

Acute cellular rejection, in liver transplant recipient, 467, 478, 479

Acute cholecystitis, 15, 15f

Acute coronary syndrome (ACS), GI bleeding in, 216–217

Acute erosive gastritis, 87

Acute fatty liver of pregnancy (AFLP), 398
    acute liver failure in, 433
    and complications of cirrhosis, 408
    defined, 401
    demography of, 402
    diagnosis of, Swansea criteria for, 404–405
    fetal testing in, 406
    and HELLP syndrome distinguished, 401, 404
    laboratory investigations in, 405–406, 406f
    LCHAD deficiency in, 398, 402–403

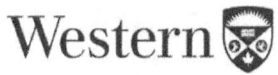

pathophysiology of, 403
prognosis in, 408
treatment of, 407–408
trimester of onset of, 409
Acute ischemic injury, to liver, 433–434, 447
Acute liver failure (ALF)
  acetaminophen hepatoxicity and, 428–430, 429f
  in acute fatty liver of pregnancy, 433
  acute ischemic injury and, 433–434, 447
  autoimmune hepatitis and, 432–433
  in Budd-Chiari syndrome, 434, 447
  causes of, 421–423, 422–423
    uncommon, 424
  complications of, 426–427
  defined, 420–421
  diagnosis of, 421
  differential diagnosis in, 425–426
  drug-induced liver injury and, 430–431, 446–447
  epidemiology of, 421
  hepatic encephalopathy and, 435–437
  liver transplantation in, 453–454
    King's College risk stratification criteria for, 425, 428
  malignant infiltration and, 434–435, 447
  mechanism of injury in, 421
  mushroom poisoning and, 446
  prognosis in, 427–428
  viral hepatitis and, 422, 431
  Wilson disease and, 432
Acute pancreatitis, 16–17, 17f
  as ALF complication, 427
Acute rejection, in liver transplant recipient, 467, 478, 479
Acute renal failure, as ALF complication, 427
Acute respiratory failure, as ALF complication, 427
Adalimumab, for treatment of IBD in pregnant patients, 299
Adenocarcinoma
  esophageal, risk factors for, 59, 60
  gastric. *See* Gastric adenocarcinoma
Adenoma

hepatic. *See* Hepatic adenoma (HA)
progression to carcinoma, sequence in, 336f
Adenomatous polyps/Adenomatous polyposis syndromes, 337. *See also* Familial adenomatous polyposis (FAP)
medication efficacy in, 357
Adjuvant therapy, for *H. pylori* eradication, 251–252
Alcohol
acetaminophen hepatotoxicity threshold and, 445
as solid organ cancer risk, 503
Alcohol-based hand sanitizers, *C. difficile* infection and, 321–322, 325
Alcoholic cirrhosis of liver, 453
Allocation of liver, for transplantation, 456
Child-Turcotte-Pugh score for, 457
MELD system. *See* Model for end-stage liver disease (MELD)
Allograft dysfunction, liver transplant rejection and, 479
Alpha-fetoprotein (AFP) screening
in pediatric FAP management, 358, 360
in pregnancy, 410
Amanita phalloides (mushroom poisoning), acute liver failure and, 446
American Society for Gastrointestinal Endoscopy (ASGE), anticoagulant and anti-platelet medication management guidelines, 211–212
Amino acids (AA), in stomach, 111–112
Aminosalicylate (5-ASA), for treatment of IBD in pregnant patients, 297
Amoxicillin, for *H. pylori* eradication, 254
adverse effects, 250
eradication rates, 250
Ampicillin, in treatment of ICP, 416
Amsterdam criteria
for HNPCC, 364
for Lynch syndrome, 361–363
Anastomotic ulcer, after Roux-en-Y gastric bypass, 183
Angiography, interventional, in NVUGIB, 150, 162

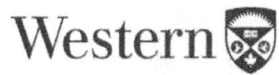

Anion-binding resins, for recurrent *C. difficile* infection, 330
Anisakis gastritis, 92
Antibiotic resistance, in anti-*H. pylori* therapy, 248
Antibiotics
  associated with *C. difficile* infection, 322
  in MHE management, 524, 525–526
Antibody testing, in *H. pylori* diagnosis, 244
Anticoagulants, and post-procedure bleeding risk
  acute bleeding, 216
  atrial fibrillation and stroke risk and, 208
  in colonoscopic polypectomy, 202
  deep vein thrombosis and, 210
  management guidelines, 211
  prosthetic cardiac valves and, 209, 210
    mechanical heart valves, 216
  reinstitution recommendations, 219
Anti-*H. pylori* IgG antibodies, 231
Anti-IL-5 mAB, for eosinophilic esophagitis, 49, 52
Antiplatelet therapy, and post-procedure bleeding risk
  acute bleeding, 215
  in colonoscopic polypectomy, 202, 203
  management guidelines, 211
  in NVUGIB, 159
    aspirin vs., 155
    high-risk patients and, 154
  reinstitution recommendations, 219
Antommarchi, Dr. Francesco, 269
APC gene, in familial adenomatous polyposis, 338f, 338–339
  APC/β-catenin pathway, 340f, 343
  mutation of, 343
  structure and function of, 339f, 343
Appendix, acute, 25, 26f
"Asian esophageal cancer belt," 58
Aspirin (ASA)
  adenomatous polyps and, 357
  and bleeding risk in colonoscopic polypectomy, 202
  in NVUGIB

after endoscopic therapy, 157
clopidogrel and ticlopidine vs., 155
future rebleeding and, 149
H. pylori and, 158
ulcer complications and, 158, 160
ulcer healing, PPIs and, 156
reinstitution recommendations, 219
Atrial fibrillation
anticoagulants and, 208
H. pylori infection and, 240
Atrophic gastritis, 83f
autoimmune metaplastic, 82
chronic, gastric acid secretion and, 122–123
multifocal, 83f, 83–84
Attenuated adenomatous polyposis coli (AAPC), 345–346
Autoimmune hepatitis, 432–433
Autoimmune metaplastic atrophic gastritis (AMAG), 82, 84
Avicenna, 268
Azathioprine (6-MP)
in treatment of IBD during pregnancy, 298
in treatment of ICP, 416

B
BabA protein, *H. pylori* infection and, 223
Bacterial gastritis, 90–91
Bacterial infection
in acute liver failure, 438–439
as ALF complication, 426
Band erosion, endoscopic treatment for, 188
Bariatric surgery
benefits of, 173, 186
complications of, 181
endoscopic treatment, 187–188
endoscopy after, 186–187
indications for, 172–173, 186
non-alcoholic fatty liver disease and, 179, 180t–181t, 181

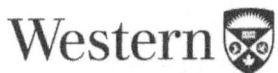

post-operative medical care, 188–194
pre- and post-operative considerations, 172
rise in, 172
types of, 176, 177f–178f
for weight reduction, 174, 174f, 175f, 175t
Barrett esophagus, *H. pylori* infection and, 240–241
B12-deficiency associated anemia, after bariatric surgery, 192–193
Bethesda criteria, for tumor tissue testing, 366
 in HNPCC, 365
 revised guidelines, 366–367
Bile ducts, cholangiocarcinoma of, 17–18, 18f
Bile secretion
 CYP7A1 enzyme and, 288–289
 disorders of, 283–284
 hepatocytes and, 281f
Bile/Bile acid (BA)
 composition of, 280f
 conjugation in intestine, 289–290
 conjugation in liver, 289
 -dependent and -independent flow, physiology of, 292, 293
 fecal elimination of, 283, 283f
 functions of, 280
 ileal reabsorption of, 283, 283f
 metabolism of, 292–293
  changes during pregnancy, 413
 reabsorption of, 290
 synthesis of
  CYP7A1 enzyme and, 288–289
  in hepatocytes, 281f
 transport proteins for, 293
 transporter defects
  diseases associated with, 281–282
  inborn errors, 294
Biliary tract obstruction, 284
 following liver transplantation, 464
Biliary tree, CT features, 8, 8f
Biliopancreatic diversion, 176, 178f

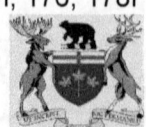

complications associated with, 185, 185f
with duodenal switch, 176, 178f
Billroth, Theodor, 269
Biologics therapy, in PTLD, 500
Biopsy, in *H. pylori* diagnosis, 247
Bismuth, for *H. pylori* eradication, 254
  adverse effects, 250
  eradication rates, 249
Bleeding
  in acute liver failure, 437
  after ERCP sphincterotomy, 205–206
  antiplatelet and anticoagulant therapy associated with, 215–216
  gastroduodenal ulcer, Forrest endoscopic classification of, 132
  gastrointestinal, in acute coronary syndrome, 216–217
  lower GI, in HIV/AIDS patients, 151
  from marginal ulcer after bariatric surgery, 188
  postpolypectomy. *See* Postpolypectomy bleeding
  post-procedural, medications and. *See under* Anticoagulants *and* Antiplatelet therapy
  upper GI. *See* Non-variceal upper GI bleeding (NVUGIB); Upper GI bleeding (UGIB)
Blood transfusion, contraindications in IgA deficiency, 145–146
Body image, after bariatric surgery, 191–192
Boerhaave syndrome, 13f–14f, 13–14
Bone, CT window width/level of, 6
Bovine lactoferrin, *H. pylori* eradication and, 251–252
Brain
  hepatic encephalopathy and, 511–512
    pathological changes, 513
  PTLD manifestations in, 497f
Budd-Chiari syndrome (B-CS), acute liver failure in, 434, 447
Budesonide, for eosinophilic esophagitis, 51–52

C
CA19-9, for cholangiocarcinoma diagnosis, 554

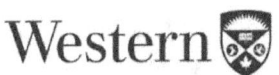

Cag pathogenicity island, *H. pylori* infection and, 224
Canada, liver transplantation survival in, 462, 462f
Cancer
  colon. See Colon cancer
  esophageal. See Esophageal cancer
  gallbladder, 15f–16f, 15–16
  gastric. See Gastric cancer
  in liver transplant recipient
    frequency, 504
    management of, 504–506
  perforated, of transverse colon, 23f
Candidiasis, gastritis and, 91–92
Carcinogenesis, multistep, in colon, 336f
Carcinoma. See Cancer; *specific carcinomas*
Cardia, gastric, 88, 104
Cardiovascular disease, following liver transplantation, 483–484
Carditis, 87–88
Catheterization, esophagogastroduodenoscopy vs., 217–218
CD_4^+ lymphocytes, in autoimmune metaplastic atrophic gastritis, 84
Central nervous system (CNS), involvement in MHE, 521
Cephalic-vagal stimulation, of gastric acid secretion, 119–120, 120f
Cerebrotendinous xanthomatosis, diet therapy for, 475
Certolizumab, for treatment of IBD in pregnant patients, 299
Chemotherapy
  for hepatocellular carcinoma, 551
  in PTLD, 500
Child-Turcotte-Pugh (CTP)score, liver allocation based on, 457
Cholangiocarcinoma, 17–18, 18f
  classification of, 552
  demography of, 551
  diagnosis of
    imaging modalities used, 553–554, 554f
    other tests, 554

imaging features of, 18
outcome predictors for, 553
pathology of, 552, 553f
risk factors for, 551–552
treatment of, 554–555
Cholangiocyte, in enterohepatic circulation, 293
Cholecystectomy, diarrhea following, 285, 285f
Cholecystitis, acute, 15, 15f
Cholecystokinin (CCK)
  gastrin and, 109, 115
  parietal cells and, 117
  receptors, 111
Cholelithiasis
  after bariatric surgery, 190
  after Roux-en-Y gastric bypass, 184
Choleretic diarrhea, following ileal resection, steatorrhea vs., 287
Choleretic effects, of UDCA, 291
Cholestasis of pregnancy, recurrent, risk factors for, 418. *See also* Intrahepatic cholestasis of pregnancy (ICP)
Cholestyramine, for recurrent *C. difficile* infection, 330
Chromosomal instability, in carcinogenesis in the colon, 336
Chronic active superficial gastritis, gastric acid secretion and, 122–123
Chronic atrophic gastritis, gastric acid secretion and, 122–123
Chronic liver disease
  natural history of, 450f
  with upper GI bleeding, management of, 144
Chronic rejection, in liver transplant recipient, 478
Church staging system, for desmoid tumors in Gardner variant of FAP, 355
Ciprofloxacin, for treatment of IBD in pregnant patients, 299
Circular rings, in eosinophilic esophagitis, 42f
Cirrhosis of liver
  alcoholic, liver transplantation in, 453
  bleeding risk and, 213

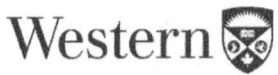

and complications in AFLP, 408
natural history of, 452f
pre-existing, acute liver failure and, 423
stages of, 452f
Clarithromycin, for *H. pylori* eradication, 253, 254
   adverse effects, 250
Clopidogrel
   aspirin vs., 155
   and bleeding risk in colonoscopic polypectomy, 202, 203
   reinstitution recommendations, 219
Clostridium difficile infection
   antibiotics associated with, 322
   clinical and endoscopic variants of, 318–319
   described, 314–315
   diagnosis and confirmatory testing, 316
   epidemiology of, 317
   in immunocompromised patient with IBD, 309
   mild, management and treatment of, 323–324
   organism characteristics in, 315, 316f
   pathogenesis of, 320–321
   prevention of, 321
   recurrent
     defined, 328–329
     risk factors for, 325
   risk factors for, 321
     recurrence of infection, 325
   severe
     complications in, 327
     guideline definitions, 326
     treatment, 327
   severe complicated
     guideline definitions, 326
     treatment, 327–328
   symptoms of, 316
   transmission of, 317
   treatment of, 322–323
     in mild disease, 323–324
     in recurrent disease, 328–331

in severe disease, 325–327
in severe disease with complications, 327–328
Clostridium difficile-associated diarrhea (CDAD), 332
with colitis, 318
Coagulopathy, in acute liver failure, 426, 437
Cognitive Drug Research Battery, 519
Colectomy, in severe complicated *C. difficile* infection, 327–328
Colestipol, for recurrent *C. difficile* infection, 330
Colitis
   C. difficile-associated diarrhea with, 318
   fulminant, 319
   pseudomembranous. *See* Pseudomembranous colitis (PMC)
Colon
   bleeding in HIV/AIDS patients, 151
   multistep carcinogenesis in, 336f
   PTLD manifestations in, 497f
Colon cancer
   genetics of, 334f
      mutations, types and mechanism of, 335
      terminology of, 335
   lifetime risk of, 334f, 345
   progression from adenoma to, sequence in, 336f
Colonoscopy, in FAP management, 358, 359
Computed tomography (CT)
   density measurements, 5–6, 6f
   of head, in FAP management, 358
   of hepatic masses, 530
      adenoma, 532, 533f
      cholangiocarcinoma, 553
      focal nodular hyperplasia, 538
      hemangioma, 11f, 543, 543f
      hepatocellular carcinoma, 548, 549, 549f
      nodular regenerative hyperplasia, 536
   scanner characteristics, 4–5, 5f
   scanning protocols and their uses, 11f–12f, 11–13
   windows in, 6
Concomitant therapy (CT), for *H. pylori* eradication, 255

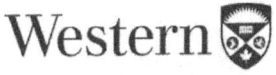

Confusion, in hepatic encephalopathy, 516
Congenital hypertrophy of the retinal pigment epithelium (CHRPE), 342, 350, 354
Contraindications, defined, 465
Contrast, in CT scanning, 7
Cosmetic/body image issue, after bariatric surgery, 191–192
Coxibs, adenomatous polyps and, 357
Crohn disease, 94
Cromolyn sodium, for eosinophilic esophagitis, 49, 52
Crowded conditions, *H. pylori* transmission in, 230
Culture, in *H. pylori* diagnosis, 244–245
Cyclosporine, for treatment of IBD in pregnant patients, 299
CYP7A1 enzyme, bile acid synthesis and, 288
Cystic fibrosis, diet therapy for, 474
Cytomegalovirus (CMV)
  gastritis, 91, 92f
  gastropathy, 98f
  in immunocompromised patient with IBD, 304
Cytoprotection, post-bleed, 161

D
D cells, gastric acid secretion and, 116
Dabigatran, procedure bleeding risk and, 212
De novo malignancy after liver transplantation
  background for, 490f, 490–491
  lymphoproliferative. *See* Post-transplant lymphoproliferative disorder (PTLD)
  as major cause of death, 492, 492f
  non-lymphoproliferative, risk factors for, 501
Death, following liver transplantation, causes of, 462
Decompensation, hepatic, 451, 451f
Deep vein thrombosis (DVT)
  anticoagulant use and, 210
  gastric adenocarcinoma and, 272, 273
  risk of recurrence, 209
Density measurements, in CT scanning, 5–6, 6f
Desmoid tumors, in Gardner variant of FAP, 355

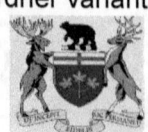

staging system for, 355
Diabetes
  following liver transplantation, 483–484
  obesity-related morbidity, resolution after bariatric surgery, 175, 175f, 175t
Diagnostic endoscopy, bleeding risk associated with, 201
Diagnostic imaging
  in cholangiocarcinoma, 553–554, 554f
  in eosinophilic esophagitis, 44–45, 45f
  in esophageal cancer, 61
  in focal nodular hyperplasia, 538f, 538–539
  in HELLP syndrome, 399–400
  in hepatic adenoma, 532, 533f
  in hepatic hemangioma, 542–543, 543f
  in hepatocellular carcinoma, 548–549, 549f–550f
  in iron deficiency anemia with obscure GI bleeding, 145
  in nodular regenerative hyperplasia, 536
  in pregnant patient with liver disease, 390
    risks to fetus, 389–390
Diarrhea
  after bariatric surgery, 193
  C. difficile-associated, with colitis, 318
  choleretic, following ileal resection, 287
  post-cholecystectomy, 285, 285f
Difaximin, for recurrent *C. difficile* infection, 329
Diffuse corporeal atrophic gastritis (DCAG), 82, 84
Disseminated intravascular coagulopathy (DIC), in paraneoplastic syndrome differential diagnosis, 275
Distension, gastric acid secretion and, 111
Dorsal motor nuclei (DMN) of vagal nerves, gastric acid secretion and, 119–120, 120f
DRESS syndrome, 447
Drug-eluting stent (DES) thrombosis, bleeding risk and, 212
Drug-induced liver injury (DILI)
  acute liver failure and, 446–447
  epidemiology of, 431
  management of, 431
  prescription drugs associated with, 430

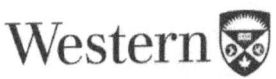

Drugs
  causing acute liver failure, 422. *See also*
    Acetaminophen hepatotoxicity; Non-acetaminophen
      hepatotoxicity
  liver injury induced by. *See* Drug-induced liver injury
    (DILI)
Dumping syndrome
  after bariatric surgery, 190
  after Roux-en-Y gastric bypass, 184
Duodenal polyps, in FAP, 351
  screening interval for, 351–352
Duodenal ulcer (DU), 81
  gastric acid secretion and, 122
  H. pylori and, 229, 233–234
Dyspepsia, symptom relief in, 229
Dysphagia, after bariatric surgery, 190

E
Eclampsia. *See* Pre-eclampsia/Eclampsia
Electroencephalography (EEG), psychometric testing vs.,
  520
Elemental diet, for eosinophilic esophagitis, 46, 52
Elimination diet, for eosinophilic esophagitis, 46, 50, 53
Embolization, transarterial, in NVUGIB, 150, 162
Endocrine cells
  in oxyntic mucosa, 105, 106f
  in pyloric mucosa, 105, 106f
Endocrine system, involvement in MHE, 522
Endoscopic findings
  after bariatric surgery, 187
  in eosinophilic esophagitis, 41, 41f–42f
  in lymphocytic gastritis, 86
  in NVUGIB, 135f
  portal hypertensive gastropathy and gastric antral
    vascular ectasia compared, 90, 152–153
  as predictor of peptic ulcer prognosis, 134, 135f
Endoscopic hemostatic therapy (EHT)
  benefits of, 149–150
  Forrest score and, 147

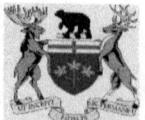

rebleeding, surgery, and mortality rates with and without, 148
Endoscopic retrograde cholangiopancreatography (ERCP)
  in cholangiocarcinoma diagnosis, 554
  sphincterotomy, hemorrhage after, 205–206
Endoscopic ultrasound (EUS)
  in cholangiocarcinoma, 554
  in pediatric FAP management, 358, 360
Endoscopic variceal ligation (EVL), bleeding risk and, 213
Endoscopy
  bleeding risk associated with, 200–201. See also Postpolypectomy bleeding; *specific procedures*
  in esophageal cancer
    diagnostic, 61
    therapeutic, 66, 67
  H. pylori infection risk with, 231
  in iron deficiency anemia with obscure GI bleeding, 145
  PPI therapy in NVUGIB prior to, 134, 134f
  reintroduction of ASA after, 157
  RUGBE registry, 136f
  of upper GI tract
    in FAP management, 358
    in NVUGIB, 141f, 141–142, 147–148
End-stage liver disease, model for. *See* Model for end-stage liver disease (MELD)
Enterochromaffin-like (ECL) cells, 105–106, 106f
  gastrin and, 109
  histamine and, 112, 115
  hyperplasia of, 116
  peptide YY and, 112
  somatostatin and, 110
Enterohepatic circulation (EHC)
  disorders of, 283–284
  efficiency of, 293
  hepatocytes in, 293
    function in zone 1 vs. zone 3, 291
  intestinal luminal circulation in, 282

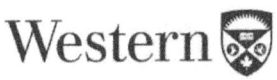

transport proteins for bile acids in, 293
Environmental multifocal atrophic gastritis (EMAG), 83f, 83–84
Eosinophilic esophagitis (EE), 36–53
  causes of, 39–40
  clinical manifestations of, 38–39
  complications of, 40–41
  demography of, 36, 37f
  diagnostic imaging in, 44–45, 45f
  differential diagnosis in, 43–44, 53
  endoscopic findings in, 41, 41f–42f
  histologic findings in, 37–38, 38f
  laboratory findings in, 44
  muscle and subserosal findings in, 45
  other conditions and, 46
  pathogenesis of, 37
  treatment of, 46–53
    limitations of medications used for, 50–51
Eosinophilic gastritis, 95
Eosinophilic gastrointestinal diseases (EGIDS), diagnostic work-up for, 43–44
Epstein Barr virus (EBV)
  in immunocompromised patient with IBD, 305
  in post-transplant lymphoproliferative disorder, 463
  in PTLD pathogenesis, 463. *See also* Post-transplant lymphoproliferative disorder (PTLD)
Eradication therapy. *See Helicobacter pylori* eradication therapy
Erosive gastropathy, 87, 96, 97, 99f
Esophageal cancer, 56–67
  classifications in
    postoperative, 65
    preoperative, 63–65
    of tumors, 57
  clinical features of, 56
  diagnostic imaging in, 61
  presenting symptoms in, 56–57
  risk factors for, 58–60
  staging of, 61–63

treatment of, resectable vs. unresectable, 65–66
Esophageal dilation, for eosinophilic esophagitis, 49–50
Esophagitis. See Eosinophilic esophagitis (EE)
Esophagogastroduodenoscopy (EGD)
  bleeding gastroduodenal ulcers and, 133
  catheterization vs., 217–218
  in chronic liver disease with upper GI bleeding, 144
  eosinophilic esophagitis and, 41
  in FAP management, 359
    for duodenal polyps, 351
  in *H. pylori* diagnosis, 247
  in IGA deficiency, 146
  in iron deficiency anemia with upper GI bleeding, 145
  in NVUGIB
    international normalized ratio and, 214–215, 215f
    planned and unplanned, 150
    PPI infusion before, 145
  PPI infusion before
    Forrest score and, 147
    in NVUGIB, 145
  in pregnant patient with liver disease, 391
Esophagus
  bleeding in HIV/AIDS patients, 151
  CT scanning in Boerhaave syndrome, 13f–14f, 13–14
  eosinophilic esophagitis, 36–53. See also Eosinophilic
    esophagitis (EE)
  esophageal cancer, 56–67
  small caliber, in eosinophilic esophagitis, 42f
Extrinsic contrast, 7

F
Familial adenomatous polyposis (FAP), 337
  AAPC variant of, 345–346
  cancer risk in, 345
  clinical features of, 343, 344f
  extracolonic manifestations of, 344, 348–349
  Gardner variant. See Gardner variant of FAP
  genetic testing in, 341–342, 357

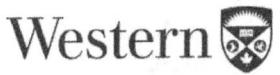

genetics of, 345. See also APC gene, in familial adenomatous polyposis
GI tract screening in, 358–359
management of, 356, 358–360
M(UT)YH gene mutations in. See MUTYH polyposis
screening guidelines, 346, 358–360
Turcot variant. See Turcot syndrome
variants of, 345–346
Families, *H. pylori* transmission within, 229–230
impact of, 230–231
Fasting state
acetaminophen hepatotoxicity threshold and, 445
intestinal luminal circulation in, 282
Fat halo, in mesenteric panniculitis, 20
Fecal antigen test, in *H. pylori* diagnosis, 244–245
Feces
bile acid elimination in, 283, 283f
transplantation of, for recurrent *C. difficile* infection, 331
Fed state, intestinal luminal circulation in, 282
Fentanyl, in treatment of ICP, 416
Fetus
factors in HELLP pathogenesis, 407
in intrahepatic cholestasis of pregnancy
clinical presentation and outcomes from, 414
complications from, 415
ionizing radiation risks to, 389–390
medication risk categories and, 416–417
testing in AFLP, 406
Fibrosis, bariatric surgery and, 181t
Fidaxomicin, for recurrent *C. difficile* infection, 330
Fine needle aspiration (FNA), for cholangiocarcinoma diagnosis, 554
Flagyl, for *H. pylori* eradication
adverse effects, 250
eradication rates, 249
Fluticasone, for eosinophilic esophagitis, 51
Focal nodular hyperplasia (FNH)
considerations in, 537
diagnostic imaging in, 538f, 538–539

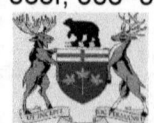

pathology of, 539, 540f
treatment of, 540–541
Food impaction/"foreign body" ingestion, differential diagnosis, 53
Forrest endoscopic classification
of bleeding gastroduodenal ulcers, 132
PPI therapy prior to EGD/EHT and, 147
Foveolae, corkscrew appearance of, 99f
Fructose intolerance, hereditary, diet therapy for, 474
Fulminant colitis, 319
Fundic gland polyps, 261
Fungal infection
in acute liver failure, 426–427, 439
in immunocompromised patient with IBD, 306–307
Furazolide, for *H. pylori* eradication, 253
Furrows, linear, in eosinophilic esophagitis, 41f

G
Galactosemia, diet therapy for, 474
Gallbladder
CT features of, 8, 8f
diseases of, 15f–16f, 15–16
inflamed, with hyperemia and wall irregularity, 8, 8f
Gallbladder carcinoma, 15f–16f, 15–16
Gardner variant of FAP, 345
desmoid tumors in, staging system for, 355
extraintestinal associations of, 348–350
Gastrectomy, 176, 177f
Gastric acid output, measuring
basic output, 119
indications for, 118
maximal/peak output, 119
post-prandial, 119
Gastric acid secretion, 107
basal output, 119
cephalic-vagal stimulation of, 119–120, 120f
functions of, 112–113
via H^+, K^+-ATPase proton pump, 113
increased, diseases associated with, 122–123

inhibitory factors, 118
intraluminal contents in, 121–122
maximum/peak output, 119
measurement of, 118–119
pathways for, 108–112
post-prandial, 119
surgically-induced, 112
Gastric adenocarcinoma, 81–82
clinical features of, 271–272
demography of, 270
history of, 268
paraneoplastic syndromes in, 272–273
risk factors for, 271
Gastric antral vascular ectasia (GAVE), and portal
hypertensive gastropathy compared, 90, 152–153
Gastric banding, 176, 177f
slippage, and gastric prolapse, 182f
weight loss and, 175t
Gastric bypass, weight loss and, 175t
Gastric cancer
H. pylori-associated, 234–235
bacterial and host factors in development of, 225–229
ulcerated, negative oral contrast CT of, 12f
Gastric carcinoid tumors (ECLomas), 116
Gastric glands, 104f, 104–105
secretions from, 106
Gastric graft-versus-host disease, 95–96
Gastric lymphoma, *H. pylori*-associated, 235
bacterial and host factors in development of, 225–229
Gastric prolapse, 182f
Gastric remnant distension, after Roux-en-Y gastric
bypass, 183
Gastric ulcer, 81–82
Gastrin/Gastrin receptors
gastric acid secretion and, 108–109, 115
H. pylori infection and, 224
negative feedback on, 115
Gastritis
acute erosive, 87

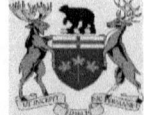

atrophic. See Atrophic gastritis
causes, classification of, 77–78
collagenous, 85–86
differential diagnosis in, 100
diffuse antral, 79, 80f
eosinophilic, 95
granulomatous, 93, 93f
H. pylori. See Helicobacter pylori gastritis
infectious, 90–92
lymphocytic, 86, 94
non-ulcer, H. pylori infection and, 237
phlegmonous/suppurative, 85
terminology associated with, 74–76
types of, 78–79
Gastritis cystica profunda (GCP), 86–87
Gastroduodenal ulcer bleeding, Forrest endoscopic classification of, 132
Gastroenterologists, H. pylori infection risk in, 231
Gastroesophageal reflux disease (GERD), H. pylori infection and, 240–241
Gastrointestinal complications, of transplant immunosuppression, 480–481
Gastrointestinal disorders, after bariatric surgery, 189–190
Gastropathy(ies)
classification of, 96
differential diagnosis in, 100
hyperplastic, 88, 96
portal hypertensive, and gastric antral vascular ectasia compared, 90
reactive (erosive), 87, 96, 97, 99f
Gastroplasty, 176, 177f
weight loss and, 175t
Gene sequencing, in FAP genetic testing, 341
Genetic testing, in familial adenomatous polyposis, 341–342
Genotype-phenotype correlations, in FAP genetic testing, 342
Glycogen storage disease, diet therapy for, 474

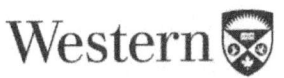

Graft non-function, following liver transplantation, 464
Graft-versus-host disease (GVHD), gastric, 95–96
Granulomatous gastritis, 93, 93f
Growth retardation, *H. pylori* infection and, 235–236

H
H^+, K^+-ATPase "proton pump," acid secretion via, 113
Hand sanitizers, *C. difficile* infection and, 321–322, 325
Hand washing, *C. difficile* infection prevention and, 321–322
Heartburn, after bariatric surgery, 190
Helicobacter pylori eradication therapy
  clinical impact of, 257–258
  clinical studies on, 253–255
  eradication confirmation, 256
  eradication prediction, 256–257
  eradication rates, 249–250, 251, 252, 253, 257
  indications for, 259
  reinfection rates, 258–259
Helicobacter pylori gastritis, 80–82, 236
  chronic, 225
  disease outcomes and, 81f
  multifocal atrophic, 84, 85f
Helicobacter pylori infection
  age at, 222
  ASA-induced ulcers and, 158
  associations with
    GI diseases, 231–232, 233–236
    negative, 240–241
    non-GI diseases, 232
    positive, 236
    special circumstances, 259
    unclear, 237–240
  clinical findings in, 241–242
  diagnosis of, 242–243
  incidence/prevalence of, 222, 223f
  in NVUGIB, future rebleeding and, 149
  organism characteristics, 222
    adhesion/colonization, 225–226

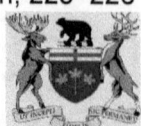

host responses and, 226–229
pathogenesis of, 223–224
pathophysiology of, 224–229
risk factors for, 229–231
testing for
  accepted indications, 243
  controversial indications, 243–244
  endoscopic, 245–246
  noninvasive/non-endoscopic, 244–245
transmission routes, 230
treatment of, 247–250
  adjuvant therapies, 251–252
  common adverse effects, 250–251
  eradication therapy, 256–259
  outcomes and considerations, 253–255
HELLP syndrome
  and AFLP distinguished, 401, 404
  clinical features of, 398f, 398–399
  complications in, 399
    treatment of, 400
  defined, 397
  demography, 397
  diagnostic imaging in, 399–400
  laboratory findings in, 399
  onset of, 409
  pathogenesis of
    fetus factors, 407
    maternal factors, 407
  pathophysiology of, 397–398
  pre-eclampsia and, 394, 398
  prognosis in, 400–401
  second trimester RUQ pain and, 403
  treatment of, 400
Hemangioma, hepatic. See Hepatic hemangioma
Hematemesis, after bariatric surgery, 190
Hematologic causes, of acute liver failure, 422–423
Hemochromatosis, diet therapy for, 474
Hemodynamic therapy, endoscopic, rebleeding risk after, 143

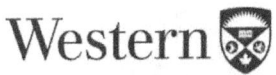

Hemorrhage. See Bleeding
Hemospray®, 150
Hemostatic therapy, endoscopic. See Endoscopic
  hemostatic therapy (EHT)
Heparin, reinstitution recommendations, 219
Hepatic adenoma (HA)
  causes of, 530
  clinical findings in, 530–531
  demography of, 530
  diagnostic imaging in, 532, 533f
  pathology of, 531f–532f, 532
  treatment of, 533
Hepatic decompensation, 451, 451f
Hepatic encephalopathy (HE)
  acute liver failure and, 435–437
  clinical findings in, 513–515
  demography of, 510
  minimal, 515–526. See also Minimal hepatic
    encephalopathy (MHE)
  overt, 515
  pathology, 512–513
  pathophysiology of, 510–512
  patient cooperation in, 514–515
Hepatic hemangioma
  clinical findings in, 542
  demography of, 541
  diagnostic imaging in, 542–543, 544f
  multiphasic CT of, 11f
  pathology of, 541, 542f
  pathophysiology of, 542
  treatment of, 544
Hepatic hydrothorax, 466
Hepatic masses, benign vs. malignant, 528. See also
    specific lesions
  differential diagnosis in, 528–529
  imaging studies of, 529–530
Hepatic scintigraphy, in focal nodular hyperplasia, 538
Hepatitis, as cause of acute liver failure, 422, 431, 446
  autoimmune hepatitis, 432–433

Hepatitis A virus (HAV) infection
 as cause of acute liver failure, 431
 treatment cautions during pregnancy, 410
Hepatitis B virus (HBV) infection
 as cause of acute liver failure, 431
 chronic, surveillance screening for HCC in, 550
 in immunocompromised individual with IBD, 302–303
 recurrence after liver transplantation, 475
 treatment cautions during pregnancy, 410
Hepatitis C virus (HCV) infection
 in immunocompromised individual with IBD, 302–303
 recurrence after liver transplantation, 475
 treatment cautions during pregnancy, 410
Hepatitis E virus (HEV) infection, as cause of acute liver failure, 431, 446
Hepatobiliary scanning, in focal nodular hyperplasia, 539
Hepatoblastoma, pediatric imaging studies of, 358
Hepatocellular carcinoma (HCC)
 alpha-fetoprotein screening and, 409–410
 at-risk persons, surveillance of, 548–549, 549f–550f
 clinical manifestations of, 547–548
 demography of, 544, 544f
 diagnostic imaging in, 548–549, 549f–550f
 histopathology of, 545f–547f
 liver transplantation in
  criteria for, 461
  stage 2 HCC, UNOS policy on, 461
 risk factors for, 545
 treatment of, 550–551
 variants of, 547
Hepatocyte
 bile acid synthesis in, 281f
 in enterohepatic circulation, 293
 function in zone 1 vs. zone 3, 291
Hepatotoxicity. *See* Acetaminophen hepatotoxicity; Non-acetaminophen hepatotoxicity
Hereditary fructose intolerance, diet therapy for, 474
Hereditary liver diseases, diet therapy for, 474–475

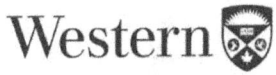

Hereditary non-polyposis polyposis syndrome (HNPCC), 337
  Amsterdam criteria for, 364
  cancer risk and mutations in, 361
  diagnosis of, 361
  epidemiology of, 360
  extracolonic cancer in, 370
  genetics of, 360
  management of, 368
  pathologic features in, 369
  polyp identification in, 368–369
  tumor tissue testing in. See Bethesda criteria, for tumor tissue testing
Herpes simplex virus (HSV)
  gastritis, 91
  in immunocompromised patient with IBD, 304–305
Hippocrates, 268
Histamine
  gastric acid secretion and, 112, 116–117, 117f
  overproduction, gastric acid secretion and, 122–123
HIV/AIDS
  GI tract bleeding in, differential diagnoses for, 151
  in immunocompromised individual with IBD, 303–304
Host immune response, in *H. pylori* infection, 227–229
Hounsfield Units (HU), 5–6, 6f
Human papilloma virus (HPV), in immunocompromised patient with IBD, 305–306
Hydrothorax, hepatic, 466
Hyperacute rejection, in liver transplant recipient, 478
Hyperemesis gravidarum, 391–392
  H. pylori infection and, 238
  medications used in, 392
  trimester of onset of, 409
Hypereosinophilia. diagnostic work-up in, 44
Hyperosmolar purgation, in MHE management, 525
Hyperparathyroidism, gastric acid secretion and, 122–123
Hyperplastic gastropathies, 88
  hypersecretory, Ménétrier's disease compared, 89

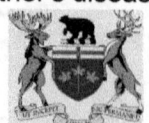

Hyponatremia, in model for end-stage liver disease, 459–460
Hypotension, in non-variceal upper GI bleeding, 130

I
IgA deficiency
 contraindications for blood transfusion in, 145–146
 management of, 146–147
IgG antibodies, anti-*H. pylori,* 231
Ileal reabsorption, of bile acids, 283, 283f
Ileal resection, 286, 286f
 choleretic diarrhea vs. steatorrhea following, 287
Ileocolic intussusception, 22, 22f
Ileocyte, in enterohepatic circulation, 293
Ileo-jejunal bypass, 176
Immunocompromised individual
 defined, 302
 GI conditions in, 302–304
 inflammatory bowel disease in
  international travel considerations, 309
  opportunistic infections, 302–309
  vaccination considerations, 310
Immunosuppressants (IM)
 after liver transplantation
  adverse effects of, 482–483
  gastrointestinal complications and, 480–481
 in IBD patients, 309
  with GI conditions, 303
  international travel considerations, 309
  with opportunistic infections, 304–309
  vaccination considerations, 310
Immunosuppression
 reduction in PTLD, 499–500
 transplant. *See* Transplant immunosuppression
Immunotherapy, for recurrent *C. difficile* infection, 331
In vitro protein truncation, in FAP genetic testing, 341
Infectious gastritis
 bacterial, 90–91
 parasitic, 92

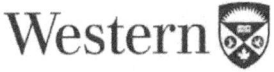

viral, 91–92
Inflammatory bowel disease (IBD)
  H. pylori infection and, 240
  in immunocompromised individual
    international travel considerations, 309
    opportunistic infections, 302–309
    vaccination considerations, 310
  in pregnant patient, 296–300
    outcomes, 297
Inflammatory response, in H. pylori infection, 226–227
Infliximab, for treatment of IBD in pregnant patients, 299
Influenza, in immunocompromised patient with IBD, 306
Inherited disorders, involving liver, 475
Inhibitory Control Test, 519
Integers, positive and negative, 5–6, 6f
International Diabetes Federation (IDF), indications for bariatric surgery, 172–173
International normalized ratio (INR), non-variceal bleeding and, 214–215, 215f
Interventional angiography, in NVUGIB, 150, 162
Intestine
  bile acid conjugation in, 289
  bile function in, 280
  luminal circulation in, 282
Intrahepatic cholestasis of pregnancy (ICP)
  clinical presentation and outcomes from, fetal and maternal, 414
  complications of, 411
  demography of, 412
  fetal complications in, 415
  genetics of, 412
  laboratory and liver biopsy findings in, 415
  pathophysiology of, 413
  prognosis in, 417–418
  risk factors in, 411–412, 413
  treatment of, 416–417
    cautions for, 411
  trimester of onset of, 409
Intraluminal contents, in gastric secretion, 121

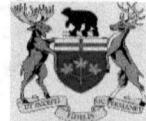

Intrinsic contrast, 7
Intussusception, ileocolic, 22, 22f
Ionizing radiation, risk to fetus, 389–390
Iron deficiency anemia
  after bariatric surgery, 192
  with upper GI bleeding, management of, 145

J
JC virus (JCV), in immunocompromised patient with IBD, 306

K
Kidney
  CT features of, 10, 10f
  hepatic encephalopathy and, 511
  involvement in MHE, treatment for, 521
  paraneoplastic syndromes involving, 274–275
King's College risk stratification criteria, for liver transplantation in ALF, 425, 428

L
Lactitol, in MHE management, 523
Lactulose, in MHE management, 523, 525
Laparoscopic adjustable gastric band, 176, 177f
  complications associated with, 182
  considerations for, 179
  weight loss after, 191
Large bowel, CT features of, 10, 10f
L-aspartate (LOLA), in MHE management, 524
Leaks, after bariatric surgery, endoscopic treatment for, 187–188
Lesar-Trelat syndrome, 273, 274f
Levofloxacin, for *H. pylori* eradication, 250, 253, 254
Lifestyle issues, in MHE management, 523
Linkage testing, in FAP, 341
Liver. *See also* Hepatic *entries*
  acute failure. *See* Acute liver failure (ALF)
  allocation for transplantation, 456
    Child-Turcotte-Pugh score for, 457

MELD system. See Model for end-stage liver disease (MELD)
bile acid conjugation in, 289
bile function in, 280
cirrhosis of. See Cirrhosis of liver
CT features of, 8, 8f
decompensation of, 451, 451f
hepatic encephalopathy and, 510–511
inherited disorders involving, 475
masses in. See Hepatic masses; *specific lesions*
PTLD of, 498f
window width/level of, 6
Liver diseases
end-stage. See Model for end-stage liver disease (MELD)
hereditary, diet therapy for, 474–475
as indications for transplantation, 468
in pregnancy. See Pregnancy, liver diseases in
recurrence after liver transplantation, 475–476
Liver resection, for hepatocellular carcinoma, 550
Liver transplantation
acute cellular rejection after, 467
in acute liver failure, 453–454
King's College risk stratification criteria for, 425, 428
with multiple organ failure, 440–441
in alcoholic cirrhosis, 453
allocation of liver for, 456
Child-Turcotte-Pugh score for, 457
MELD system. See Model for end-stage liver disease (MELD)
assessment protocol for, 454
clinical findings following, 464
complications of, 472–473, 480–481
contraindications for, 465, 470–471
de novo malignancy after
background for, 490f, 490–491
lymphoproliferative. See Post-transplant lymphoproliferative disorder (PTLD)
as major cause of death, 492, 492f

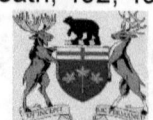

non-lymphoproliferative, risk factors for, 501
death following, causes of, 462–463, 492, 492f
hemodialysis for, prognostic significance of, 466–467
for hepatocellular carcinoma, 551
  criteria for, 461
  in stage 2 HCC, UNOS policy on, 461
indications for, 450, 466, 468–469
long-term considerations after, 483–485
patient considerations in, 450, 454–455
post-transplant lymphoproliferative disorder and, 463
referral tips, 453
and retransplantation, MELD score and, 467
survival following
  in Canada, 462, 462f, 490f, 490–491
  with deceased donor, 455f
  with living-related donor, 456f
  short- vs. long-term, 455, 490f, 490–491
treatment cautions during pregnancy, 411
UNOS listing criteria for, 476–477
Living-related donor, liver transplantation using
  evaluation protocol, 471
  survival following, 456f
Local modalities/Loco-regional therapies, for
    hepatocellular carcinoma, 550
London Health Sciences Center (LHSC), liver transplant
    recipient survival rates, 455f–456f
Long-chain 3-hydroxyacyl-CoA dehydrogenase (LCHAD)
    deficiency
  in AFLP, 398, 402–403
  in HELLP, 398
Lower GI bleeding (LGIB), in HIV/AIDS patients, 151
Low-molecular weight heparin (LMWH), reinstitution
    recommendations, 219
Lung
  involvement in MHE, treatment for, 521
  window width/level of, 6
Lung bases, CT features, 7, 7f
Lymphocytic gastritis, 86, 94
  histologic findings in, 86, 98f

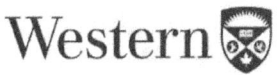

Lymphoma
  gastric. *See* Gastric lymphoma, *H. pylori*-associated
  of small bowel, 19f, 20
Lynch syndrome, 361
  diagnostic criteria for, 361–362
  extracolonic cancer surveillance guidelines in, 372–373
  screening and management guidelines for, 371–372

M

Magnetic resonance imaging (MRI), of hepatic masses, 529
  adenoma, 532
  cholangiocarcinoma, 553
  focal nodular hyperplasia, 538, 538f
  hemangioma, 543
  hepatocellular carcinoma, 548–549, 550f
  nodular regenerative hyperplasia, 536
Malignant infiltration, as cause of acute liver failure, 434–435, 447
Marginal ulcer (MU) bleeding, after bariatric surgery, endoscopic treatment for, 188
Mastic (chewing) gum, 252
MDR3 (ABCB4) gene mutations, 412, 413
Medications
  fetal risk categories
    for treatment of cholestatic disorders in pregnancy, 416–417
    for treatment of IBD, 296
  management after bariatric surgery, 189
  in MHE management, 523–525
Membranous nephropathy (MN), 274–275
Ménétrier's disease (MD)
  acid secretion in, 89
  in gastropathy differential diagnosis, 100
  and hyperplastic, hypersecretory gastropathy compared, 89
Mental state, grading in HE patients, 513–515
Meperidine, in treatment of ICP, 416
Mepolizumab, for eosinophilic esophagitis, 49, 52

Mesenteric panniculitis, 20–21, 21f
Metabolic bone disease, after bariatric surgery, 193
Metabolic causes, of acute liver failure, 422–423
Metabolic function, of bile, 281
Methotrexate, for treatment of IBD in pregnant patients, 298
Metronidazole
  in MHE management, 524
  for treatment *C. difficile* infection
    mild form, 323
    recurrent form, 329
    severe complicated form, 328
  for treatment of IBD in pregnant patients, 299
Microsatellite instability (MSI)
  Bethesda criteria and, 364
  in carcinogenesis in the colon, 336, 364
Midazolam, in treatment of ICP, 417
Minimal hepatic encephalopathy (MHE), 515–526
  blood findings in, 516–517
  clinical findings in, 515–516
  defined, 515
  diagnostic algorithm for, 518
  management options for, 522–526
  pathophysiology, 515z
  psychometric testing in, 519–520
  treatment of, 520–522
    reasons for, 522
Mismatch repair (MMR)
  colon cancer and, 335
  in Lynch syndrome, 364
  Turcot syndrome and, 353
Model for end-stage liver disease (MELD), 457, 458f
  hyponatremia and, 459–460
  liver allocation system, 459, 465
  predictive value of, 458
  score/score testing
    frequency of, 460
    predictive value of, 458
    and retransplantation, 467

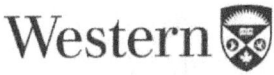

UNOS modification, 460–461
Modifier genes, colon cancer and, 335
Montelukast, for eosinophilic esophagitis, 49, 52
Muir-Torre syndrome, 370
Multi-detector CT scanners, 4–5, 5f
Multiphasic IV contrast CT, uses for, 11, 11f
Multiple organ failure syndrome (MOFS), in acute liver failure, 426–427, 439–441
Mushroom poisoning, acute liver failure and, 446
Mutations, types and mechanism, in colon cancer genetics, 335
MUTYH polyposis
  genetic testing in, 357
  genetics of, 347
  management of, 348
  phenotype in, 347–348
Mycobacterium avium-intracellulare gastritis, 91, 94f
Mycobacterium tuberculosis gastritis, 91
Myocardial infarction (MI), *H. pylori* infection and, 239

N
Napoleon Bonaparte, 268
National Comprehensive Cancer Network (NCCN), extracolonic cancer surveillance guidelines in Lynch syndrome, 372–373
National Institute for Health and Clinical Excellence (NICE), indications for bariatric surgery, 172–173
National Institutes of Health (NIH), indications for bariatric surgery, 172–173
Neomycin, in MHE management, 524
Nephropathy, membranous, 274–275
Neural mediation, of gastric acid secretion, 116
Neurotransmitters
  hepatic encephalopathy and, 512
  in MHE
    management, 526
    pathophysiology, 515
Nodular regenerative hyperplasia (NRH)
  causes of and associations with, 534

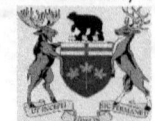

clinical findings in, 534
demography of, 534
diagnostic imaging in, 536
pathogenesis (speculated) of, 536
pathology of, 534–535, 535f
synonyms for, 533
treatment of, 536
Non-acetaminophen hepatotoxicity
liver transplantation and, 425, 428
treatment of, 445
Non-alcoholic fatty liver disease (NAFLD), bariatric surgery and, 179, 180t–182t, 181
Non-contrast CT, uses for, 11
Non-melanoma skin cancer (NMSC), in liver transplant recipients, 463–464, 501–502
Non-skin solid organ tumors, in liver transplant recipients, 463, 502
Non-ulcer gastritis (NUD), *H. pylori* infection and, 237
Non-variceal upper GI bleeding (NVUGIB)
adverse prognostic variables in, 143, 162–163
case example/discussion of, 127–128, 153–160
clinical manifestations of, 126–127
demography of, 126
endoscopic evaluation and management of, 127
estimation of volume depletion in, 128
hypotension and, 130
international normalized ratio and, 214–215, 215f
mortality in high-risk patients, 137t
odds ratio in, 131, 132, 137t
persistent/recurrent
clinical endpoints in, 144, 161–162
endoscopy predicting, 134, 135f
risk factors, 131, 132, 162
scoring systems predicting, 131
physical findings in, 129
registry on, 136f
Rockall Risk Score in, 142
surgery in, 151, 162

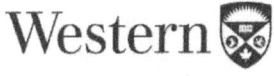

treatment options, 138. *See also under*
  Esophagogastroduodenoscopy (EGD)
 clip vs. combination therapy, 140–141, 141f
 endoscopy, 141f, 141–142
 meta-analysis of, 138t–140t
NSAIDs
 and bleeding risk in colonoscopic polypectomy, 202
 H. pylori infection and, 234–235
 in NVUGIB, future rebleeding and, 149
 reinstitution recommendations, 219
Nuclear imaging studies, of hepatic masses, 529–530
Number Connection Test (NCT), 519
Nutritional deficiency risk
 after biliopancreatic diversion, 185
 after Roux-en-Y gastric bypass, 184
 after sleeve gastrectomy, 183
Nutritional support
 after bariatric surgery, 188–189
 in eosinophilic esophagitis, 46, 50, 52
 in esophageal cancer, 67
 in MHE management, 525–526

O
Obstruction, biliary tract, 284
Octreotide therapy, for NVUGIB, 147
Odds ratio, in non-variceal upper GI bleeding, 131, 132, 137t
Once-daily regimens, in anti-*H. pylori* therapy, 248–249
Oncogenes, colon cancer and, 335
Oncologic causes, of acute liver failure, 422–423
Opportunistic infections, in inflammatory bowel disease, 302–309
Oral contraceptives, intrahepatic cholestasis of pregnancy and, 414, 417
Oral contrast CT, positive and negative, 12f, 12–13
Orthotopic liver transplantation, adverse effects of immunosuppressants after, 482–483
Osteomas, in FAP, 349, 350
Overt hepatic encephalopathy (OHE), 515

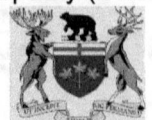

Oxalate nephrolithiasis, after Roux-en-Y gastric bypass, 184
Oxyntic glands, 104, 104f, 105, 105f
   endocrine cells and, 105, 106f

P

Palliative treatments, in unresectable esophageal cancer, 66–67
Pancreas
   CT features of, 9, 9f
   imaging studies, in FAP management, 358
Pancreatitis
   acute, 16–17, 17f
   H. pylori infection and, acute and chronic, 224–225
Panniculitis, mesenteric, 20–21, 21f
Papules, whitish, in eosinophilic esophagitis, 42f
Paraneoplastic syndromes
   defined, 272
   differential diagnosis of, 275
   in gastric adenocarcinoma, 272–273
   involving kidney, 274–275
   involving skin, 273–274, 274f
   treatment of, 275
Parasitic infections, in immunocompromised patient with IBD, 306–307
Parasitic infectious gastritis, 92
Parietal cells
   gastric acid secretion and, 108
   inhibitors of, 114, 117, 117f
Patterson-Kelly syndrome, esophageal cancer and, 59, 60
Pbeumococcal infection, in immunocompromised patient with IBD, 308–309
PCR, in *H. pylori* diagnosis, 245
Péan, Jules Emile, 269
Pepsin secretion, 106–107
Pepsinogens, 106–107
Peptic ulcer/Peptic ulcer disease (PUD). *See also* Non-variceal upper GI bleeding (NVUGIB)

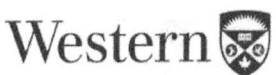

after bariatric surgery, 193–194
bleeding outcomes, effects of PPIs on, 137f
H. pylori-associated, 233
   bacterial and host factors in development of, 225–229
   therapeutic options, 260–261
poor prognosis for, factors predicting, 133–134, 135f
Peptide YY (PYY), gastric acid secretion and, 112
Peptides, gastric acid secretion and, 110–111
Perforated carcinoma, of transverse colon, 23f
Peripheral vein thrombosis (PVT), gastric adenocarcinoma and, 272–273
pH, outcomes in GI disorders, 225, 234, 247
Phlegmonous gastritis (PG), 85
Phospholipid transport, inborn errors of, 294
Plummer-Vinson syndrome, esophageal cancer and, 59, 60
Pneumatosis intestinalis, 24, 25f
Pneumocystis jiroveci (PCJ), in immunocompromised patient with IBD, 307
Polypectomy, colonoscopic, bleeding risk associated with. *See* Postpolypectomy bleeding
Polyposis syndromes
   adenomatous, 337. *See also* Familial adenomatous polyposis (FAP)
   characteristics of, 337
   hamartomatous, 337
   hereditary GI, 337
   M(UT)YH gene mutations in. *See* MUTYH polyposis
Polyps
   adenomatous, 357. *See also* Familial adenomatous polyposis (FAP)
   duodenal, in FAP, 351–352
   fundic gland, 261
Portal hypertension, treatment cautions during pregnancy, 411
Portal hypertensive gastropathy (PHG), 97, 99f
   and gastric antral vascular ectasia compared, 90, 152–153

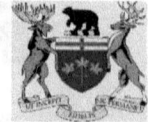

Positron emission tomography (PET) scan, of hepatic
    masses, 530
  adenoma, 532
  cholangiocarcinoma, 554, 554f
  focal nodular hyperplasia, 539
  hemangioma, 543
  hepatocellular carcinoma, 549
Postpolypectomy bleeding
  conditions associated with, 202–203
  risk factors for, 204
  therapeutic agents associated with, 202–203
Post-transplant lymphoproliferative disorder (PTLD), 463,
    493–494
  clinical manifestations of, 496, 497f
  diagnosis of, 498f, 498–499
  management of, 499–501
  pathogenesis of, 495–496
  prognosis in, 499
    negative factors, 496
  risk factors for, 494–495
Prednisolone, in treatment of ICP, 416
Prednisone, for eosinophilic esophagitis, 52
Pre-eclampsia/Eclampsia
  clinical features of, 394–395
  defined, 392
  demography of, 392–393
  diagnostic investigations in, 395–396, 396f
  fetal considerations in, 393, 395
  maternal considerations in, 394–395
  pathophysiology of, 393–394
  risk factors for, 393
  treatment of, 396–397
  trimester of onset of, 409
Pregnancy
  following liver transplantation, 484–485
  inflammatory bowel disease in, 296–300
    outcomes, 297
  liver diseases in, 388–418. *See also* Acute fatty liver of
    pregnancy (AFLP)

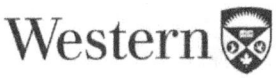

changes seen during
  hepatic physiology, 388
  signs and laboratory values, 389–390
  general approach to, 388–391
  non-pregnancy associated, 388. *See also specific diseases*
  occurrence of, 388
  pregnancy associated, 388. *See also specific diseases*
  treatment cautions, 410–411
  testing for, after bariatric surgery, 191–192
Primary sclerosing cholangitis (PSC), in liver transplant recipient, 504
Probiotics
  H. pylori eradication and, 251
  in MHE management, 524, 525–526
  for recurrent *C. difficile* infection, 330–331
Propofol, in treatment of ICP, 417
Prostaglandins
  gastric acid inhibition and, 118
  gastric acid secretion and, 110
Prosthetic cardiac valves
  mechanical, anticoagulation and, 216
  thromboembolism risk and, 209, 210
Proton pump, H^+, K^+-ATPase, acid secretion via, 113
Proton pump inhibitor (PPI) therapy
  with anti-*H. pylori* therapy, 234, 247–248
    adverse effects, 250
    eradication rates, 249–250, 257
  and ASA-induced ulcer healing, 156
  benefits of, 149
  benzimidazole, mechanism of action, 114
  effect on outcomes in PUD bleeding, 137f
  for eosinophilic esophagitis, 47–49
  before esophagogastroduodenoscopy, in NVUGIB, 145
  in high-risk patients, mortality and, 137t
  in NVUGIB prior to endoscopy, 134, 134f
  oral forms, 147
  prior to EGD/EHT, Forrest score and, 147

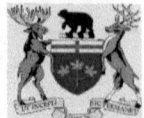

Prurigo chronica multiformis, *H. pylori* infection and, 237f, 238
Pseudomembranous colitis (PMC), 316f–317f, 319, 332
  C. difficile infection and, 321
Psychiatric disorders, after bariatric surgery, 189
Psychometric Hepatic Encephalopathy Score (PHES), 519
Psychometric testing
  EEG vs., 520
  in minimal hepatic encephalopathy, 519–520
Pulmonary embolus (PE), gastric adenocarcinoma and, 272
Purgation, hyperosmolar, in MHE management, 525
Pyloric glands, 104f, 104–105
  endocrine cells and, 105, 106f

R
Radiation, ionizing, risk to fetus, 389–390
Rapid urease testing (RUT), in *H. pylori* diagnosis, 245
Reabsorption, of bile acids, 290
Reactive (erosive) gastropathy, 87, 96, 97, 99f
  histologic findings in, 97, 98f–99f
Recipient survival, following liver transplantation
  from deceased donor, 455f
  from living-related donor, 456f
Recurrent abdominal pain, in adolescents, *H. pylori* infection and, 237
Registry on non-variceal upper GI bleeding and endoscopy (RUGBE), 136f
Regurgitation, after bariatric surgery, 190
Reitan Test, 519
Rejection, after liver transplantation
  acute cellular, 467, 478, 479
  chronic, 479
  hyperacute, 478
Renal proximal tubular cell, in enterohepatic circulation, 293
Repeatable Battery for the Assessment of Neuropsychological Status (RBANS), 520

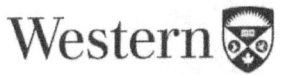

Resection
  hepatic, for hepatocellular carcinoma, 550
  ileal. See Ileal resection
Retained antrum syndrome, gastric acid secretion and, 122
Rifabutin, for *H. pylori* eradication, 250
Rifampin, for *H. pylori* eradication, 253
Rifaximin, in MHE management, 524
Risk factors
  for atrial fibrillation and stroke, 208
  for *C. difficile* infection, 315
  for cholangiocarcinoma, 551–552
  for esophageal cancer, 58–60
  for gastric adenocarcinoma, 271
  for *H. pylori* infection, 229–231
  for hepatocellular carcinoma, 545
  in intrahepatic cholestasis of pregnancy, 411–412, 413
  for non-variceal upper GI bleeding, 131
  for postpolypectomy bleeding, 204
  for post-transplant lymphoproliferative disorder, 494–495
  for post-transplant non-lymphoproliferative *de novo* malignancy, 501
  for pre-eclampsia/eclampsia, 393
  for recurrent cholestasis of pregnancy, 418
  for recurrent deep vein thrombosis, 209
  for thromboembolism, 200, 206–207, 209, 210
Rockall Risk Score, in NVUGIB prognosis, 142, 146
Roux-en-Y gastric bypass, 173, 176, 177f
  complications associated with, 183–184
  considerations for, 179
  weight loss after, 191

S
Saccharomyces boulardii, for recurrent *C. difficile* infection, 331
S-adenosyl–L-methionine (SAM), 412
"Sandwich sign," small bowel imaging, 19f, 20
Scintigraphy, in focal nodular hyperplasia, 539

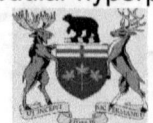

Secretagogues, 114
  acetylcholine, 116
  gastrin, 115
  neural mediation, 116
Secretin, gastric acid inhibition and, 118
Secretion, 107
  functions of, 112–113
  gastric acid. *See* Gastric acid secretion
  from gastric glands, 106–107
  regulation of, 114–118, 117f
Sequential therapy, for *H. pylori* eradication, 253, 255
Sexual function, following liver transplantation, 484–485
"Shock liver" syndrome, 433–434
Sigmoid volvulus, 23f, 24
Sigmoidoscopy, in FAP management, 358, 359
Single phase IV contrast CT, uses for, 11
Sirolimus-mTOR inhibitor, 464, 505–506
  liver transplant recipient and, 464
Skeletal muscle, hepatic encephalopathy and, 511
Skin
  paraneoplastic syndromes involving, 273–274, 274f
  PTLD manifestations in, 497f
Skin cancer, non-melanoma, 463–464
Sleeve gastrectomy, 176, 177f
  complications associated with, 183
  considerations for, 179
Small bowel
  bleeding in HIV/AIDS patients, 151
  CT features, 10, 10f
  diseases of, 19f, 20–22, 21f–23f, 24, 25f
  hepatic encephalopathy and, 510
  imaging studies of, in FAP management, 358
Small intestinal bacterial overgrowth (SIBO), 284–285
Smoking
  H. pylori infection and, 254, 259
  eradication therapy failure and, 242, 256, 257
  peptic ulcer disease and, 233
Soft tissue, window width/level of, 6
Solid organ cancers, in liver transplant recipients, 503

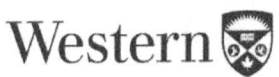

non-skin tumors, 463, 502
Somatostatin (SST)
　gastric acid secretion and, 110
　H. pylori infection and, 224
　for NVUGIB, 147
Sphincterotomy, hemorrhage after, 205–206
　preventive factors, 206
　venous thromboembolic events, high-vs.low-risk patients, 206–207
Spigelman staging system, and screening for duodenal polyps in FAP, 351–352
Spleen, CT features, 9, 9f
Squamous cell carcinoma, esophageal, risk factors for, 58–59, 60
Staging
　of desmoid tumors, in Gardner variant of FAP, 355
　of duodenal polyps in FAP, 351–352
　of esophageal cancer, 62–63
　　AJCC groupings, 61–62
　　modalities used in, 62
Steatohepatitis, bariatric surgery and, 180t
Steatorrhea, following ileal resection
　choleretic diarrhea vs., 287
　pathophysiologic changes causing, 287–288
Steatosis
　bariatric surgery and, 180t
　following liver transplantation, 484
Stent placement, GI bleeding and, 216–217
Steroid therapy
　for eosinophilic esophagitis, 47–49, 51–52
　for IBD in pregnant patients, 298
Stoma, after bariatric surgery, 187
　stenosis of. *See* Stomal stenosis
Stomach
　amino acids in, 111–112
　bleeding in HIV/AIDS patients, 151
　Crohn disease of, 94
　CT features of, 10, 10f
　gastritis, 74–96

gastropathies, 96–100
ulcerated gastric carcinoma of, 12f
Stomal stenosis
after Roux-en-Y gastric bypass, 183
after vertical banded gastroplasty, 183
Stone formation, bile function in, 281
Stroke risk, anticoagulants and, 208
Stroop Test, 520
Suppressor genes, colon cancer and, 335
Suppurative gastritis (SG), 85
Swansea criteria, for diagnosis of AFLP, 404–405

T
Technetium-99m, in imaging studies of hepatic masses
focal nodular hyperplasia, 539
hemangioma, 543
Tetracycline, for *H. pylori* eradication
adverse effects, 250
eradication rates, 249
Thromboembolism, risk factors for, 200
after sphincterotomy, 206–207
deep vein thrombosis and, 209–210
prosthetic cardiac valves and, 209
Thrombosis, late stent, bleeding risk management, 212
Thrombotic thrombocytopenic purpural hemolytic uremic syndrome (TTP/HUS), in paraneoplastic syndrome differential diagnosis, 275
Thyroid exam, pediatric imaging studies, in FAP management, 358
Ticlopidine, aspirin vs, 155
Transarterial embolization (TAE), in NVUGIB, 150, 162
Transplant immunosuppression
adverse effects of, 482–483
gastrointestinal complications of, 480–481
Transplantation
fecal, for recurrent *C. difficile* infection, 331
hepatic. *See* Liver transplantation
Travel, immunosuppression in IBD patients and, 309
Trousseau syndrome, 272

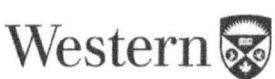

Tuberculosis, in immunocompromised patient with IBD, 307–308
Tumor markers (CA19-9), for cholangiocarcinoma diagnosis, 554
Tumor node metastasis (TNM) staging, in esophageal cancer, 62–63
Turcot syndrome, 345, 353
 defined, 352
Tyrosinemia, diet therapy for, 474

U
UDCA, choleretic effect of, 291
Ulcerated gastric carcinoma, negative oral contrast CT of, 12f
Ultrasound (US)
 endoscopic
  in cholangiocarcinoma, 554
  in pediatric FAP management, 358, 360
 of hepatic masses, 529
  adenoma, 532
  cholangiocarcinoma, 553
  focal nodular hyperplasia, 538
  hemangioma, 542–543
  hepatocellular carcinoma, 548
  nodular regenerative hyperplasia, 536
United Network for Organ Sharing (UNOS)
 listing criteria for liver transplantation, 476–477
 MELD exceptions and, 460–461
 stage 2 hepatocellular carcinoma policy, 461
Upper GI bleeding (UGIB)
 chronic liver disease with, management of, 144
 in elderly vs. younger patients, 151
 in HIV/AIDS patients, differential diagnoses, 151
 iron deficiency anemia with, management of, 145
 non-variceal. *See* Non-variceal upper GI bleeding (NVUGIB)
Urea breath test, in *H. pylori* diagnosis, 245, 247
Urease production, *H. pylori* infection and, 223, 246
Ursodeoxycholic acid (UCDA), in treatment of ICP, 416

benefits of, 416–417

V
VacA exotoxin, *H. pylori* infection and, 223–224
Vaccination considerations, for immunocompromised individual with IBD, 310
Vancomycin, for treatment of *C. difficile* infection
  mild form, 323, 324
  recurrent form, 329, 331
  severe complicated form, 328
Varicella zoster virus (VZV), in immunocompromised patient with IBD, 305
Vascular causes, of acute liver failure, 422–423
Vertical banded gastroplasty, 176, 177f
  complications associated with, 183
Viral infection, as cause of acute liver failure, 422, 431
Vitamin B12 deficiency, *H. pylori* infection and, 238–239
Vitamin therapy, *H. pylori* eradication and, 251
Volume depletion, estimation in non-variceal upper GI bleeding, 128
Vomiting, prolonged, after bariatric surgery, 190

W
Warfarin, reinstitution recommendations, 219
Weight reduction
  after bariatric surgery, 191
  bariatric surgery for, 174, 174f, 175f, 175t
Wilson disease
  as cause of acute liver failure, 432
  diet therapy for, 474
  treatment cautions during pregnancy, 410
Window level (WL), 6
Window width (WW), 6

X
Xanthomatosis, cerebrotendinous, diet therapy for, 475

Z
Zollinger-Ellison syndrome (ZES)

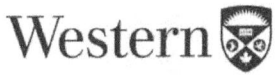

after bariatric surgery, 194
gastric acid secretion and, 122
in gastropathy differential diagnosis, 100

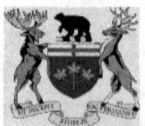

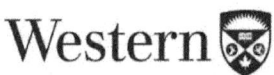

www.ingramcontent.com/pod-product-compliance
Lightning Source LLC
Chambersburg PA
CBHW071352170526
45165CB00001B/7